Basic and Clinical
Immunology

9

99

)

-- OCT 2004

For Churchill Livingstone

Publisher Timothy Horne
Project Editor Jim Killgore
Designer Sarah Cape
Project controller Kay Hunston
Editor Jane Ward

Basic and Clinical
Immunology

Mark Peakman MB BS PhD MRCPath

Senior Lecturer in Immunology,
King's College School of Medicine and Dentistry;
Honorary Consultant Immunologist,
King's College Hospital,
London

Barts and The London.

Diego Vergani MD PhD FRCPath

The Richard Crispin Professor of Immunology,
University College School of Medicine,
Institute of Hepatology;
Honorary Consultant Immunologist,
University College Hospital,
London

Illustrated by

Robert Britton and Ethan Danielson

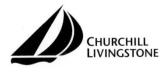

**CHURCHILL
LIVINGSTONE**

NEW YORK EDINBURGH LONDON MADRID MELBOURNE SAN FRANCISCO AND TOKYO 1997

CHURCHILL LIVINGSTONE
Medical Division of Pearson Professional Limited

Distributed in the United States of America by Churchill
Livingstone Inc., 650 Avenue of the Americas, New York, N.Y.
10011, and by associated companies, branches and representatives
throughout the world.

First published 1997

Standard edition ISBN 0 443 04672 7

International Student Edition first published 1997
International Student Edition ISBN 0 443 05780 X

British Library Cataloguing in Publication Data
A catalogue record for this book is available from the British Library.

Library of Congress Cataloging in Publication Data
A catalog record for this book is available from the Library of
Congress.

Medical knowledge is constantly changing. As new
information becomes available, changes in treatment,
procedures, equipment and the use of drugs become
necessary. The authors and the publisher have, as far as it is
possible, taken care to ensure that the information given in
this text is accurate and up to date. However, readers are
strongly advised to confirm that the information, especially
with regard to drug usage, complies with current legislation
and standards of practice.

The
publisher's
policy is to use
**paper manufactured
from sustainable forests**

Produced by Longman Asia Ltd, Hong Kong
NPCC/01

Preface

'Immunology is an invention of the devil.'

From the outset, this book was intended as a text combining the basic science components required to understand the role of immunity in disease with an account of the major diseases classified under the umbrella of clinical immunology. The book would thus naturally span the curricula of most medical or paramedical courses, from basic to applied. From technical, medical, dental and science students at all levels, we had both perceived a glaring need for such a text. But as if any stimulus was required for us to see the project to completion, an article appeared in a popular news magazine for doctors whilst the book was being planned, asking several regular contributors for their most hated words. 'Immunology' made its appearance as 'an invention of the devil, who is making it up as he goes along because he is not too clear about this stuff either.' The article went on to compare immunology to a Rube Goldberg or Heath Robinson cartoon: for example, the light is turned on when you trip over a chair, startling the cat, who leaps against the door which swings shut, knocking a picture off the wall which strikes the light switch as it falls. And as a final evidence that immunology was truly demonic, a conversation with an expert physician, encountered at an international conference, was recounted in the same article. 'I hope you understand all this stuff', he had said to the journalist, 'they didn't teach it when I was in medical school and I never figured it out.' We hope that this book goes some way towards redressing the balance.

It would have been impossible to be authoritative about every aspect of clinical immunology. For this reason, we have consulted friends and colleagues with the relevant expertise to advise us, and to these we are indebted: Fred Dische, Adrian Eddleston, John Fabre, Jonathan Frankel, Elizabeth Higgins, Rob Higgins, William Hirst, Giorgina Mieli-Vergani, Lindsay Nicholson and Anton Pozniak. We are also grateful to colleagues who provided photographic material for illustrations, notably Nat Cary, Fred Dische and Magnus Norman, Jane Evanson, Stella Knight, Jonathan Frankel, Elizabeth Higgins, Patrick O'Donnell, Bernard Portmann and John Salisbury.

London
1997

M.P.
D.V.

Contents

Symbols used in the diagrams

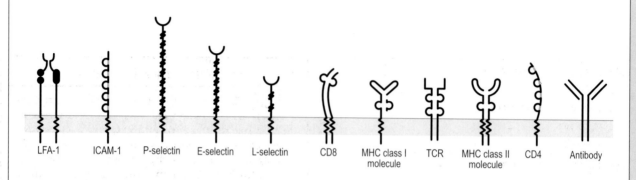

LFA-1   ICAM-1   P-selectin   E-selectin   L-selectin   CD8   MHC class I molecule   TCR   MHC class II molecule   CD4   Antibody

Antigen presenting cell

Basophil

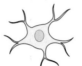

Dendritic cell

Monocyte

Class I MHC molecule with TCR and associated antigen

Macrophage

Megakaryocyte

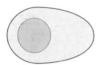

Plasma cell

Eosinophil

Class II MHC molecule with TCR and associated antigen

Erythrocyte

Mast cell

Lymphocyte

Neutrophil

Symbols used in the text

Immunology in-depth

Focus on clinical immunology

Anatomy and cells of the immune system

Pluripotent haemopoietic stem cells

There are two important clinical implications of the process by which one cell type gives rise to all elements of the blood. First, individuals whose pluripotent haemopoietic stem cells are irretrievably damaged, for example by exposure to irradiation arising from the 'Chernobyl' nuclear disaster, can be fully reconstituted by transplantation of compatible bone marrow containing stem cells from a healthy donor. Second, cancer arising in a stem cell during a critical phase of its development may result in cancerous white blood cells (leukaemia) of more than one lineage circulating in the blood — so called 'biphenotypic' leukaemias.

The immune system resembles other elements of mammalian physiology in being composed of specialised cells that function within discrete, organised anatomical structures. To understand its role in host defence, it is necessary first to become familiar with the anatomy of the immune system — both gross and microscopic.

CELLS OF THE IMMUNE SYSTEM

The bone marrow is the source of the precursor cells that ultimately give rise to the cellular constituents of the immune system, save for one brief period during fetal life when the liver is also a site of immune cell development. The production of immune cells is one component of **haemopoiesis**, the process by which all cells that circulate in the blood arise and mature. An important underlying principle of haemopoiesis is that there is a single precursor cell that is capable of giving rise to all blood cell lineages, ranging from platelets to lymphocytes (Fig. 1.1). This cell is known as the **pluripotent haemopoietic stem cell**: it is to the bone marrow what the queen bee is to the hive. Immunology concentrates upon the roles of white blood cells in host defence: these include the granulocytes (neutrophils, eosinophils, and basophils), monocytes and lymphocytes.

GRANULOCYTES

The granulocyte/monocyte lineage gives rise to precursors that mature within the bone marrow and are released into the blood. The granulocytes constitute approximately 65% of all white cells and derive their name from the large numbers of granules found in their cytoplasm. The appearance of these granules under the light microscope following conventional staining provides a further subdivision. Granules with intense blue staining are found in basophils, which make up 0.5–1% of granulocytes; red-staining granules are present in eosinophils (3–5%); while neutrophils (90–95%) have granules that remain relatively unstained (Fig. 1.2a–c). The term '**polymorphonuclear cell**', describing the multilobed nuclei of granulocytes, has become synonymous with neutrophils, which constitute by far the majority of granulocytes, but eosinophil nuclei may have a similar appearance. Granulocytes circulate in the blood and migrate into the tissues particularly during inflammatory responses. The exception to this rule is the **mast cell**, which is fixed in the tissues. Mast cells and basophils share many common features, yet their derivation is different: the basophil is of the same lineage as neutrophils and eosinophils, whilst mast cells arise from an as yet unidentified precursor possibly in the spleen, thymus or lymph node.

MONOCYTES AND DENDRITIC CELLS

Monocytes form between 5 and 10% of circulating white blood cells and have a short half-life, spending approximately 24 hours in the blood. They enter the extravascular pool and become resident in the tissues, where they are termed **macrophages**. Whilst each macrophage was thought to derive from a single monocyte, there is now evidence that macrophages may also arise following division of immature forms of monocytes. Monocyte and macrophage morphology is highly variable, but in broad terms they are larger than

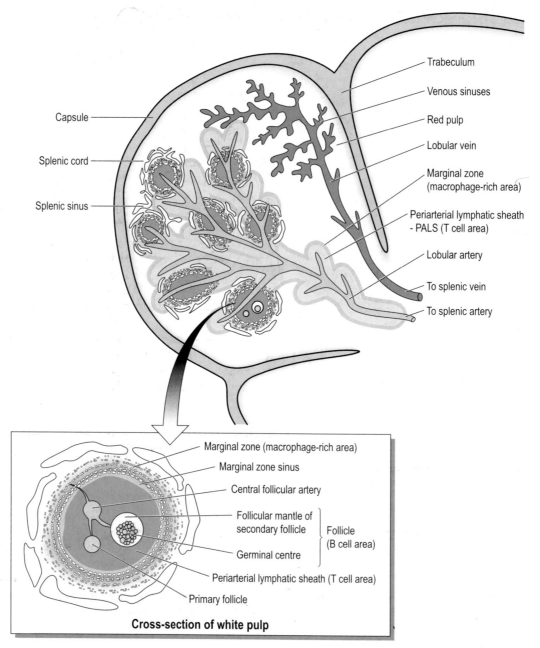

Fig. 1.6 **Structure of the spleen.**

Organs of the immune system
- Primary lymphoid organs (bone marrow and thymus) are sites of development and maturation of immune response cells.
- Secondary lymphoid organs (lymph nodes, spleen, mucosa-associated (MALT) and gut-associated (GALT) lymphoid tissue) organise the immune response.
- White blood cells become further specialised in secondary organs.
- Lymphocytes recirculate through blood, secondary lymphoid organs and lymphatics in a process of organised immune surveillance.

CHAPTER 2

Innate immunity I: physical and humoral protection

FREEDOM FROM THE BURDEN OF DISEASE

The Latin *immunis*, meaning *free from burden*, has provided the English term immunity; it is often used in non-scientific contexts such as diplomatic immunity, crown immunity and so on. In biology, the burden is disease — caused by a variety of viruses, fungi, bacteria, protozoa, worms and toxins — and the physiological role of the immune system is to keep it at bay.

A broad definition of the immune system would be that it evolved to be able to identify **self**, and thus recognise **non-self**. The ability to make such a distinction is relatively primordial: sea anemones also have the capacity to recognise and react to non-self. The immune system in humans is often challenged by non-self, including pathogens such as those described above as well as organs transplanted from unrelated donors. Protection from these is afforded by a variety of cognitive and destructive processes, the understanding of which forms the basis of immunology.

Immunity to pathogens has several layers of complexity. We do not all catch the 'bug' that is 'going around'; we do not all suffer a cold with the same intensity; some of us happily harbour microbes that could prove lethal to others. However, there are some general principles about immunity that we can deduce from our own common experience.

Some facts are obvious: if you have an open wound or burn, it is important to maintain cleanliness and protect the exposed tissues from becoming infected, since loss of physical barriers lowers immunity. Wound infections may be dealt with adequately by the immune system without the need for antibiotics, and this protection is present at any age. By comparison, we consider the newborn to be at greater overall risk of infection: they have less immunity. Other well-recognised truths relate to the infections of childhood. If you have measles, chicken pox or mumps as a child, you are extremely unlikely to suffer the same illness again. However, immunity to mumps does not stop a child catching measles. We can conclude that we are born with some immunity and that the rest may be acquired during life; some immune responses can be specific for a microbe: they may be learned and retained in an 'immunological memory'.

TYPES OF IMMUNITY

Innate immunity

Immunity present at birth is termed innate. The innate immune system is the main, first-line defence against invading organisms. Its characteristics are that it is present for life, has no specificity and no memory. (An exception, to be discussed later, is the protective antibodies that babies acquire from their mothers.) The lack of specificity has led to the use of the term non-specific immunity. Innate responses are most useful in protection against:

- pyogenic ('pus-forming') organisms, e.g. *Staphylococcus aureus*, *Haemophilus influenzae*
- fungi, e.g. *Candida albicans*
- multicellular parasites, e.g. worms such as *Ascaris*, the roundworm.

Innate immunity has three components: physicochemical, humoral and cellular.

Physical barriers (Fig. 2.1) are the **skin** and **mucosae**, **secretions**, which continually wash and cleanse mucosal surfaces, and **cilia**, which help the removal of debris and foreign matter. Immunologically active factors present in mucosal secretions, in blood and in the cerebro-spinal fluid (the *humors*) are termed humoral. The most important of these is **complement**, the others being additional **opsonins** (an opsonin aids digestion of bacteria by neutrophils), such as C-reactive protein, and proteolytic **enzymes** (e.g. lysozyme). Cellular components are the **neutrophil**, the **eosinophil** and the **mast cell**, as well as the **NK cell**.

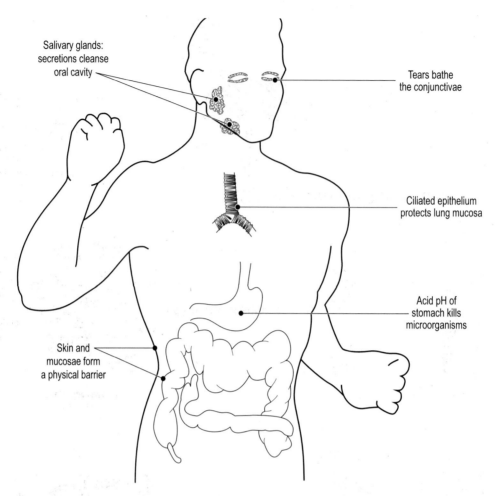

Salivary glands:
secretions cleanse
oral cavity

Tears bathe
the conjunctivae

Ciliated epithelium
protects lung mucosa

Acid pH of
stomach kills
microorganisms

Skin and
mucosae form
a physical barrier

Fig. 2.1 **Physicochemical barriers to infection which form the first line of innate defence against infection.**
Secretions such as saliva and tears also contain antibacterial enzymes such as lysozyme.

Acquired immunity

In contrast, some types of immune response are not present at birth but are gained as part of our development. The acquired or specific immune response is the antithesis of innate immunity. It is absent at birth and has specificity and memory; hence it may also be termed **adaptive**.

Paralysis of one component of either of these two forms of immunity can have a profound effect on the host defence against infection.

Contrasting characteristics of innate and acquired immunity

Innate immunity

- Characteristics: non-specific, is present at birth and does not change in intensity with exposure.
- Components: mechanical barriers, secreted products and cells (granulocytes, NK cells).
- Protects from: bacteria, fungi, worms.

Acquired immunity

- Characteristics: specific responses, acquired from exposure and increases in intensity with exposure.
- Components: secreted products and cells (lymphocytes).
- Protects from: bacteria, including intracellular infection, viruses and protozoa.

COMPLEMENT

Complement was described at the turn of the century during studies on the nature of immune reactions to bacteria in serum. Serum removed from animals that have been infected with a microorganism can subsequently agglutinate (clump together) and then lyse the same bacteria in a test tube (Fig. 2.2). Lysis, but not agglutination, is inhibited by pre-heating the serum at 56°C for 30 minutes. The lysing activity can be reconstituted using fresh serum from an animal not previously exposed to the bacteria. Therefore, a heat-labile factor without specificity for an organism is essential for its lysis. Agglutination and lysis were inhibited by pre-heating the serum at more than 60°C.

Several conclusions may be drawn from this evidence: (1) there is an inducible serum factor, fairly heat

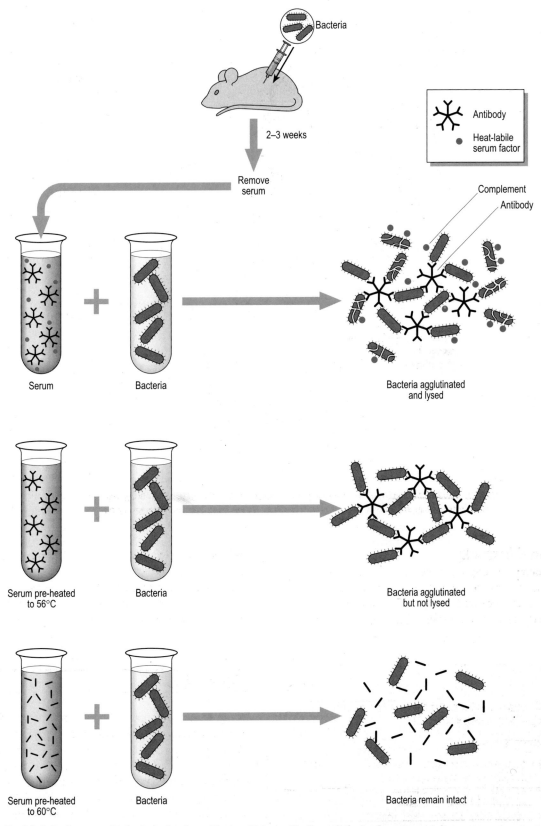

Bacteria

2–3 weeks

Remove
serum

Antibody

Heat-labile
serum factor

Complement
Antibody

Serum

Bacteria

Bacteria agglutinated
and lysed

Serum pre-heated
to 56°C

Bacteria

Bacteria agglutinated
but not lysed

Serum pre-heated
to 60°C

Bacteria

Bacteria remain intact

Fig. 2.2 Animals exposed to bacteria develop antibody, which specifically agglutinates the same organism.
Lysis is achieved through the action of a heat-labile serum factor which *complements* the action of antibody.

stable, that is specific for an organism and capable of agglutinating but not killing it; (2) another serum factor, heat labile, is not able to identify an organism but may help in its destruction. The first factor (1) was originally termed **antibody** and is specific for the target which induces it (the **antigen**), in this case a foreign organism. Since it is capable of specific reactions, antibody is part of the acquired/specific/adaptive immune

---

🔍 Antibody

Antibody is a glycoprotein produced by lymphocytes following stimulation with a macro-molecule (usually termed the antigen). An example of an antigen would be a protein coating the surface of a bacterium or virus. Antibody is a sophisticated glycoprotein that occurs in several different types with differing functions, but it is sufficient for the present to view it simplistically as a molecule with a shape like the letter 'Y'. The two smaller arms are identical to each other and each carries the ability to bind antigen; the trunk of the Y has specialised sites for interaction with complement proteins or specific receptors on cells. Granulocytes and mast cells, for example, bear receptors for antibody. Through interaction with complement and cells, antibody can give the innate immune system a specificity that, on its own, it does not possess. This serves as a reminder that the innate and acquired immune systems work best in concert.

Table 2.1 **Terminology of the complement system**

State of component	Nomenclature
Precursor molecules	Capital C followed by a number for the classical and common pathways, e.g. C1, C2 Capital letter followed by number for the alternative pathway, e.g. B1
Fragments	Small letter suffix, e.g. C4a, Ba
Inactivated components	Letter i prefix, e.g. iC3b
Active state	Bar over symbols, e.g. C4bC2a

system and will be considered in detail later (see box: 'Antibody' and p. 36). The serum factor (2) is **complement**, a group of heat-labile serum proteins that *complement* antibody in the destruction of organisms.

Complement is a protein cascade (cf. the kinin and clotting cascades) composed of more than 40 proteins including regulatory factors. The components are made in the liver, though some local production at sites of inflammation may be undertaken by macrophages. Complement has three pathways: the **alternative** and **classical** pathways, which are both capable of igniting the third pathway, known as the **common** or **membrane attack pathway**.

COMPLEMENT PROTEINS

The majority of complement proteins are soluble, although some are membrane bound. The soluble proteins circulate in an inactive state, and each must be activated sequentially for the reaction to proceed. Each activated molecule can catalyse the conversion of several molecules of the next component in the sequence; this gives the cascade the key attribute of amplification. The overall serum concentration of complement proteins is 3–4 g/l.

Several biological activities appear as a consequence of complement activation, the main ones being cell or bacterial **lysis**, the production of **pro-inflammatory mediators**, which amplify and perpetuate the process, and **solubilisation** of antigen–antibody complexes.

The confused and ever-changing terminology of the complement system was partly to blame for its past unpopularity with students and clinicians. In recent years the World Health Organization has proposed a standard nomenclature to obviate this (see Table 2.1). The precursor molecules, the fragments derived from

enzymatic cleavage of the parent molecule, the inactivated component and the active state of isolated or integrated complement components are all clearly defined in the same way for every component of the pathways.

COMPLEMENT ACTIVATION

Activation of the complement system occurs through two distinct pathways, **classical** and **alternative**, which converge for the terminal complement sequence, which provides most of the biological activity (Fig. 2.3). Classical and alternative pathways are composed of two distinct enzyme cascades that culminate in the cleavage of C3 and C5. Cleavage of C3 produces important biological consequences, while breakdown of C5 achieves the same and, in addition, provides the triggering stimulus to the final common pathway. The classical and alternative pathways bear striking resemblances, particularly in terms of protein structure (e.g. C2 and B), which is thought to arise from gene duplications occurring during the evolution of the cascade (see the box: 'Complement genes'). The two pathways are, however, triggered by different substances and through different initiation mechanisms.

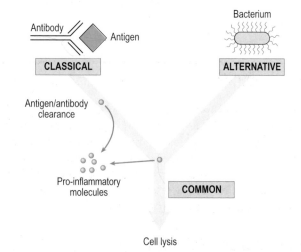

Fig. 2.3 **Overview of complement activation pathways.**
The final common pathway may be activated via the classical or alternative routes, which are intiated by antigen–antibody complexes and bacteria, respectively. Three main results of activation are clearance of complexes, release of biologically active mediators and direct cell lysis.

Complement genes

Gene duplication is thought to account for the striking similarities in the structure of proteins in the classical and alternative pathways. A further example of gene duplication is found in the region on human chromosome 6 that encodes some of the complement proteins, where there are two adjacent loci encoding C4. Approximately 35 different forms (alleles) of the C4 gene have been described, each encoding slightly different proteins. This is termed gene polymorphism and, although it is not a feature of all complement genes, it was used to settle the question of the relative contributions of macrophages and liver cells to the synthesis of complement proteins in the circulation. This was elegantly clarified by studies on C4 in the circulation of patients before and after liver transplantation. In post-transplant patients, the complement components have totally converted to the type of the liver donor, indicating the liver as the site of synthesis of circulating complement factors.

Complement

- Complement comprises a large number of serum proteins that are mainly made in the liver.
- Complement forms protein cascades, each activated component catalysing the activation of several molecules of the next component: causing amplification of the response.
- The consequences of complement activation are cell lysis, production of pro-inflammatory mediators and solubilisation of antigen–antibody complexes.
- There are three pathways: the alternative and the classical pathways both activate the third common or membrane attack pathway.

COMPLEMENT PATHWAYS

The two parallel initial pathways of complement both activate the third common pathway. In evolutionary terms, the alternative pathway is relatively primitive and a part of the innate immune system whilst the classical pathway, which is relatively recent, combines with antibody to initiate activation and is, therefore, an adjunct to the acquired immune system.

THE CLASSICAL PATHWAY

The classical pathway is activated by an interaction between antigen and antibody, forming a so-called **immune complex**. Antibodies can bind to, or 'fix', complement only after reacting with their antigen. The

formation of the complex provokes a conformational change in the antibody molecule that discloses a site for binding of the first complement component **C1**. C1 is a multimeric compound composed of six molecules termed **C1q**, and two each of **C1s** and **C1r**. C1q is an elongated protein with a rod-like stem composed of a triple helical structure and a globular head resembling a tulip (Fig. 2.4). It is the globular head that binds antibody. Six C1q molecules arrange themselves in a 'bunch' and the four C1r and C1s molecules attach in a calcium-dependent interaction. When antibody binds to two or more heads of C1q, C1r is cleaved to give an active molecule C$\overline{\text{1r}}$, which cleaves C1s. C1s extends the activation process by cleaving the next complement component **C4** to C4b, which continues the reaction process, and C4a, which has other biological properties (see below).

Cleavage of C4 to C4b reveals an internal thioester bond, which is swiftly inactivated by binding water molecules unless it can form covalent bonds with cell surface proteins or carbohydrates. Should this happen, C4b becomes relatively stable and binds to **C2** in a

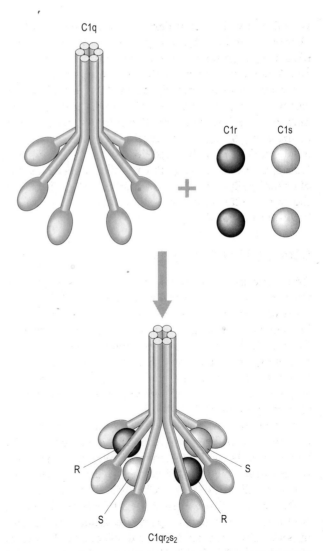

Fig. 2.4 **'Tulip' structure of the C1q hexamer with dimers of C1r and C1s in place.**
The globular heads of the C1q molecules bind antibody.

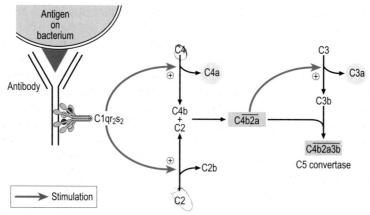

Fig. 2.5 **Activation of the classical pathway.**
Antigen–antibody complexes bind C1q. The C1qrs complex cleaves C4 and C2 to form the classical pathway C3 convertase $\overline{C4b2a}$. Following C3 cleavage, the C5 convertase is formed. Biologically active fragments C4a and C3a are generated. C3b alone has other actions and may also 'drive' forward activation of the alternative pathway.

magnesium-dependent reaction (Fig. 2.5). This illustrates one of the important forms of control over the complement cascade, namely that enzymatically active molecules are unstable and tend to degrade rapidly unless a solid surface, usually that of a target such as a bacterium, is available.

The C2 is itself then cleaved by C1s to form the complex $\overline{C4b2a}$, known as the **classical pathway C3 convertase**. **C3** is a similar molecule to C4, having an internal thioester bond. Two fragments derive from C3 cleavage. The smaller of these, C3a, has powerful biological properties; the larger, C3b, displays the labile binding site that allows the molecule to bind to membranes close to, but distinct from, $\overline{C4b2a}$. The proximity of C3b to $\overline{C4b2a}$ leads to the generation of the last enzyme of the classical pathway, $\overline{C4b2a3b}$ (the **classical pathway C5 convertase**) which cleaves **C5**, a component of the membrane attack pathway.

In addition to antigen–antibody complexes, the activation of the classical pathway can be initiated by aggregated immunoglobulins and by non-immunological stimuli such as DNA and C-reactive protein.

THE ALTERNATIVE PATHWAY

Activation of the alternative pathway proceeds in a different manner from that of the classical pathway, since it appears to be based on a 'tickover' mechanism. To illustrate the tickover concept, the analogy with an automatic car proposed by Lachmann is helpful. If an engine is idling or 'ticking over', any movement of the throttle will accelerate the engine and cause the car to move. Similarly, in the alternative pathway, there is a continuous, slow reaction sequence that is insufficient to produce any measurable effect. Activators of the alternative pathway are substances that act on the throttle. Availability of C3b is the essential requirement for activation of the alternative pathway to proceed;

this requirement is again fulfilled by the internal thioester bond, which undergoes continuous low-grade hydrolysis. Free C3b binds **factor B** and the C3bB complex becomes the substrate of a circulating enzyme, **factor D**, which, by removing from C3bB the fragment Ba, generates $\overline{C3bBb}$ (Fig. 2.6). This complex, the **alternative pathway C3 convertase**, can cleave C3, detaching C3a from C3b which can reinitiate the activation process.

How do the alternative pathway activators work? Such activators are insoluble polysaccharides (e.g. the sugar inulin) and the surfaces of cells of non-self origin. This primitive discrimination between self and non-self is partly a result of the abundance of natural inhibitors

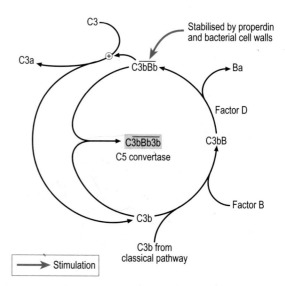

Fig. 2.6 **Alternative pathway activation.**
C3 'tick-over' generates C3b, C3bB and $\overline{C3bBb}$, which in turn cleaves C3. The tick-over is accelerated if the active enzymes are stabilised on bacterial cell walls, or if more C3b is produced from the classical pathway. The alternative pathway C5 convertase C3bBb3b is generated.

(see below) on the surface of autologous (self) cells. Bacteria and other organisms provide a surface for C3b and C3bBb deposition and protection from the destructive action of circulating regulatory factors I and H, allowing the pressure on the throttle to increase. Further impetus is given by properdin, or **factor P**, which stabilises C3bBb and renders it more efficient. Positive feedback is provided here, since C3bBbP generates more C3b, which is capable of forming more enzyme. The complex C3bBb3b, analogous to C4b2b3b, is the **alternative pathway C5 convertase**, initiating the membrane attack pathway sequence.

THE MEMBRANE ATTACK PATHWAY

This final common complement pathway (Fig. 2.7) generates one more biologically active component, C5a, but more importantly leads to the formation of the 'killer molecule' of the system. This is known as the **membrane attack complex** (**MAC**), since it provokes membrane damage. The cleavage of C5 by the classical or alternative pathway convertases gives the smaller fragment C5a and the larger C5b split product, which continues the reaction sequence by binding to **C6** and inducing it to express a labile reactive site for **C7**. The C5b67 complex is highly lipophilic and binds

to membranes, where it lies as a high-affinity receptor for **C8**. C8 has three chains (α, β, γ) of which the γ inserts into the membrane, anchoring the C5b678 complex. C5b678 binds and polymerises **C9**, forming the MAC, the final component of the system. As many as 12–15 C9 molecules may cluster around one C5b678 complex, inserting into and traversing the membrane bilayer (Fig. 2.8). Holes are made in the membrane, and if a sufficient number are created death results through osmotic lysis.

CONTROL MECHANISMS

Complement activation is kept in check by a variety of control mechanisms. The importance of such regulation is clear from the severity of the pathological states that result from congenital or acquired deficiencies of control proteins (see Ch. 19). We have already seen that lability of the active molecules is an inherent control and hinted at the presence of control proteins. Dilution of activated molecules within biological fluids also lessens their potential impact. More specific regulation is provided by circulating or membrane-bound proteins. The classical pathway is controlled in its initial stage by **C1-inhibitor** (also known as C1 esterase), a protein in the blood that blocks the enzymatic function of activated C1 by combining with it in a virtually irreversible stoichiometric complex. In the circulation, **factor I** is an enzyme that degrades C3b while **factor H** binds C3b and accelerates the destructive action of factor I (Fig. 2.9, p. 17). Factor I is also able to restrain activation of the classical pathway by destroying C4b. This destructive process is enhanced if C4b is complexed with a protein called **C4-binding protein** (C4bp). Two circulating proteins with a similar function are **protein S** and **SP-40,40**. Both are capable of binding the C5b67 complex to form an inactive moiety, preventing membrane insertion and formation of the MAC. Finally, a circulating enzyme, **carboxypeptidase N**, cleaves the carboxy-terminal arginine from C3a, C4a and C5a and the resulting molecules (termed, for example, C5a-des arg) are inactivated.

Other regulatory proteins are membrane bound. **Membrane attack complex inhibitory factor** (MACIF) — also known as **CD59** — exemplifies membrane-bound control proteins. (CD is the abbreviation for **cluster of differentiation**, and CD numbers are widely used to identify surface molecules in the immune system. An outline of the CD system is given in the box: 'The CD classification', p. 18.) CD59 is designed to avoid bystander damage: the accidental insertion of MACs destined for a bacterium into the cell wall of a lymphocyte or other host cell. CD59, contitutively expressed on mammalian cells, interferes with the MAC insertion, thus preventing cell lysis. **Decay accelerating factor** (DAF), a transmembrane glycoprotein found on most blood cells, competes for C4b, thus inhibiting formation of the classical pathway C3 convertase.

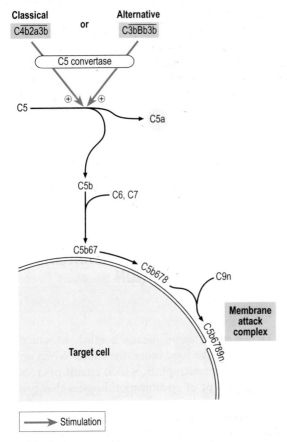

Classical
C4b2a3b

or

Alternative
C3bBb3b

C5 convertase

C5

$\oplus$ $\oplus$

C5a

C5b

C6, C7

C5b67

C5b678

C9n

C5b6789n

Target cell

Membrane attack complex

⟶ Stimulation

Fig. 2.7 The final common pathway.
The C5 convertases generate C5b and the pro-inflammatory C5a. C5b67 binds the target cell membrane and with addition of C8 and a C9 polymer the membrane attack complex forms.

simple to see how the presence of CRs 1, 3 and 4 on neutrophils can result in more efficient engulfment.

CELL RECRUITMENT AND ACTIVATION

The low-molecular-weight fragments C4a, C3a and C5a are known as **anaphylatoxins**. This name derives from their putative role in a clinical syndrome **anaphylaxis** (see p. 139) in which they activate mast cells and basophils directly through specific receptors. C5a and, to a lesser extent, C3a are also **chemotactic**, a term used to describe the ability to attract cells, in this case neutrophils (see p. 127).

CELL LYSIS

Complete complement activation through either pathway occurring on cell surfaces leads to cell lysis. Typical targets could include bacteria and enveloped viruses, but host erythrocytes, platelets and lymphocytes may also become victims in certain pathological conditions.

Complement pathways

- Classical pathway is activated by antigen–antibody complexes, aggregated immunoglobulins and by stimuli such as DNA and C-reactive protein.
- Alternative pathway has a continual slow reaction that only produces effects if it is activated by insoluble polysaccharides and the surface of non-self cells in the presence of C3b.
- Both the classical and alternative pathways produce a C5 convertase which initiates the membrance attack pathway.
- The final product of the complement cascades is the MAC (membrane attack complex), which forms holes through cell membranes causing lysis and cell death.
- Control is achieved by the lability of the components, by dilution and by specific regulatory proteins.
- Regulatory proteins can be circulating or membrane bound; the latter include the complement receptors, which are found on cells of the immune system itself.

REMOVAL OF IMMUNE COMPLEXES

Immune complexes of antibody and antigen are forming in the circulation continuously in small numbers, with periodic increases during infections or inflammatory episodes. These are potentially harmful, since they can become deposited in vessel walls or tissues and incite complement activation, with all the pro-inflammatory effects that that entails. Larger complexes, composed of a lattice of antibodies and antigens (Fig. 2.10), are more likely to become insoluble and fixed in the tissues. Complement has two key protective functions to prevent such damage: the ability to maintain immune complexes in solution and the ability to expedite their

---

The CD classification

Lymphocytes, monocytes, granulocytes and other cells have surface receptors and molecules that are vital in a whole range of immunological functions: cell–cell signalling, cell activation, hormone–receptor signalling and many others. The surfaces of immune cells are literally covered with such proteins. Different cells with particular functions have distinct surface proteins, whilst other molecules will be common to several cell types. A major breakthrough in defining surface molecules came in the 1970s, with the discovery of monoclonal antibodies. In a nutshell, monoclonal antibodies are proteins tailormade to bind to a specific target. They are usually raised by injecting the target protein into mice. Researchers in the 1970s and 1980s raised monoclonal antibodies by injecting mice with crude extracts made from various types of immune cell. Some of the monoclonal antibodies generated were able to bind to structures on the surfaces of the target cells. These could be used as tools to distinguish populations of lymphocytes with different functions, as well as identifying neutrophils and monocytes.

By the mid-1980s, however, so many monoclonal antibodies were being produced around the world in so many laboratories that confusion reigned: how did we know whether the surface molecule recognised by monoclonal antibody A produced in Atlanta was the same as that recognised by monoclonal antibody B produced in Baltimore? An international workshop, now meeting regularly, was established. Monoclonal antibodies were exchanged by researchers and panels of experts sat to judge whether the antibodies recognised the same target protein. Because several different antibodies (a cluster) could recognise the same surface protein, and because surface proteins indicated the differentiation of a cell (e.g. granulocyte or lymphocyte), the monoclonal antibodies were assigned a number according to the cluster of differentiation to which they bound. A cluster of differentiation is, therefore, a surface molecule found on cells according to their lineage and differentiation and identifiable by one or more monoclonal antibodies. A comprehensive list of commonly used CD numbers is given in Appendix 1.

---

removal from the circulation. The covalent binding of C3b to antibody in a complex inhibits lattice formation and maintains solubility. In addition, C3b-coated complexes attach to cells' CR-1, a phenomenon termed immune adherence. The main cells involved are erythrocytes, on which CR-1 is present at relatively low density. By virtue of their high numbers in the circulation, however, erythrocytes express over 85% of circulating CR-1. These cells act as a buffer, constantly restoring the number of complexes to an acceptably low level. Once bound, immune complexes are transported on red cells to the liver and spleen, where they are released and taken up by resident macrophages.

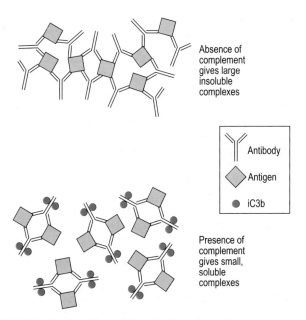

Absence of complement gives large insoluble complexes

Antibody

Antigen

iC3b

Presence of complement gives small, soluble complexes

Fig. 2.10 Lattice formation and the role of complement in immune complex solubilisation.
Since antibodies are divalent (two antigen-binding arms), large antigen–antibody complexes form. C3b binds antibody and forms a complex that stoichiometrically inhibits other antibodies from binding. Soluble complexes can be transported to the spleen and liver for clearance by red blood cells bearing C3b receptors (CR1).

OTHER FACTORS IN HUMORAL IMMUNITY

Other proteins may play a role in the innate immune response. One such is **C-reactive protein** (CRP), so named because of its property of binding to the C-polysaccharide of the pneumococcus. CRP is produced in the liver and binds phosphorylcholine moieties, which constitute a major component of bacterial cell wall teichoic acid. Having bound, CRP can activate complement through the classical pathway, independently of antibody. One of the most striking features of CRP, however, is that its blood levels rise 10–100 fold within hours of the start of an infective or inflammatory process. Since it has a relatively short half-life, it has, therefore, become extremely useful in monitoring infective or inflammatory processes, and particularly their response to treatment.

Fibronectin is a circulating protein capable of binding bacteria, particularly staphylococci and streptococci. Since it also binds macrophages and monocytes, it enhances clearance of these organisms. Fibronectin levels decline during infection and, like CRP, it is also used in disease monitoring, particularly in premature babies in whom the innate immune system is especially important.

Lysozyme is a bactericidal enzyme secreted in saliva, tears and other body fluids, as well as being present in neutrophil granules. It cleaves bacterial cell wall proteoglycans at a precise point, breaking the bonds between N-acetylglucosamine and N-acetylmuraminic acid.

Biological results of activation of the complement system

- Opsonisation involves coating the walls of pathogens with protein that can then attract and bind to phagocytic cells.
- Cell recruitment, e.g. C5a attracts neutrophils.
- Cell activation, e.g. mast cells and basophils, directly by C3a, C4a and C5a.
- Cell lysis follows completion of the complement cascade on the surface of a target cell.
- Removal of immune complexes prevents a harmful build-up of pro-inflammatory molecules.

Other proteins of the innate system

- C-reactive protein binds components of the bacterial cell wall and can then activate complement independently of antibody.
- Fibronectin binds bacteria and monocytes and macrophages, thus enhancing clearance.
- Lysozyme is a bactericidal enzyme found in body fluids and neutrophil granules.
- C-reactive protein and fibronectin levels can be used to monitor the effect of treatment on infective and inflammatory processes.

Innate immunity II: cellular mechanisms

There are several elements to the cellular immune system that are present and functional at birth, constituting the innate cellular immune system. The granulocytes — neutrophils, eosinophils and basophils — are all present in the blood and have the capacity to migrate into the tissues. Migration of these cells into tissues is unidirectional and may be rapidly up-regulated as required. The mast cell is resident in the tissues, particularly at epithelial surfaces and is characterised by the presence of abundant intracellular granules. A fifth circulating cell type involved in innate immunity, the NK cell, has a more specialised function in immune surveillance against viral infection and possibly against tumour cells. In view of their ontologic structural and functional similarities with the lymphocyte, NK cells will be dealt with in a later chapter (p. 107).

Neutrophils, eosinophils and basophils are involved in different areas of the immune response. Neutrophils are adapted to the killing and removal of bacteria and fungi and are key cells in this process, whilst eosinophils have a predominant role in the control of infection with multicellular parasites, such as worms. Basophils and mast cells have a less well-defined physiological role in immunity. It is possible that they represent a somewhat vestigial part of the immune system. Whatever their *raison d'être*, mast cells are involved in the pathogenesis (i.e. the mechanism of pathological tissue damage) of the clinical syndrome known as allergy, a common and debilitating immune-mediated disorder. Whilst the functional activity of granulocytes and mast cells varies with the cell type, all four of these different cells discharge some of their functions through the release of granules. As we have seen with the complement system, it is artificial to make strict divisions between the innate and acquired immune systems. Granulocytes and mast cells have their innate functions in the immune response modified and given more direction by one element of the acquired immune system, namely specific antibody (see previous chapter and p. 36).

The sequence of events that leads from a granulocyte in the resting state to the completion of its role in an immune response includes signalling, activation, migration from the blood and effector function. Migration into tissues is not a random, but rather a directed process. It involves adhesion between receptors on the granulocyte surface and their ligands on the membranes of endothelial cells, which provide the gateway to the tissues. The adhesion molecules involved are also employed for migration by lymphoid cells.

In the present chapter the mechanisms through which granulocytes become activated, their adhesive and migratory properties and the toxic effector molecules that they generate will be discussed. In Chapter 8, it will be possible to see the way in which these responses dovetail with other elements of the immune system to provide protection from pathogens. In the case of the mast cell, in the present section we will outline the mechanisms and effects of cell activation, whilst in Chapter 10 we will see the mast cell in the context of the pathological tissue damage which results in the clinical condition of allergy.

NEUTROPHILS

The neutrophil has a distinctive appearance, with its polymorphic nucleus and neutral staining granules. The multilobed nucleus is important for the cell to make rapid transit from the blood through tight gaps in the endothelium. The neutrophil is abundant in the circulation, present at a concentration of 2×10^9 to 7×10^9 per litre. The half-life in blood is 6 hours and in the tissues 1–2 days. In health, few neutrophils will be seen in the tissues. The blood and bone marrow form an abundant pool of cells, and neutrophils are recruited and called to sites of infection and inflammation as and when required. In the presence of bacterial or fungal infection, the neutrophil is activated to kill the offending organism.

NEUTROPHIL GRANULES

Neutrophils have two main types of granule: the first appear during their development in the bone marrow (primary or azurophilic granules) and the second group appears later (secondary or specific granules); secondary granules are three times more common in the cytoplasm. Granule contents, and the functions associated with them are shown in Table 3.1.

Both primary and secondary granules may be released intracellularly or extracellularly following fusion with the plasma membrane. Granules are mobilised in response to several stimuli: the products of bacterial cell walls, complement proteins, the leukotriene group of lipid mediators and small bioactive peptides called cytokines. **N-formylated peptides** (for example, N-formyl-methionyl-leucylphenylalanine (FMLP)) are bacterially derived and bind to receptors on the neutrophil surface. The ability of neutrophils to respond to bacterial proteins is clearly a major advantage for their innate responses. Activation products from **complement**, such as iC3b, also bind to specific surface membrane receptors. **Leukotrienes** (LT) are biologically active products of the lipooxygenase pathway of arachidonate metabolism and some, such as LTB_4, have potent stimulatory effects on neutrophils (see box: 'Arachidonic acid metabolites in inflammation'). Finally, **cytokines** such as neutrophil activation protein-1, NAP-1, also known as interleukin-8; tumour necrosis factor-α, (TNF-α) and granulocyte–monocyte colony stimulating factor (GM-CSF) have potent effects on neutrophils (for an introduction to cytokines, see boxes: 'Cytokines' & 'General properties of cytokines').

Within the primary granules are important antibacterial effector molecules. Myeloperoxidase is part of a microbicidal system (see p. 29). Collagenase and elastase break down fibrous structures in the extracellular matrix, facilitating progress of the neutrophil through the tissues. Cathepsin G is cidal to a range of Gram-positive and Gram-negative organisms, as well as some *Candida* species. Cathepsins B, D and E are also bactericidal.

The secondary granules contain pre-formed receptors and an assortment of proteins, not all of which have a clearly defined function as yet. It is noteworthy that the secondary granules contain pre-synthesised receptors for some of the molecules capable of activating them (Table 3.1). As secondary granules are released at a site on the neutrophil surface, therefore, the pole of the membrane which is involved shows an increase in specific receptors, enhancing the directional nature of the response. This may be particularly important in the process known as chemotaxis, the directed movement of cells (see p. 27).

Other granule contents are also critical in the innate immune response. Lactoferrin decreases cell surface charge, enhancing cell adhesion; it may also help in the generation of the hydroxyl radical, $^{\bullet}OH$, a microbicidal toxin (see p. 29).

NEUTROPHIL ACTIVATION

Neutrophils are activated by numerous stimuli: some of the most described molecules involved include the complement component C5a, LTB_4, FMLP and interleukin-8 (IL-8). Each of these are likely to be released at sites of infection and inflammation. To make their contribution to the inflammatory process, neutrophils must migrate to the relevant site in the tissues. This requires some organisation: the affected organ must signal the focus of injury and the neutrophil must bind and adhere specifically to that tissue.

The interface between tissues and blood is formed by endothelial cells. Tissue signals are given out by endothelial cells lining the post-capillary venules, where blood flow is at its slowest. Tissue damage, whether it is caused by infection or other injury, results in the release of mediators, such as histamine from mast cells (see p. 30), with profound effects on vessel walls. The resulting dilatation of vessels, with increased 'leakiness' and further reduction of the rate of blood flow facilitates neutrophil access to the site. Neutrophils have a tendency even in the resting state to adhere lightly to the endothelium, in a process termed 'rolling'. This slows their movement right down, but more specific mechanisms are required for the neutrophil to actually stop and exit the blood. Substances (e.g. cytokines) released from damaged tissues or bacteria (e.g. cell wall products) have a direct effect on the endothelial cells, causing them to become 'sticky', so that neutrophils will adhere firmly. These processes, of rolling and then adhesion, involve a group of molecules broadly termed **adhesion molecules**. Stickiness results from the increased expression of a family of adhesion molecules on

Table 3.1 Contents and function of neutrophil granules

Function	Primary granules	Secondary granules
Microbicidal mechanisms		Respiratory burst complex (cytochrome b_{558}, flavine adenine dinucleotide (FAD) and quinolones)
Microbicidal enzymes	Myeloperoxidase, lysozyme	Lysozyme
Proteinases	Collagenase, elastase, cathepsin G	Collagenase
Acid hydrolases	Cathepsins B, D, E	
Receptors		N-formyl-methionyl-leucylphenylalanine (FMLP) receptors, leukocyte function associated antigen-1 (LFA-1), Mac-1 (CR-3: receptor for iC3b)
Others		Lactoferrin; histaminase; vitamin B_{12}-binding proteins

Arachidonic acid metabolites in inflammation

Following the activation of several different types of cell (especially the mast cell (see p. 30), but also macrophages, granulocytes and lymphocytes), lipids in the cell membrane are converted de novo into inflammatory mediators that have potent effects on the vasculature and on inflammatory cells such as the neutrophil. There are three different classes of such lipid mediators, all deriving from precursor membrane phospholipids and being converted by the action of the enzyme phospholipase A2 (see Fig. 3.1).

The first major lipid mediator to be described was **prostaglandin D$_2$** (PGD$_2$), derived from the cyclooxygenase pathway of arachidonic acid metabolism. This binds receptors on smooth muscle in the vascular endothelium, leading to vasodilatation. This increases blood supply and slows leukocytes passing through the tissues, allowing them to migrate from the blood. Other types of prostaglandin (e.g. PGE$_2$ and PGF$_2$, produced by macrophages) also have potent pro-inflammatory effects.

The second major group of mediators are termed the **leukotrienes** and are formed when arachidonic acid is converted through the lipooxygenase pathway. Mast cells synthesise LTB$_4$, LTC$_4$, LTD$_4$ and LTE$_4$, whilst the neutrophil synthesises LTB$_4$. These mediators also cause vasodilatation, as well as extravasation of fluid into the tissues.

The third lipid-derived mediator, **platelet-activating factor** (PAF) is produced by mast cells and also has the effect of relaxing vascular smooth muscle.

Perhaps one of the major driving forces behind the research in this field has been the knowledge that the lipid derivatives released as a result of these inflammatory reactions have a profound effect on smooth muscle in the lung, causing bronchial constriction. This is manifest as tightness of the chest and wheezing, symptoms of the chronic chest condition called **asthma**.

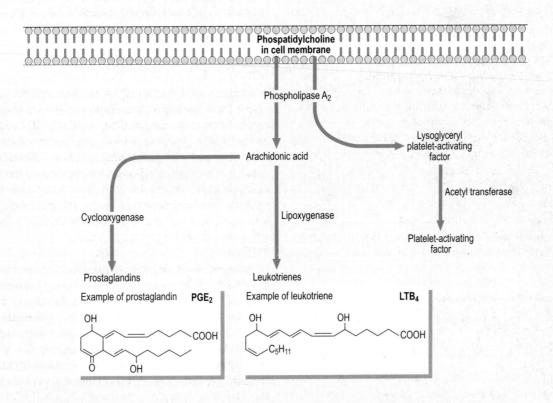

Fig. 3.1 **Biosynthetic pathways of lipid mediators, the leukotrienes, prostaglandins and platelet-activating factor, and their typical structures.**

the endothelium; at the same time, the counter-ligands for these are up-regulated on the rolling neutrophils. Similar stimuli up-regulate the ligands and counter-ligands on the different cell types, so that adhesion is a concerted process. These adhesion molecules are found on all leukocytes and a variety of other cells. The interaction between complementary molecules on neutrophils and endothelial cells results in adhesion of the neutrophils and the opportunity for them to enter the tissue.

Cytokines

Cytokines are small-molecular-weight soluble factors released by cells (cyto-) to communicate with and influence the function (-kines) of other cells through specific surface receptors. The definition is rather broad and, as you will note, has no mention of immunology. This is because it has become clear that factors which were thought to be released solely by immune cells and to have specific immunological effects, have subsequently been shown to be released by a variety of cell types and to have a wide range of effects on a variety of cell types. Studies in the 1970s and 1980s indicated that the immune system communicated and discharged effector functions using soluble factors. These were usually named by their function: MAF for macrophage-activating factor; MIF for migration-inhibition factor; NAF for neutrophil-activating factor; interferon because it interferes with viral replication, etc. As for CD numbers, the rapid growth of this area of immunological studies led to confusion: several research groups might each use a different name to describe a different effect of the same soluble factor. The question also arose: was MAF in Massachusetts the same as MAF in Manchester? Some attempt to clarify these issues was made by changes in nomenclature. Factors produced by lymphocytes were called **lymphokines**; factors produced by monocytes **monokines**. As soon as it became clear that these distinctions could not be upheld (i.e. that other cells than these can secrete these factors), the general term **cytokines** became more widely used. The advent of molecular biology has established a secure future for soluble immunological mediators. At a winter meeting held in the Swiss town of Interlaken, it was decided to call factors that are released by white blood cells and act on white blood cells **interleukins**. By current convention, once an effect is described, the factor that mediates it must be identified, sequenced and its gene also identified. Through this approach, interleukins 1 to 17 have so far been identified.

General properties of cytokines

Cytokines are typically of 15–20 kDa molecular mass. There appears to be a family of cell surface receptors with similar structure. This holds for different cytokines and across different species. There are several important features of cytokines:

- Each cytokine has many different effects on different cells: this property is called **pleiotropy**.
- A cytokine can have a direct effect on the cell which releases it: this **autocrine** function is well described and serves as a feedback mechanism.
- Cytokines can also have effects on cells immediately around them: this is a **paracrine** function.
- In addition, they may act like hormones and have **endocrine** effects on cells and organs remote from the site of release.
- Cytokines often induce the release of other cytokines.
- One final property is that of **synergism**: cytokines may act in concert to achieve an effect greater than the summation of their individual actions.

affinity for sugar moieties); the selectins have diverse roles in cell adhesion. Currently, there are three well-described selectins, P-selectin, E-selectin and L-selectin (Fig. 3.2a; Table 3.2). The 'P', 'E' and 'L' stand for platelet, endothelium and leukocyte, respectively, indicating the predominant cell type expressing each selectin. P-selectin is also found on endothelium. P-selectin and E-selectin bind a sialylated carbohydrate residue which is constitutively expressed on neutrophils (CD15s). L-selectin binds specifically with a glycoprotein cell adhesion molecule (GlyCAM-1) on the endothelium.

Integrins

The integrins are heterodimers; in other words the functional unit is composed of two different polypeptide molecules, in this case termed the α and β chains. There are two families of integrins, defined according to the structure of the β chain. The β_2 integrins are important in adhesion in all leukocytes including lymphocytes: these will be discussed here (Table 3.3). The β_1 integrins are a family of adhesion molecules of

ADHESION MOLECULES

Broadly speaking, there are three main families of surface proteins whose prime role appears to be intercellular adhesion, and these are defined on the basis of shared structural features (Fig. 3.2): the **selectin** and **integrin** families and a third group, the **intercellular adhesion molecules** (ICAMs).

As more molecules involved in adhesion are being defined, so the classification and terminology tries to keep pace. Many, but not all, of the molecules are named using the CD nomenclature.

Selectins

Selectins were named because their N-terminal domain resembles various lectins (lectins are molecules with

Table 3.2 **The selectins**

CD designation	Selectin type	Cell type expressed on	Ligand and its site
CD62	P-selectin	Endothelium	Sialyl Lewis X (CD15s) on neutrophils
CD62E	E-selectin	Endothelium; platelets	Sialyl Lewis X (CD15s) on neutrophils
CD62L	L-selectin	Neutrophil	GlyCAM-1 on endothelium

Note: sialyl Lewis X (CD15s) is a carbohydrate moiety on leukocytes, especially neutrophils; GlyCAM-1, glycoprotein cell adhesion molecule-1

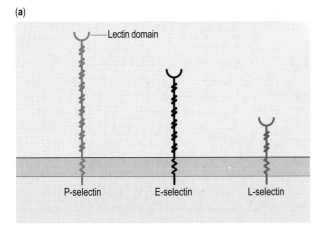

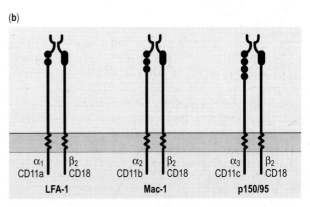

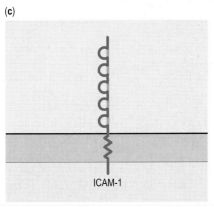

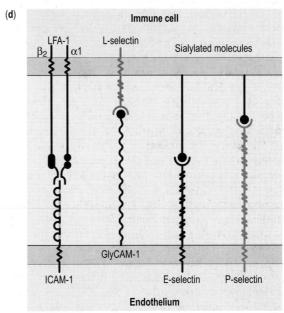

Fig. 3.2 **Adhesion molecules.**
(**a**) The selectins have N-terminal domains that are homologous to a variety of sugar-binding lectins. (**b**) The β_2 integrin family have similar structures with α and β chains that are non-covalently associated. (**c**) The ICAMs have a domain structure similar to immunoglobulin. (**d**) Interaction between these molecules (modified with permission from Springer 1990 Nature 346: 426–427).

particular importance in T cell function: these will be discussed in a later section (see p. 80).

The β_2 integrins have a common β chain and three different α chains, which share 25–65% amino acid sequence homology (Fig. 3.2b). Using the CD nomenclature, the common β_2 chain of 750 amino acid residues is CD18, the α chains (1100 residues) are CD11a, CD11b and CD11c. The heterodimer combination CD11a/CD18 is leukocyte function associated antigen-1 (LFA-1) and is found on lymphocytes, monocytes and neutrophils. CD11b/CD18 is known as Mac-1 (for macrophage-1) or complement receptor-3 (CR-3) and

is present mainly on granulocytes and monocytes. CD11c/CD18 is referred to as p150/95, the numbers referring to the molecular weights of the α and β chains, but it is more correctly termed complement receptor-4 (CR-4).

Intercellular adhesion molecules (ICAMs)

The ligands for the integrins are shown in Table 3.3. In the context of neutrophil adhesion, the most important interactions are between Mac-1 and CR-4 with ICAMs on the surface of endothelial cells. ICAMs are single-chain molecules that form part of the immunoglobulin

Table 3.3 **The integrins**

CD designation	Integrin	Cell type expressed on	Ligand and its site
CD11a/CD18	Leukocyte function associated antigen-1 (LFA-1)	Neutrophils; lymphocytes; monocytes	ICAM-1 and ICAM-2 on endothelium
CD11b/CD18	Macrophage-1 (Mac-1); complement receptor-3 (CR-3)	Neutrophils; monocytes; some lymphocytes	ICAM-1 on endothelium; iC3b following complement activation
CD11c/CD18	p150/95; complement receptor-4 (CR-4)	Tissue macrophages (to a lesser extent neutrophils and monocytes)	iC3b; C4b

gene superfamily of molecules (see p. 37), in that they have a structure comprising five immunoglobulin-like domains (Fig. 3.2c). ICAM-1 is expressed on a variety of cells involved in immune processes, as well as on endothelium; since the majority of leukocytes express integrins, this provides a mechanism to facilitate cell–cell contact, for example between a B lymphocyte and a T lymphocyte. ICAM-1, as well as its physiological role as the ligand for integrins, is also the receptor for rhinoviruses, which cause the common cold.

NEUTROPHIL MIGRATION

Neutrophils permanently express L-selectin (so-called 'constitutive' expression) and endothelial cells constitutively express P-selectin, whilst E-selectin expression requires induction and protein synthesis. The interaction between selectins and their ligands is a weak adhesive force, but it provides the first step in neutrophil migration. The selectin interaction is sufficient to induce some neutrophils in the blood to slow down and move along the margin of the endothelium. This **margina-**

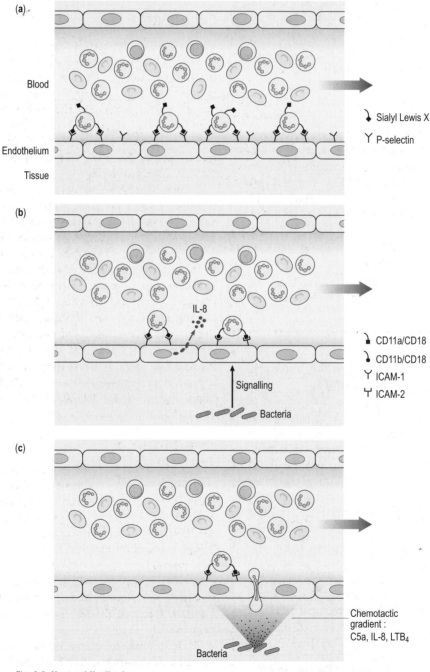

Fig. 3.3 **Neutrophil adhesion.**
(**a**) Margination and rolling of neutrophils, due to weak interactions between constitutively expressed molecules on these cells and endothelium. (**b**) Activation of neutrophils and endothelium causes expression of integrins and ICAMs, and the neutrophil stops. (**c**) Permeation of the neutrophils through the endothelium (diapedesis).

tion is probably continuous, and the marginating pool of neutrophils proceeds along the endothelium in a process termed **rolling** (Fig. 3.3a). The selectin-mediated adhesion is not strong enough to counter the forces of normal blood flow, but in post-capillary vessels the neutrophils can slow down sufficiently to permeate the tissues if a further adhesive mechanism is applied.

This increase in neutrophil–endothelium adhesion is only achieved if activating signals are generated for both cells; for example, signals might include iC3b, FMLP, LTB$_4$ and various cytokines, including IL-8, all of which activate neutrophils and endothelial cells. There is some evidence to suggest that such mediators work optimally when loosely bound to sialylated carbohydrates on the endothelial surface: they are thus in a position to 'catch' rolling neutrophils. Neutrophil activation has two effects. First, there is a **functional up-regulation** of the adhesion molecules such as LFA-1 and Mac-1 already on the neutrophil surface. This is a poorly understood process, presumably involving conformational changes that greatly increase the affinity of these molecules for their ligands on the endothelium. Second, the secondary granules release fresh adhesion molecules from their granules onto the neutrophil surface.

On the endothelial side, ICAM-2 is constitutively expressed on the endothelium and, along with ICAM-1, it is also induced by various mediators, particularly cytokines such as interferon-γ, IL-1 and TNF, all likely to be released at sites of inflammation (for a summary of the functions of different cytokines, see Appendix 2).

The induction of the integrin/ICAM system locally in inflamed tissues increases neutrophil–endothelium

affinity by many times, enabling neutrophils to stop 'rolling' and pass through the endothelium at that site (Fig. 3.3b). The neutrophil is drawn to the point of highest concentration of the activating signals, providing it with the direction required to travel to the inflammatory focus. The act of passing through the endothelium is referred to as **diapedesis**.

The whole process of margination, rolling and diapedesis can be likened to a motorway with several lanes of traffic. If a driver wishes to be able to exit he must be in the slow lane to be ready for the slip-road, whilst the speed of flow makes exiting from the fast lanes much more difficult.

CHEMOTAXIS

Chemotaxis is defined as the directed movement of a cell along a gradient of increasing concentration of the attracting molecule (termed a chemoattractant). It is a property used by neutrophils when they migrate to the site in the tissues where the concentration of chemotactic factors is highest: in other words, the epicentre of the inflammatory process. The most potent chemotactic factors are the C5a complement component, FMLP, IL-8 and LTB$_4$.

Neutrophils have a constant process of random movement akin to the Brownian motion of molecules in the gaseous phase. When a chemotactic factor binds at one pole of the cell, two processes take place: there is granule release, to up-regulate receptors for the chemotactic factors at that pole; and the neutrophil extends its membrane and cytoplasm into thin, foot-like processes known as pseudopodia (Fig. 3.4). After extending, the leading pseudopodium anchors itself and the remainder of the cytoplasm is drawn up. A new pseudopodium is extended and the process repeated; the motion can best be described as resembling that of a caterpillar. Pseudopodia are rich in microtubules, actin, myosin and actin-binding protein, which forms the actin into a lattice structure.

PHAGOCYTOSIS

The ability to ingest and kill microorganisms is a key component in host defence. Neutrophils have the capacity to ingest more than one bacterium or fungus at once in the process of phagocytosis, and this is equally applicable to other macromolecular structures. When large numbers of phagocytes are involved in an infective process, an abscess filled with pus (dead or dying neutrophils) may form; if the process is inflammatory but not infective, for example around a foreign body implanted in the tissues, a so-called 'sterile' abscess may form.

Phagocytosis is comparatively ineffective in the absence of **opsonins**, the co-factors that coat microorganisms and enhance the ability of neutrophils to engulf them (opsonisation). Receptors for the opsonins are present on the neutrophil surface, forming a bridge between cell and organism, but opsonins are also

---

When neutrophils fail us

Nothing has been more graphic in illustrating the critical role of normal neutrophil function in maintaining a physiological balance of immunity than the elucidation of genetic abnormalities in which one component of the neutrophil is missing or impaired. In all of these abnormalities, recurrent bacterial and fungal infections lead to failure to thrive, organ damage and premature death.

For example, several cases have been described of a condition in which the secondary granules are absent. The affected children suffer lung and skin infections, the main organisms involved being *Staphylococcus aureus* and *Candida albicans*. In a slightly more common abnormality, the respiratory burst fails, usually because of the absence of part of the cytochrome b_{558}. Again, pus-forming organisms and fungi cause frequent and prolonged infections of bone, skin and lungs. In another condition, the common β chain of the integrins is not synthesised. The resulting failure of leukocyte adhesion severely impairs immunity in the tissues, giving rise to repeated infections and premature death (**leukocyte adhesion deficiency syndrome, LAD**).

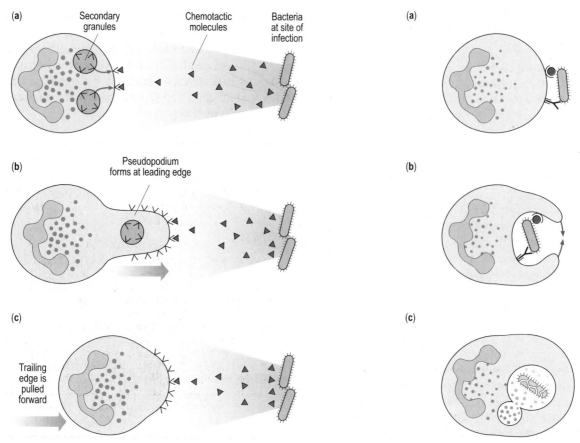

(a)

Secondary granules

Chemotactic molecules

Bacteria at site of infection

(b)

Pseudopodium forms at leading edge

(c)

Trailing edge is pulled forward

Fig. 3.4 **Neutrophil chemotaxis.**

(a)

(b)

(c)

Fig. 3.6 **Phagocytosis.**
(**a**) Opsonised bacterium binds to neutrophil. (**b**) Pseudopodia extend around the bacterium. (**c**) Bacterium is engulfed inside a phagosome to which granules fuse and release their contents.

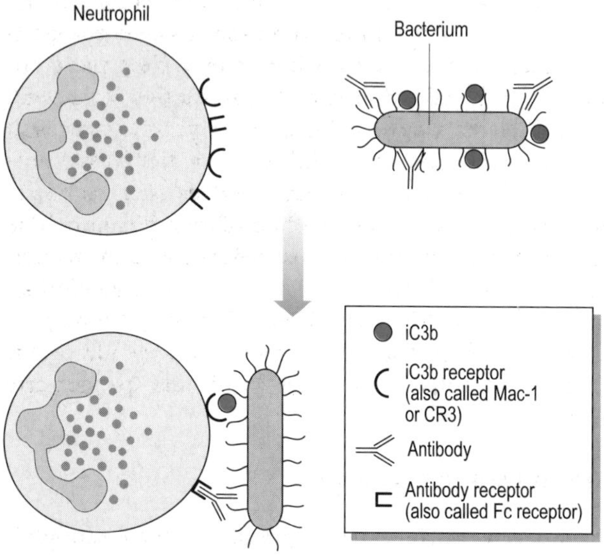

Neutrophil

Bacterium

- ● iC3b
- C iC3b receptor (also called Mac-1 or CR3)
- Antibody
- C Antibody receptor (also called Fc receptor)

Fig. 3.5 **Opsonisation.**
Opsonins coat microorganisms and enhance the neutrophils' ability to engulf them.

Phagocytosis is achieved using pseudopodia. These are extended to surround an organism or particle and eventually meet and fuse to form an enclosed vacuole termed a **phagosome**. The intracellular phagosome can now be fused with neutrophil granules, releasing their digestive and toxic contents to attack the phagosome contents (Fig. 3.6). Occasionally, granule contents may be discharged into the external milieu, for example if a particle is too large to engulf, leading to tissue damage; this process is termed 'reverse phagocytosis'.

NEUTROPHIL KILLING

Killing bacteria and fungi is a critical, life-saving step. In some disorders, killing is impaired and although the ability to phagocytose may remain intact, the individual suffers recurrent, often fatal infections. Killing is the end result of complex mechanisms: in simple terms there are two microbicidal routes: one **oxygen-dependent** and the other **oxygen-independent**. The oxygen-independent mechanisms are those alluded to earlier; microbicidal enzymes such as lysozyme and the cathepsins. There are two oxygen-dependent mechanisms: the **respiratory burst** and the **hydrogen peroxide–myeloperoxidase–halide system**. The best-known is the respiratory burst, so-called because of its use of

potent activators of neutrophils (Fig. 3.5). The best opsonins are the complement component C3b, C-reactive protein and antibody. The role of antibody, raised against a particular organism, is a good example of the specific immune system giving direction to the innate.

Oxygen-dependent mechanisms to produce toxic metabolites

The respiratory burst

1. *Generation of superoxide anion*

$$O_2 + electron \rightarrow O_2^-$$

(It is not clear where the electron comes from: probably a $NADPH \rightarrow NADH + H^+$ reaction.)

2. *Generation of hydrogen peroxide*

$$HO_2 + O_2^- + H^+ \xrightarrow{\text{superoxide dismutase}} O_2 + H_2O_2$$

3. *Generation of singlet oxygen*

$$H_2O_2 + OCl^- \rightarrow {}^1O_2 + H_2O + Cl^-$$

4. *Generation of hydroxyl radical*

$$O_2^- + H_2O_2 \rightarrow O_2 + OH^- + {}^\bullet OH$$

The hydrogen peroxide–myeloperoxidase–halide microbicidal system

$$H_2O_2 + 2Cl^- + H^+ \xrightarrow{\text{myeloperoxidase}} H_2O + Cl_2 + OH^-$$

oxygen. There are two approaches to understanding the respiratory burst: one is simply to identify the toxic metabolites it generates to kill bacteria and the second is to elucidate the process by which they are generated.

The main toxic metabolites that have been identified are:

- superoxide anion O_2^-
- hydrogen peroxide H_2O_2
- singlet oxygen ${}^1O_2$
- hydroxyl radical ${}^\bullet OH$.

The other approach is more complex and attempts to understand the chemical processes which generate these toxic metabolites. Unfortunately, this approach has a heavy reliance upon daunting chemical equations (see box: 'Oxygen-dependent mechanisms to produce toxic metabolites').

The main constituents of the respiratory burst complex, found in the secondary granules, are a membrane-bound complex of three components: **flavin adenine**

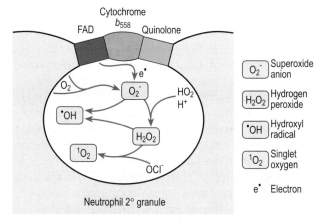

Fig. 3.7 Respiratory burst in secondary granules generates toxic molecules to kill bacteria.

dinucleotide (FAD), quinolone and a unique cytochrome, **cytochrome b_{558}** (Fig. 3.7).

In the hydrogen peroxide–myeloperoxidase–halide system, H_2O_2 generated by the respiratory burst, myeloperoxidase from the primary granules and a halide such as Cl^- combine to give chlorine and hydroxyl ions, both toxic to microorganisms.

Neutrophils

- The neutrophil is an essential component of the cellular innate immune system, involved in killing bacteria and fungi.
- A pool of neutrophils continuously rolls along the endothelial surface of blood vessels tethered by weak cell–cell interactions mediated by specific receptors.
- Following activation of both neutrophil and endothelium, specialised adhesion molecules halt neutrophil rolling and facilitate their entry into the tissues.
- Neutrophils move towards chemical attractants, and engulf microorganisms by phagocytosis.
- Killing is mediated by oxygen-dependent and oxygen-independent routes: the most important involves the generation of a respiratory burst.

EOSINOPHILS

The eosinophil comprises some 3–5% of all granulocytes in the circulation. This statistic hides the reality, however, since several hundred times more eosinophils are present in the tissues, where they collect preferentially at epithelial surfaces and may survive for several weeks. The distinctive staining of eosinophils is a result of the granule contents, mainly cationic (i.e. basic) proteins with affinity for acid aniline dyes such as eosin, and this remains the best method of identification. The main role of eosinophils in host defence is in protection against multicellular parasites such as worms (helminths), which is afforded by the release of toxic, cationic proteins. Outside the tropics, however, they are important for their contribution to allergic disease, particularly asthma.

EOSINOPHIL GRANULES

There are two main types of granule in the eosinophil: specific and primary. The specific granules predominate and contain the cationic proteins, of which there are four main types. **Major basic protein** (MBP; so-called because it is the most abundant cationic protein), **eosinophil cationic protein** (ECP) and **eosinophil neurotoxin** are all potently and exquisitely toxic to helminths, while ECP also has some bactericidal properties. **Eosinophil peroxidase** is distinct from myeloperoxidase in neutrophils but catalyses a similar reaction (see box: 'Oxygen-dependent mechanisms to produce toxic metabolites').

The primary granule contents remain poorly characterised. Other granule-like structures have been seen that are in fact lipid vesicles, which may provide swift release of LTC_4 and LTD_4. LTC_4 and another mediator, platelet activating factor (PAF), to produce changes in airway smooth muscle and vasculature, which are important in allergic reactions (see below).

EOSINOPHIL ACTIVATION

Like neutrophils, eosinophils are activated by a variety of mediators for which they have receptors. Specific receptors for C3b/C4b (CR-1), iC3b (CR-3), C5a and LTB_4 are present on the membrane, as are others for several different classes of antibody. Ligand binding to any of these may activate the cell. Again, as for the neutrophil, the involvement of antibody in eosinophil reactions adds specificity. Of particular interest in this regard are receptors for the antibody classes known as IgE, which has a role in allergy, and IgA, which has a role in protection of mucosal surfaces. Receptors are also present for the cytokines IL-3 and IL-5, which promote the development and differentiation of eosinophils, and for GM-CSF, which also acts on other cells as the name suggests. IL-5 is an essential and sufficient growth factor for eosinophils and may also be produced by them.

EOSINOPHIL ADHESION

Eosinophils appear to have a similar mechanism of migration to that of neutrophils, employing similar surface molecules. The selective migration of eosinophils over neutrophils in certain pathological conditions is difficult to explain, but eosinophils alone appear to possess **very late antigen-1** (VLA-1, a member of the integrin family), which binds **vascular cell adhesion molecule-1** (VCAM-1) on the endothelium.

EOSINOPHILS IN HOST DEFENCE

Although in vitro studies demonstrate that eosinophils are capable of phagocytosis and intracellular degranulation, in vivo they probably employ complement and antibody-guided local release of toxic cationic proteins onto the surface of helminths. There is increasing evidence that their defensive properties overlap with those of the acquired immune response. Eosinophils can synthesise and express on their surface CD4 and HLA-DR (see p. 86) which are associated with antigen-specific cell-mediated responses. This evidence, taken with their longer life compared with neutrophils, ability to secrete cytokines and maintain and perpetuate a state of cell activation, indicates that they are a markedly more sophisticated cell than the neutrophil.

Eosinophils

- The eosinophil contains several cationic proteins that are vital in host defence against helminthic parasites.
- At a more sophisticated level, eosinophil responses are under cytokine control and may involve interaction with lymphocytes.
- Eosinophils are a feature of the infiltrate in tissues involved in allergic responses, though their role remains unclear.

MAST CELLS AND BASOPHILS

Mast cells and basophils share many features in common, but it should also be noted that at least two types of mast cell exist in the rat, according to the tissue in which they are found, and that site-specific differences probably also exist in humans. The two main features of these cells are the histamine-containing granules and the possession of high-affinity receptors for IgE (contrasting with the low-affinity type on eosinophils).

MAST CELL AND BASOPHIL GRANULES

Mast cell and basophil mediators are categorised as preformed and as those synthesised de novo (Table 3.4; Figs 3.8 and 3.9). The best known is **histamine**, a low-molecular-mass amine (111 Da) with a blood half-life of less than 5 minutes and which constitutes 10% of the cell's weight. Injected into the skin, histamine

Table 3.4 **Mast cell and basophil mediators**

Mediators	Actions/comments
Pre-formed mediator	
Histamine	Vasodilatation
	Vascular permeability ↑
	Smooth muscle contraction in airways
Protease enzymes	Mainly tryptic enzymes (cf. pancreatic trypsin)
	Digestion of basement membrane causes ↑ vascular permeability
	Digestion of connective tissue to ↑ cell migration
	Cleavage of C3 → C3a
Proteoglycans	Mainly heparin in mast cells
	Mainly chondroitin sulphate in basophils
	Responsible for distinctive blue staining
	Anticoagulant activity
Chemotactic factors	Eosinophil chemotactic factor of anaphylaxis
	Neutrophil chemotactic factor
Synthesised de novo	
Platelet activating factor (PAF)	Vasodilator
LTB_4, LTC_4, LTD_4	Eosinophil activators
	Neutrophil chemoattractants
	Platelet activators
	Vascular permeability ↑
	Bronchoconstrictors
Prostaglandins (mainly PGD_2)	Vascular permeability ↑
	Bronchoconstrictors
	Vasodilators

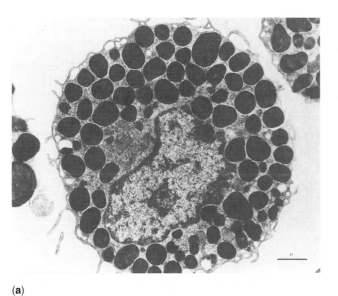

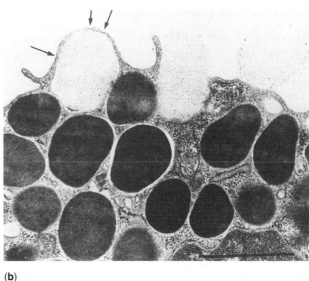

(a)   (b)

Fig. 3.8 **Granule release from mast cells.**
Electron micrographs of a normal mast cell (**a**) and a mast cell 20 seconds after activation (**b**). The release of granules (arrowed) results in a loss of electron density. (Reproduced with permission from Upjohn Inc.)

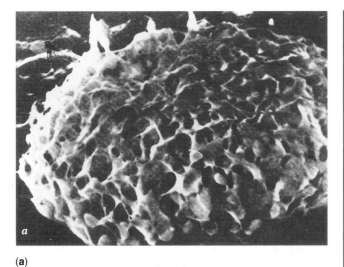

(a)

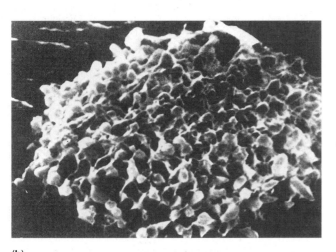

(b)

Fig. 3.9 **Granule release from mast cells.**
Scanning electron micrograph of a resting (**a**) and a degranulating (**b**) mast cell. (Reproduced with permission from Upjohn Inc.)

Histamine

Histamine has two receptors. The H_1 receptor mediates the vascular and bronchial smooth muscle effects and is blocked by drugs such as mepyramine and terfenadine, which form the basis of many proprietary antihistamines used for allergic reactions such as hay fever. The H_2 receptor mediates gastric acid secretion and is blocked by the now famous drugs cimetidine and ranitidine, which have revolutionised treatment of gastric and duodenal ulceration.

The consequences of mast cell and basophil degranulation depend upon the site of release. In contact with the airways, histamine induces smooth muscle contraction, a process that underlies the airway obstruction seen in asthma. At other mucosal sites, there may be tear formation, nasal discharge (coryza), conjunctival redness, gritty eyes and itching. Widespread activation of mast cells and basophils with release of mediators into the circulation results in the state termed **anaphylaxis** — a syndrome of circulatory shock and collapse with low blood pressure and chest tightness leading to arrested breathing and death unless treated.

induces the typical 'wheal and flare' or 'triple' response. Initially there is reddening (erythema) of the skin at the site as arterioles dilate and post-capillary venules contract. This is followed by increased vascular permeability, with leakage of plasma fluid into the tissues causing swelling (wheal). Finally, histamine acts directly on local axons to induce more widespread vascular changes distant from the injection site (flare).

MAST CELL AND BASOPHIL ACTIVATION

Activation of mast cells and basophils by the antibody class IgE is an important feature of allergic disease that will be dealt with subsequently (Ch. 10). The anaphylatoxins C3a, C4a and C5a activate basophils and may activate lung mast cells, while FMLP probably acts on basophils alone.

Mast cells and basophils

- Mast cells and basophils are similar in structure and appear to serve similar roles in the tissues and blood, respectively.
- Mast cell and basophil granule products, particularly histamine and the leukotrienes, have profound effects on blood vessels and bronchial smooth muscle.
- The effect of release of mast cell and basophil granules differs according to the stimulus and site, producing anything from a localised wheal and flare to anaphylactic shock.

Acquired immunity: antigen receptors

The nature of the acquired immune system is quite distinct from that of innate immunity. Before the development of an acquired immune response, the host immune system is in a state of ignorance and naivety towards the provoking stimulus, which might be, for example, a virus or bacterium. During the first encounter between host and microbe, the immune system begins to 'identify' and 'learn' distinctive structural features of the microorganism. This enables a process of specific recognition. Effector responses (e.g. killing, neutralisation of toxins) can now be initiated, giving the host protection. At the same time, a memory bank of the most effective components of the immune response to that microbe can be laid down. Thus, in future responses to the same organism, host defences can be mobilised more quickly, with a greater initial force. In the acquired immune response, then, we can see the cardinal features of **specificity**, **memory**, and **variable intensity**.

In general, the innate and acquired immune responses do not become activated independently. They perform optimally when complementing each other. In particular, antibodies generated through acquired immunity are capable of directing components of the innate immune system (e.g. complement, neutrophils, mast cells) onto relevant targets.

ANTIGENS AND ANTIBODIES

ANTIGENS

Antigens may be defined as structures which **gen**erate an **anti**- response by the immune system. If we take as an example of an antigen a core viral protein (Fig. 4.1), the immune system has three elements that are used in the binding and recognition of this antigen:

- antibodies
- T cell receptors
- MHC molecules.

Antibodies are generated by B lymphocytes and plasma cells. They are large glycoprotein structures with recognition sites for part of an intact antigen (in general, intact antigens are larger than the size of the antigen-binding site of the antibody). The antibody–antigen interaction is shape dependent: imagine the antigen as the jelly and the antibody-binding site as the jelly mould. The shapes are sometimes termed conformations, and antibody binding is, therefore, conformation dependent. Antibodies can bind antigens that are free in solution, so-called soluble antigens. Alternatively, the antigen may be fixed on the surface of a cell or tissue. The part of the antigen with which the antibody interacts is termed an **epitope**. This region of the antigen determines which antibody will bind and may also be referred to as an **antigenic determinant**.

T cell receptors are the second type of receptor for antigen; they are found on T lymphocytes and, like antibodies, are large glycoproteins. However, there are some important differences between the two. T cell receptors interact not with whole intact antigens, but with a short segment of amino acids (**peptide antigen**) derived from the intact antigen by proteolysis. Within a

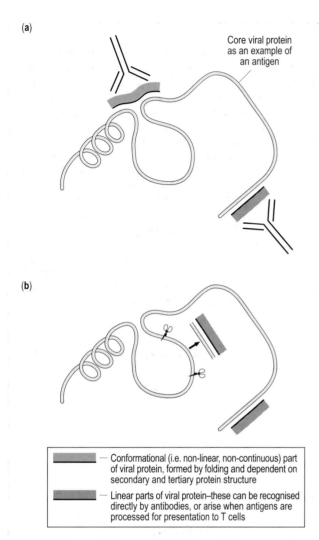

(a)

Core viral protein
as an example of
an antigen

(b)

— Conformational (i.e. non-linear, non-continuous) part
of viral protein, formed by folding and dependent on
secondary and tertiary protein structure

— Linear parts of viral protein–these can be recognised
directly by antibodies, or arise when antigens are
processed for presentation to T cells

Fig. 4.1 Viral core protein as an example of an antigen.
(**a**) Antibodies see 'shapes' derived from the conformational or
linear parts of the antigen. (**b**) T cells and MHC molecules bind
short peptides that are essentially linear in structure and can be
derived from any part of a molecule.

particular antigen, this is termed the **T cell epitope**. A
further difference is that the T cell receptor cannot
interact with soluble peptide antigen directly; the antigen must be held and presented by other glycoprotein
molecules. These 'other molecules' are the third
element of the immune system which binds antigen:
the **major histocompatibility complex (MHC)
molecules**. MHC molecules hold the peptide antigen
enclosed within a groove. What is recognised by the
T cell receptor, therefore, is the combination of shapes
formed by the peptide antigen and the walls of the
groove in the MHC molecule.

Antigens, whether intact or short peptides, interact
with these three types of receptor through non-covalent
forces, such as hydrogen bonding, electrostatic attraction and van der Waals forces. The interaction is typically reversible, and obeys the laws of mass action.
Taking antibody–antigen interactions as an example:

$$\text{antigen} + \text{antibody} \rightleftharpoons \text{antigen–antibody complex}$$

There is a dynamic equilibrium between the dissoci-
ated antigen and antibody and the antigen–antibody
(or 'immune') complex. The strength, or **affinity**, of
the interaction can be defined as the concentration of
antigens allowing half the antibodies to be complexed
and half to remain in solution. This concentration is
expressed in moles and is called the **dissociation constant** (K_d). The smaller the number, the higher the
affinity. In general, of the three immune molecules
designed to bind antigen, antibody has the highest
affinity for antigen (estimated to be as high as 10^{-11} M
for binding to natural antigens), with MHC molecules
having a lower affinity for peptides (approximately
10^{-6} M) and the T cell receptor a lower affinity still for
the peptide–MHC complex.

Because of their characteristic structure, with two
'arms', antibodies have at least two sites for binding
antigen. In some cases, this number is even higher
(e.g. one type of antibody, IgM, has five 'arms' and,
therefore 10 sites). Antibodies have a flexible hinge
between the arms and, therefore, may be able to use
more than one binding site in certain circumstances,
for example when an antigen repeats itself as part of the
coat of a bacterium. This increases the overall strength
of binding, compared with when a single site is used.
The overall strength of attachment is termed the
avidity.

ANTIBODIES

Antibodies, i.e. those soluble glycoproteins that exhibit
antigen-binding ability, belong to a group of large polypeptides termed the **immunoglobulins**. The term
immunoglobulin derives from the facts that they have
an immune function and they are identifiable in the
fraction of serum proteins termed the globulins (see
box: 'Electrophoretic separation of serum proteins' and
Fig. 4.2). All antibodies are immunoglobulins; not all
immunoglobulin molecules necessarily have demonstrable antigen-binding (i.e. antibody) function. However, the terms antibody and immunoglobulin are
frequently used interchangeably.

Antibodies have a range of functions and uses, both
biological and as clinical tools:

1. In host defence:
   - targeting of infective organisms
   - recruitment of damaging host effector
     mechanisms
   - neutralisation of toxins
   - removal of foreign antigens from the
     circulation
2. In clinical medicine:
   - specific anti-pathogen antibody levels used in
     diagnosis/monitoring a disease
   - pooled antibodies administered passively for host
     therapy/protection
3. In laboratory science: antibodies are used in a vast
   range of diagnostic and research applications.

Electrophoretic separation of serum proteins

Red and white blood cells circulate in a fluid enriched with many different proteins. This fluid is termed plasma. If blood is taken and allowed to clot, the fluid remaining after removal of the clot containing the combination of cells and fibrin is termed **serum**. One of the earliest methods to be used for the separation and analysis of the different components of serum was **electrophoresis** (Fig. 4.2a). This can be carried out in a gel (e.g. agarose) or on a paper filter across which an electric field is applied. Proteins migrate within the field according to their charge: this migration is in turn influenced by the pH, and the optimum separation conditions are achieved in buffer at pH 8.6. Once separated, the proteins can be stained in the gel or filter. Albumin is a major constituent of serum proteins and at this pH migrates fast as a negatively charged molecule towards the anode. Other proteins follow at different speeds and form discrete zones, termed α and β. The Greek letters are used as prefixes for numerous serum proteins (e.g. β_2-microglobulin), on the basis of the zone to which they migrate. The term globulin relates to the globular, rather than linear, nature of many of the serum proteins.

Early studies indicated that most antibodies migrate cathodally, to a region termed γ, giving rise to the term gamma-globulins. Some immunoglobulins (notably those of the IgA class) migrate to the β region. The facts that there are several different immunoglobulin isotypes and that all antibodies differ slightly in the structure of their antigen-binding sites means that antibody molecules vary in their migration speed under electrophoresis. This leads to a 'spread-out' pattern of globulins in the β and γ regions, in contrast to the discrete band for albumin (Fig. 4.2b).

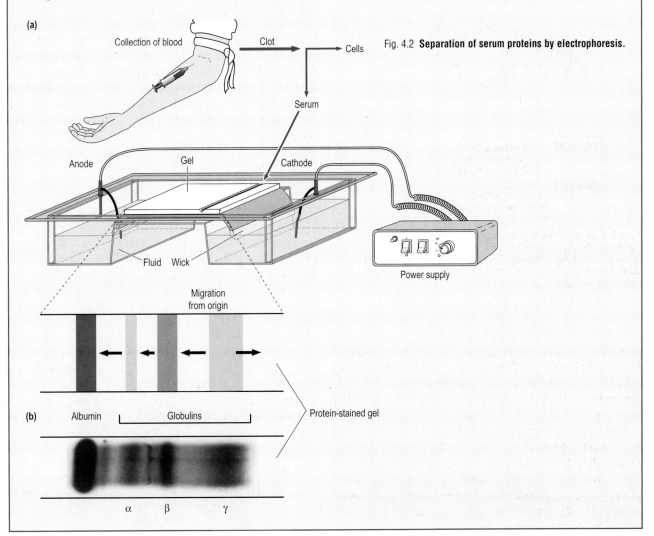

Fig. 4.2 **Separation of serum proteins by electrophoresis.**

Antibodies activate a number of immune effector functions that have an important role in host defence against disease:

- complement activation

- stimulation of phagocytosis and killing by polymorphonuclear cells
- recruitment of killer cells with receptors for antibody
- activation of mast cells.

THE MANY ROLES AND USES OF ANTIBODIES

What is the purpose of antibody binding to antigen? In protection against pathogenic (i.e. damaging) organisms, binding of an antibody molecule to the intact microbe allows the recruitment and direction of host antibacterial effector mechanisms, such as complement and polymorphonuclear cells. The classical complement pathway cannot 'recognise' a foreign organism. Antibodies act as a guidance system, focusing effectors such as complement onto appropriate targets. In this way, antibodies provide target specificity for the innate immune system. Antibody can also bind and neutralise bacterial toxins.

In the wider context of clinical medicine, antibodies are useful diagnostic tools (e.g. measurement of levels of antiviral or antibacterial antibodies can tell us of contact with an infectious organism). Perhaps by far the biggest revolution associated with antibodies has taken place in laboratory science, where the manufacture of antibody molecules 'to order' has been applied most widely (see p. 42).

There are several characteristic features of antibodies. First, they have two modes of expression: they may be synthesised and displayed on the surface of B lymphocytes where they serve as antigen receptors, or they may be exported as soluble proteins by plasma cells (remember plasma cells are end-differentiated B lymphocytes). Second, because of their unique conformation, each antibody monomer has two identical antigen-binding sites. Third, the distinctive gene complex that codes for antibodies enables antibody structure to vary enormously, to the extent that each individual can potentially construct over 10^{11} different antigen-binding sites. Fourth, after the shape of the antigen-binding site has been selected in a particular B cell, other parts of the immunoglobulin molecule can be modified to give the antibody molecule different effector functions. Some of these effector functions (notably complement activation) only occur when the antibody has actually bound antigen, preventing inadvertent initiation of the cascade.

IMMUNOGLOBULINS

STRUCTURE

The typical immunoglobulin molecule has a molecular mass of some 150–200 kDa and is made up of four polypeptide chains (Fig. 4.3). Two of the chains are relatively lighter in mass than the others: hence the terms **heavy** (H) and **light** (L) chains. The two light chains (approximately 23 kDa) in each molecule are identical to each other; the two heavy chains (50–80 kDa) are also identical. Hence the formula of an immunoglobulin molecule might be written Heavy$_2$Light$_2$ or H_2L_2. There are two alternative types of light chain, denoted by the Greek letters κ and λ. An individual immunoglobulin molecule either has two κ chains (in approximately two-thirds of cases) or two λ chains (the remaining third). There can be up to five major heavy chain types, termed α, δ, ε, γ and μ (see below). Again, in each individual immunoglobulin molecule, the two heavy chains used will be identical.

When the structures of different antibody molecules are compared, several facts become apparent. Each heavy chain and each light chain has a relatively stable segment, which varies little between different molecules, as well as a zone in which the amino acid sequence varies enormously from antibody to antibody (see box: 'Variability and hypervariability in antibodies' and

Antigens and antibodies

- Acquired immunity has specificity, memory and a variable response.
- The molecular target of the acquired immune response is termed the antigen: the precise part of the antigen bound by an immune molecule is termed the epitope.
- Antigens are bound and recognised by antibodies, T cell receptors and MHC molecules.
- Antibodies are soluble glycoproteins termed immunoglobulins and can vary substantially in the range of possible antigen-binding sites. Because each molecule has at least two sites, multiple binding to large antigens is possible, increasing the avidity, or strength, of the attachment.
- Antibodies target foreign antigens, neutralise toxins and activate immune effectors: complement, mast cells, NK cells and phagocytes.
- Antibodies are displayed on the surface of B cells or circulate as soluble proteins.
- Antibodies are used in clinical and research science as diagnostic tools.

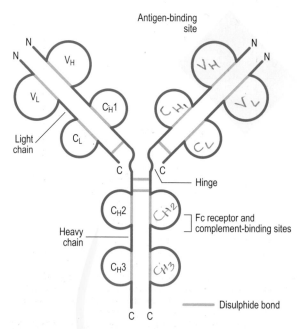

Fig. 4.3 **Typical structure of an immunoglobulin molecule.**

Fig. 4.4). The relatively constant, or **C regions**, hold the effector functions of the molecule, such as complement activation. The variable, or **V regions**, include the antigen-binding sites; the variability is critical for generating the potential to bind to more than 10^7 different antigen structures. The genetic basis for this variability is discussed below (p. 43).

To form the full antibody molecule, the two heavy chains are linked together by two interchain disulphide bonds. Each heavy chain then has a light chain attached to it, again by an interchain disulphide bond.

Variability and hypervariability in antibodies

Analysis of the amino acid sequences of several different immunoglobulin molecules reveals that some areas frequently use the same or similar stretches of amino acids, or at least the variability is small. In contrast, some areas demonstrate much greater variability, and at some points on the molecule a peak of variation in the choice of amino acids is seen. The variability can be plotted as histograms (so-called Wu and Kabat plots; Fig. 4.4). The regions of variability, of which there are three in each heavy and light chain, are termed **hypervariable** or **complementarity-determining regions** (**CDRs**; because they form a surface complementary to the three-dimensional surface of the antigen). Not surprisingly, this diversity is generated for a specific purpose: the CDRs come together after the folding of the immunoglobulin molecule into its tertiary structure and form the binding site for antigen. This explains the structural basis for the enormous variability available for recognition by antibody of a vast array of antigens.

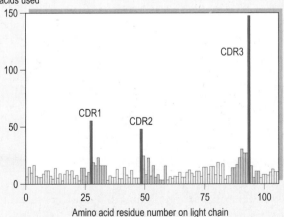

Number of different amino acids used

Fig. 4.4 **Diversity in antigen binding.**
This is dependent upon variation in the antibody structure and this diversity can be assessed by counting the number of different amino acids used at each position in a range of antibody molecules. This is called a Wu and Kabat plot and shows regions of the molecule where there is hypervariability between different antibodies (CDRs). (Modified with permission from Kabat 1980 Journal of Immunology 125: 963.)

The carbohydrate content of the glycoproteins varies between 2 and 12% and there are specific glycosylation sites. Within the heavy and light chains, there are intrachain disulphide bonds. These serve to bend segments back onto themselves, creating regions called **domains** within the heavy and light chains. This gives the immunoglobulin molecule a very distinctive structure. All immunoglobulin domains contain two layers of β-pleated sheet with three or four strands of antiparallel polypeptide chain. When first discovered, the domain structure and its genetic basis were considered highly distinctive. Subsequently, many molecules in the immune system (MHC molecules, adhesion molecules, T cell receptors and cellular co-receptors) have been shown to share a similar domain structure, giving rise to the term **immunoglobulin supergene family** to highlight this structural similarity.

In an immunoglobulin molecule the domains are named according to which chain (H or L) they are in, and numbered. Therefore, the light chain is referred to as having one V_L and one C_L domain (Fig. 4.5), while the heavy chain has a V_H and either three or four C_H domains (C_H1–4). The V_L and V_H domains combine to form the antigen-binding site. The C_H domains contain the major effector functions, such as the complement-binding site and the location for interaction with receptors on polymorphonuclear cells and mast cells. There is a **hinge region** in the middle of the molecule, which allows some freedom to the two arms bearing the antigen-binding sites. This flexibility enables antibody monomers to maximise the chances of binding two antigens at one time.

The immunoglobulin molecule can be cleaved with different enzymatic treatments (Fig. 4.6). The enzyme papain cleaves at the hinge region, breaking the two interchain disulphide bonds between the heavy chains in the process, to produce three fragments. Two of the fragments are identical and retain antigen-binding ability. These are termed **Fab fragments** (for fragment antigen binding) and have a molecular mass of about 45 kDa. The other fragment is larger (55 kDa) and has no antigen-binding site but retains the effector functions (e.g. binding to cell surface receptors). This fragment is also crystallisable and is termed the **Fc fragment** (for fragment crystallisable: numerous cells express surface receptors for immunoglobulin molecules, and since these interact with this portion of the molecule, they are termed **Fc receptors**). Cleavage of the immunoglobulin molecule with pepsin leaves the heavy–heavy interchain disulphide bond intact. Therefore, the two Fab fragments are linked, into a **F(ab')₂ fragment** with two antigen-binding sites, but no effector functions remaining.

As stated above, the part of the antibody molecule that holds the effector functions can be varied, for different roles. This is achieved through variation in the genes encoding the H chains. There are five different major types of H chain gene, giving rise to H chains denoted by a Greek letter: α, δ, ε, γ and μ, with the

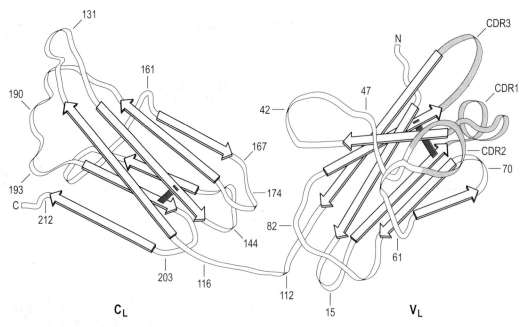

Fig. 4.5 Immunoglobulin domains in a human light chain.
The V and C regions each fold independently. The white arrows represent β-pleated sheets; the dark pink bars are intrachain disulphide bonds; and the CDR1, CDR2 and CDR3 variable regions are coloured in light pink. The last group together form the antigen-binding site. (Adapted with permission from Edmundson et al 1975 Biochemistry 14: 3953–3961.)

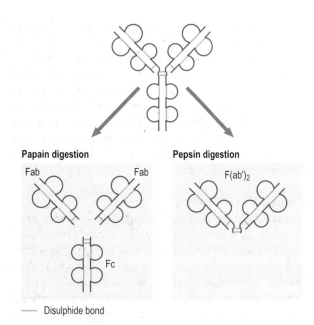

Fig. 4.6 Cleavage of antibody molecules to give Fab and Fc fragments.
Papain digestion produces two antigen-binding fragments (Fab) and one fragment that activates complement and binds to Fc receptors (Fc). Pepsin digestion produces a single F(ab')₂ fragment with two antigen-binding sites.

γ chains being further subdivided into γ_1, γ_2, γ_3 and γ_4 and the α chains into α_1 and α_2. When referring to the whole immunoglobulin molecule, **Ig** is used for short: the presence of the different heavy chains gives rise to the major **classes** of immunglobulins: **IgA, IgD, IgE, IgG** and **IgM**. The IgG molecules can be further subdivided into the IgG1, IgG2, IgG3 and IgG4 subclasses and IgA into the IgA1 and IgA2 subclasses.

All of these immunoglobulin molecules have the same basic structure, of heavy and light chain constituents. Variations in the heavy chains, giving rise to the different classes and subclasses, confer distinctive functions, and these will now be examined in more detail.

IMMUNOGLOBULIN CLASSES AND SUBCLASSES

Immunoglobulin G (IgG)

IgG is the most abundant immunoglobulin, having an average serum concentration of 10 g/l in an adult. The IgG molecule has three constant domains in the heavy chain (C_H1–3) (Table 4.1). IgG occurs as a monomer and can be subdivided into four subclasses. The variability between the four IgG subclasses is mainly located in the hinge regions and functional domains (Fig. 4.7). The IgG subclasses vary in their relative ability to perform some of the effector functions and also in their serum concentration (Table 4.2). It is not yet clear how IgG subclass selection takes place. However, some facts are known about their relative importance. For example, IgG responses to bacterial polysaccharides are predominantly made by the IgG2 subclass. IgG2 responses may, therefore, be important in combating capsulated bacteria. IgG is one of the major activators of the classical complement pathway; IgG1 and IgG3 being the main contributors amongst the subclasses. Binding of C1q to IgG in its native state is very weak; binding is greatly increased when the IgG is complexed to antigen. C1q interacts with the C_H2 domain.

Table 4.1 **Physical properties of immunoglobulins**

	IgG	IgA	IgM	IgD	IgE
Usual structural form	Monomer	Monomer (circulating IgA) Dimer (secretory IgA)	Pentamer	Monomer	Monomer
Accessory chains		J chain polyimmunoglobulin receptor (secretory chain)	J chain		
Subclasses	IgG1, IgG2, IgG3, IgG4	IgA1, IgA2			
Heavy chain	γ	α	μ	δ	ε
Number of domains in heavy chain	3	3	4	3	4
Molecular mass (kDa)	150	160 (monomer); 385 (secretory)	950	180	190
Adult serum concentration (g/l)	6–12	1–4	0.5–2	0.04	0.003
Half-life (days)	23	6	5	3	2.5
Proportion found in circulation (%)	50	50	80	75	50

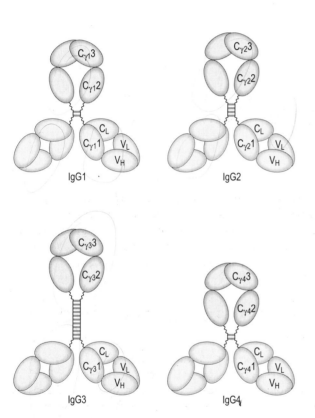

Fig. 4.7 **The four subclasses of human IgG.**
IgG3 has a distinctive extended hinge region.

— Disulphide bond

Table 4.2 **Properties of IgG subclasses**

	IgG1	IgG2	IgG3	IgG4
Proportion total IgG (%)	65	20	10	5
Activation of complement	++	+	++	–
Placental transfer	++	++	++	++
Binding to:				
Fc$_\gamma$RI	++	–	++	+
FC$_\gamma$RII	++	–	++	–
Fc$_\gamma$RIII	++	–	++	–
Major antibody responses:				
e.g. tetanus	++	+	+	++
e.g. bacterial polysaccharides	+	++	+	+

Table 4.3 **Receptors for IgG**

Receptor	Present on	Interacts with
Fc$_\gamma$RI (CD64)	Monocytes, neutrophils	IgG1, IgG3, IgG4
Fc$_\gamma$RII (CD32)	Neutrophils, eosinophils	IgG1, IgG3
Fc$_\gamma$RIII (CD16)	Neutrophils, NK cells	IgG1, IgG3

There are three cellular receptors for the Fc portion of IgG, termed Fc$_\gamma$RI, II and III (Table 4.3). These are used to bind, recruit and activate cells such as polymorphs, mononuclear phagocytes and NK cells. The Fc$_\gamma$ receptors are also important in the active process of placental transfer of IgG from the mother to the fetus. This is an important feature of the late stages of pregnancy since it confers some specific protection on the newborn during the period when its own immune system is immature.

Immunoglobulin A (IgA)

IgA is the next most abundant immunoglobulin molecule. It is distinctive in two ways. First, it can occur not only as a monomer but also as a dimer, in which two IgA molecules are joined by a short peptide (the **J chain**). The second distinctive feature is that IgA is the major immunoglobulin secreted onto the external surfaces. It is an important aspect of host defence that mucosal surfaces, which are warm and moist, are protected from unwanted microbial growth, and this is achieved through the presence in secretions (e.g. saliva, bronchial fluid, gut secretions, tears, etc.) of **secretory IgA**. Although IgA is detected abundantly in serum (usually in the monomeric form), secretory IgA (dimeric) is found in saliva, lung fluids, gastrointestinal secretions, tears, breast milk and vaginal secretions. Secretion is achieved through the attachment of dimeric IgA to a molecule (termed the polyimmunoglobulin receptor, poly-IgR) synthesised by epithelial cells lining mucosal surfaces. The IgA–poly-IgR complex is endocytosed, transported through the epithelial cell and secreted into the lumen. At this point the

IgA–poly-IgR complex is cleaved, releasing IgA and a remnant of poly-IgR, termed the **secretory chain**, of approximately 70 kDa. The importance of this process is highlighted in patients with selective IgA deficiency, in whom severe, intractable infections of the major mucosal surfaces (gastrointestinal, upper and lower respiratory tracts) are common (see p. 266). As the major secretory immunoglobulin, it can be assumed that IgA has an important role in protection against bacterial, viral and protozoal infections of mucosae. As such, it is capable of activating complement through the alternative pathway and is also an effective opsonin, reacting with $Fc_{\alpha}R$ on monocytes and neutrophils.

Immunoglobulin M (IgM)

IgM is somewhat distinctive, occurring primarily as a pentamer composed of five IgM monomers joined by the J chain (Fig. 4.8). Monomeric IgM molecules have the same basic structure as the other immunoglobulin molecules. IgM is the first immunoglobulin synthesised in an antibody response (the so-called primary response; see below, Fig. 4.9). As a pentamer it has multiple functional domains and is, therefore, a potent activator of complement. In theory, it also has 10 potential antigen-binding sites. To utilise several of these at once, the IgM molecule can become flexed (resembling a crab) so that when reacting with repeating epitopes on a cell or bacterial surface several of the antigen-binding sites may be used. This is an important property: as the first antibody to be produced in response to an antigen challenge, many IgM antibodies do not have the high affinity of later, more refined antibody responses (see below). However, by utilising multiple binding sites, an enhancement of binding can be achieved at lower antibody affinity, a major advantage in the primary response.

Immunoglobulin D (IgD)

IgD is the least well characterised of the immunoglobulins from a functional viewpoint. Serum concentrations are extremely low, and it is unlikely that in this soluble form it has any major function as an immune effector. However, surface expression of IgD is evident at a relatively immature stage of the B cell cycle, and the signalling provided by this receptor on interaction with antigen in a lymphoid follicle is a critical part of B lymphocyte activation.

Immunoglobulin E (IgE)

IgE is the largest immunoglobulin monomer, having four C_H domains. It is present in the serum of healthy individuals at extremely low levels (in the mg/l range). IgE levels rise in response to parasitic infections and in individuals who are atopic or patients with type I (immediate) hypersensitivity (allergy; see p. 131). These distinctive pathological states are related by the main effector function of IgE, which is to bind and activate mast cells. Mast cells bear 10^4–10^6 high-affinity IgE receptors, $Fc_{\varepsilon}RI$, per cell. In the interstitium, mast cells will thus acquire surface IgE. The interaction between this and specific antigen causes mast cell activation, with potent localised, and occasionally generalised, vascular effects. In physiological terms, the generation of these types of itchy, hypervascular responses is probably important in defence against parasitic infections (e.g. worms). A low-affinity receptor, $Fc_{\varepsilon}RII$ (CD23), is present on B lymphocytes and eosinophils. Interaction between $Fc_{\varepsilon}RII$ on B lympho-

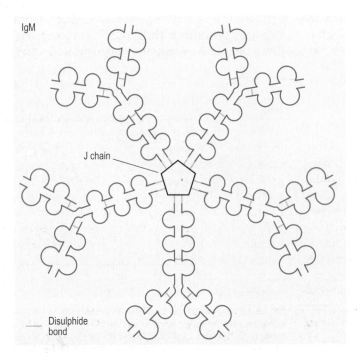
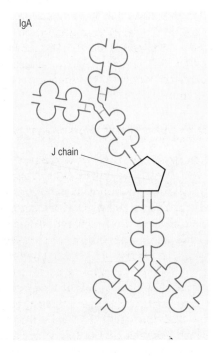

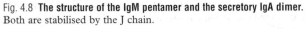

Fig. 4.8 **The structure of the IgM pentamer and the secretory IgA dimer.** Both are stabilised by the J chain.

Immunoglobulins

- The basic molecule is composed of two light and two heavy chains connected by interchain disulphide bonds. Within the chains, distinctive motifs (domains) are formed by intrachain disulphide bonds.
- Many immunological molecules have similar domain structures: the immunoglobulin supergene family.
- Antibodies contain regions that are highly variable in their amino acid content in different molecules: these zones form the antigen-binding site.
- Antibodies also have relatively constant parts; on the heavy chain these hold different functional properties, such as the ability to activate complement.
- Different heavy chains give rise to different classes of immunoglobulin: IgA, IgD, IgE, IgG and IgM.

cytes is an important part of the regulation of IgE production.

IMMUNOGLOBULIN EXPRESSION

B CELL SURFACE EXPRESSION

A short extension of immunoglobulin molecules at the carboxy-terminus during synthesis enables insertion into the B lymphocyte surface membrane. Surface-expressed antibody has an important role in B lymphocyte activation, as we have already mentioned in relation to surface IgD on immature B cells. Binding of antigen to surface immunoglobulin is an early event in the B lymphocyte cell cycle. In the case of mature B lymphocytes, interaction with surface immunoglobulin of the other classes leads to internalisation of the antigen. Complex antigens may then be broken down (processed) and presented to T lymphocytes (see p. 86). Through this process, antigen-specific B lymphocytes can activate T lymphocytes, leading to a concerted immune response.

ISOTYPES, ALLOTYPES AND IDIOTYPES

Many of the studies performed to characterise immunoglobulins have been performed by raising antibodies against the immunoglobulins: here the immunoglobulin has itself become the antigen. Immunoglobulin molecules have numerous distinctive structural features, and the differences and similarities between immunoglobulins are reflected in their antigenic properties. These antigens can be divided as follows. Some are present on all of the molecules of a particular immunoglobulin class or heavy or light chain type in a species and are called **isotypes**. For example, the ε heavy chain has antigens peculiar to IgE molecules, which are present on all of the IgE molecules in the members of that species. Other parts of immunoglobulins have

genetically determined differences between individuals. These are termed **allotypes** and are denoted by the chain affected (e.g. Gm, Em allotypes). Finally, we have to remember that the most distinctive part of an individual immunoglobulin is the antigen-binding site seated in the hypervariable region. To take the analogy of the jelly and the jelly mould again; in three-dimensional terms, the jelly mould (i.e. antibody) is as distinctive as the jelly (i.e. antigen). Injection of a human antibody into a mouse should result in the production of some murine antibodies recognising parts of the antigen-binding site. Indeed, this is the case, and such determinants in that human antibody are termed **idiotypes**. Idiotypes are antigenic determinants in the antigen-binding site (the hypervariable regions, or CDRs) and as such can only be identified by raising an antibody response to them. The antigenic epitope within the antigen-binding site is termed an **idiotope**, and a collection of idiotopes is the idiotype. It appears that anti-idiotype antibodies are a normal feature of the antibody repertoire, and it has been proposed that interaction between anti-idiotypes and the idiotypes on antibody molecules has a role in regulation of the immune response (see p. 105).

PRIMARY AND SECONDARY ANTIBODY RESPONSES

When antigen not previously encountered is injected into an animal, and the antibody response measured, several observations can be made. The antibody response is detected 5–10 days after antigen challenge, rises over the next 10–20 days, and then declines to a low level without ever completely disappearing. If the same antigen is administered again several weeks later, the antibody response is more rapid, hits a higher peak level, and declines, but to a higher baseline level than previously seen (Fig. 4.9). These two responses, therefore, differ qualitatively and quantitatively, and

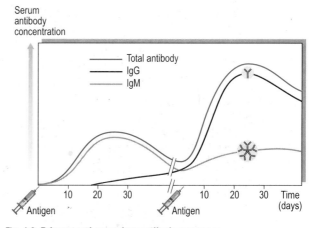

Fig. 4.9 Primary and secondary antibody responses.
Administration of an antigen at day 0 is followed by a primary antibody response, comprising predominantly IgM, at about 10 days. Rechallenge with the *same* antigen some weeks later causes a much more rapid rise in antibody levels and to a higher peak; this time the response is predominantly IgG (secondary response).

are termed primary and secondary. If a different antigen is given at the second challenge, a primary response to that antigen is seen. The secondary response is, therefore, **antigen-specific**, and demonstrates **acquisition of memory** in the immune response. There is also a higher **intensity** to the secondary response.

The qualitative differences between primary and secondary responses extend further than just the speed of appearance of antibody. The primary response is seen predominantly as antibody of the IgM class. IgG antibody specific for the same antigen begins to appear towards the end of the primary response. The secondary response, however, is predominantly IgG class antibody. There is another feature of the IgG in the secondary response: it has a higher affinity for antigen than antibody in the primary response. The genetic and cellular basis for switching from IgM to IgG class antibody is discussed below. The generation of high-affinity antibodies will also be discussed in greater depth, but in simplistic terms it can be viewed as the application of Darwinian evolutionary principles to B lymphocyte survival: those B cells with the highest affinity for an

antigen in short supply compete most effectively and undergo positive selection.

HAPTENS

Some molecules are too small of themselves to generate an antibody response when administered to an animal. However, if coupled to a larger protein (a **carrier**), these small molecules may elicit production of antibodies that are able to bind the small molecule directly, in the absence of the carrier. Such molecules are termed **haptens**. Much of the early work on the nature of antigen–antibody binding was carried out using hapten–carrier systems.

CLONALITY IN ANTIBODY RESPONSES

Plasma cells — the end stage of B lymphocyte differentiation — produce and secrete immunoglobulin. More specifically, a single plasma cell produces a single antibody, with one heavy chain type, one light chain type and one conformation of antigen-binding region. This

---

🔍 Generation of monoclonal and polyclonal antibodies

Monoclonal antibodies were 'invented' by George Köhler and César Milstein at Cambridge in 1975. Ironically, the two ended their article in Nature doubting whether their discovery was of any value in future science. In 1984, they were awarded the Nobel Prize for what is unquestionably one of the single most important contributions to the biosciences. B lymphocytes are removed from the spleens of mice immunised with an antigen (Fig. 4.10). These B cells are then fused with a tumour cell line to provide a hybrid with the best of both worlds: specific antibody production and immortality. The hybridoma is grown, and antibody appearing in the culture fluid is tested to see whether it binds the antigen of interest. Since each hybridoma is derived from a single B lymphocyte, the immunoglobulin that it produces is monoclonal. Selected hybridoma cells can be grown in culture for many years and the monoclonal antibody purified in large quantities. Thus, an antibody can be raised to almost any antigen imaginable, providing the ultimate tool for many aspects of laboratory research and clinical science.

Antibodies raised in larger mammals (rabbits, guinea-pigs, sheep, donkeys, horses) can also be of great use. Here the antigen is administered and then the animal is bled some 2–3 weeks later. The serum obtained contains a high concentration of antibodies to the antigen of interest. These **polyclonal antisera** can also be applied widely in the laboratory. They were also used for one of the earliest attempts at manipulating immunity to the advantage of humans. Horse serum, obtained from animals injected with diphtheria toxin, was used successfully to combat the toxin-mediated effects of diphtheria infection in the early part of this century.

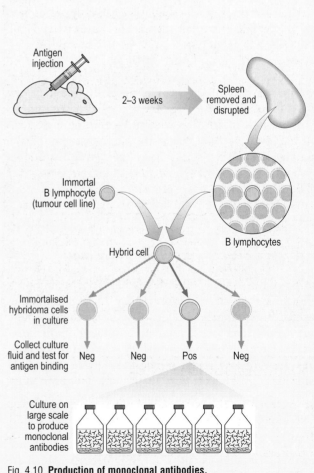

Fig. 4.10 **Production of monoclonal antibodies.**

is a **monoclonal antibody**, unvarying in its amino acid sequence. Most antibody responses to complex macromolecular antigens involve the targeting of multiple epitopes on the antigen. Each epitope may be targeted by more than a single antibody molecule. Thus, many clones of plasma cells, and many antibody types, are produced in a typical antibody response. Such a response is termed **polyclonal**. Antibody responses to a large macromolecular antigen are not evenly distributed throughout the antigen; some areas are targeted more frequently than others and are termed the **dominant epitopes**.

Monoclonal immunoglobulins are only identifiable in any quantity in two circumstances. The first is a clinical condition in which a neoplastic tumour of plasma cell origin leads to the expansion of a single clone of cells, producing a single immunoglobulin molecule (a disease termed myeloma, see p. 294). The second is when such a neoplastic tumour is fused with a B lymphocyte to give an immortalised, antibody-producing clone of B lymphocytes; such a manoeuvre is central to monoclonal antibody technology (see box: 'Generation of monoclonal and polyclonal antibodies').

Immunoglobulin expression

- Immunoglobulins on the surface of B lymphocytes bind antigen, which is then internalised, broken down and a portion is presented to T lymphocytes to activate their response to the antigen.
- Immunoglobulins can be characterised by their own ability to act as antigens: *isotypes* are epitopes that are present on all molecules of a class or chain type in a species; *allotypes* vary between individuals, *idiotypes* reflect variation in the antigen-binding sites of the immunoglobulin.
- Primary antibody responses are slow, mainly IgM and decline to low levels. Repeated exposure to the antigen at a later time elicits a more rapid response to a higher peak level that declines to a higher baseline level; this secondary response is predominantly IgG.
- Each plasma cell produces a single antibody; tumours formed from a single plasma cell will produce large quantities of this monoclonal antibody. A population of plasma cells will respond to different epitopes on macromolecular antigens giving rise to many clones of plasma cells and many antibody types: a polyclonal response.

IMMUNOGLOBULIN GENES

It is clear that the immunoglobulins are quite distinctive molecules. When examining the genes that encode these complex glycoproteins, we are looking for the explanation to some key characteristics.

- The immunoglobulin molecule has four chains; two identical heavy and two identical light chains.

- Each chain contains both highly variable *and* essentially constant regions.
- Antibody is IgM class in the primary response and IgG or other classes in the secondary response.
- Different heavy chains can be selected for an immunoglobulin molecule, hence modifying its effector function without altering antigen binding.
- During the generation of an antibody response, there is an increase in overall affinity for antigen.
- Potential binding capacity exceeds 10^{11} different antigen 'shapes', implying an equivalent number of different antibody molecules.

To summarise these points, it could be said that the genetic system for antibodies is required to generate enormous **diversity** for antigen binding at one end of the molecule and a limited choice of functional characteristics at the other. Two theories could easily explain such a model. One, favoured for many years because it did not require a rewriting of the genetics textbooks, stated that a separate gene existed for every different antibody molecule. In other words, there were 10^{11} different genes for 10^{11} different antigen-binding molecules. The other explanation was that a limited number of genes were available, but that they could combine randomly; such chance associations offered diversity. When the immunoglobulin genes were eventually identified, they were indeed limited in number, confirming the second hypothesis. However, the number was actually *too* limited to account for the enormous diversity achieved; additional mechanisms for the **generation of antibody diversity** were subsequently identified.

At a basic level, the organisation of genes for an immunoglobulin molecule can be viewed as follows. Each chain (heavy and light) is encoded by a gene complex. Within the complex are groups of genes (termed segments) that encode the variable regions (V genes), and genes that encode the constant regions (C genes) of each chain. Other genes are responsible for joining these two (J genes), or make an additional contribution to the generation of diversity (D genes). The genes are known by the capital letter V, C, J or D, suffixed by the name of the chain and a number (e.g. $V_\kappa 3$, $J_\lambda 2$, $C_\lambda 6$, $C_\gamma 1$, etc.) (Fig. 4.11).

LIGHT CHAIN GENES

The κ and λ light chain genes are on chromosomes 2 and 22, respectively, in humans (Fig. 4.12). The sequence of genes runs V to J to C, from the 5' to 3' end of the chromosome (there is no D segment for

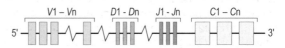

Fig. 4.11 Representation of the overall organisation of immunoglobulin genes.
The number of different genes in each gene segment is given by *n*.

κ chain gene

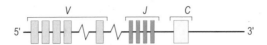

λ chain gene

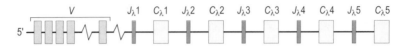

Fig. 4.12 **Map of the human κ and λ chain genes.**

light chains). For the κ chain genes, there are some 250 V_κ gene segments, four J_κ segments and one C_κ segment. In theory, then, there is the potential for $250 \times 4 \times 1 = 1000$ different combinations of these gene segments to form 1000 different κ light chains. The λ chain gene segments comprise some 30 V_λ and five C_λ gene segments, each C gene being accompanied by its own J_λ gene. The potential diversity in the λ genes is, therefore, 30×5, or 150, different light chains.

HEAVY CHAIN GENES

The human heavy chain genes, on chromosome 14, have a similar basic structure to the light chains, with two differences (Fig. 4.13). First, additional diversity is achieved by the presence of a small number of diversity (D) gene segments. Second, the different constant region gene segments encoding the heavy chain isotypes ($C_\gamma 1$–4, $C_\alpha 1$–2, C_μ, C_δ and C_ε) are located together, downstream from the V_H, D_H and J_H segments, rather than on separate chromosomes.

V_H gene segments fall into approximately eight families, each with numerous members, which are not always functional (some are pseudogenes), so that the total number of functional V_H genes is estimated at 250–1000. There are approximately 12 D_H and four J_H gene segments. The maximum diversity achievable from this range of genes is, therefore $1000 \times 12 \times 4 = 48\,000$. When combined with a κ light chain, for example, the total potential diversity of molecular structure in an immunoglobulin molecule is $1000 \times 48\,000 = 48$ million. Since an alternative would be to combine with a λ chain, there is an additional potential diversity of $150 \times 48\,000 = 7.2$ million making a combined range of 55.2 million potential molecules. This process of

forming different antibody specificities through combining different genes randomly is termed **combinatorial diversity**.

GENERATION OF IMMUNOGLOBULIN DIVERSITY

We have seen how, by careful manipulation of a large pool of genes encoding different parts of the immunoglobulin molecule, an enormous range of different immunoglobulin structures can be created (Fig. 4.14). However, there are two other manipulations which add to the diversity. First, there is a 'deliberate' imprecision in the joining together of D_H and J_H, V_H to $D_H J_H$ and V_L to J_L segments. Remembering that three nucleotides (a codon) in the gene are required per amino acid, loss or retention of whole codons when two genes join together determines whether an amino acid is present or not. Loss or addition of single nucleotides can lead to frame-shift mutations, altering the meaning of the whole of the genetic code after the join. This phenomenon is termed **junctional diversity** and is thought to increase the total potential diversity of immunoglobulin structure to approximately 10^{11}. Combinatorial and junctional diversity tend to focus the changes introduced into the hypervariable regions (CDRs), which are mainly encoded from the joining regions of the genes.

In 1983, a further discovery identified the second, additional mechanism by which antibody diversity is broadened. It was found that parts of the variable regions of different antibodies differed by a single amino acid residue, or their genes differed by a single nucleotide sequence, from the version of that gene encoded in the germline (i.e. non-rearranged DNA). This finding implied a single mutation. Subsequently, it was shown

Immunoglobulin heavy chain genes

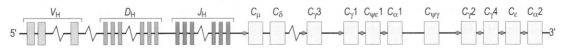

● Switch site

ψ Pseudogene

Fig. 4.13 **Organisation of the human heavy chain genes.**

(a)

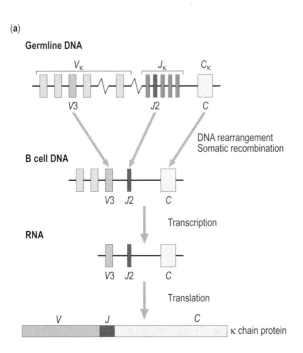

Fig. 4.14 **The overall scheme of gene rearrangements to achieve a final immunoglobulin chain.**
(**a**) For an immunoglobulin light chain. (**b**) For a heavy chain, with or without class switching.

(b)

Heavy chain gene assembly

- Switch site

that such differences appeared *after* antigenic stimulation and, therefore, *after* the initial gene rearrangements occurring in that cell. This process has been termed **somatic hypermutation**. It may involve the substitution, deletion or addition of a single nucleotide, occurring after gene rearrangement, but presumably when the cell is undertaking the class switch between the primary and secondary responses. The process of somatic hypermutation introduces an additional diversity and is frequently focused in and around the CDRs. Somatic mutation is an enigmatic process about which little is

known: it does not occur in other B cell genes, and even within the immunoglobulin molecule appears to be confined to the variable regions of the genes.

The mechanisms for the generation of antibody diversity are summarised in Table 4.4.

CLASS SWITCHING

In the process of assembling the different gene segments necessary to make an immunoglobulin molecule composed of two light and two heavy chains, random

Table 4.4 **Contribution of the different mechanisms of generation of diversity for immunoglobulin molecules and TCRs**

Mechanism	Immunoglobulin		TCR αβ		TCR γδ	
	Heavy chain	Light chain	α	β	γ	δ
Number of variable (*V*) segments	250–1000	250	50–100	50–100	8	10
Number of diversity (*D*) segments	12	0	0	2	0	2
D segments read in all three reading frames	Rare	–	–	Frequent	–	Frequent
Joining (*J*) segments	4	4	50–100	12	2	3
Potential *V* segment combinations	62 500–250 000		2500–10 000		80	
Total potential repertoire including allowance for junctional diversity	$\approx 10^{11}$		$\approx 10^{16}$		$\approx 10^{18}$	

Adapted with permission from Davis & Bjorkman 1993 Nature 334: 395.

combinations of the different component genes produce an enormous potential diversity. At this point in the development of B lymphocytes, the cells are able to express the rearranged immunoglobulin on the cell surface. Invariably, at this stage, the surface immunoglobulin (sIg) is a monomer of the IgM class. As we shall see in a later chapter, the rearrangement of immunoglobulin genes into sIgM is a very early event in the B cell life cycle and is independent of any encounter with antigen. When sIgM binds specific antigen, the B cell may become activated. One of the results of such activation is the transformation into a B cell with surface IgG, IgA or IgE, as an alternative for IgM. This process of class switching must be carried out without the B cell changing its antigen specificity: it would be no good the B cell being activated for expressing anti-X and becoming a cell capable of an anti-Y response. What has been achieved by the process of class switching, however, is to modulate the functional capabilities of the antibody produced, according to whether IgG, IgA, IgE or IgM is chosen. Here we see the genetic and molecular basis for the qualitative change in the antibody repertoire seen when a primary response (mainly IgM) becomes a secondary one (mainly IgG).

It remains largely unclear precisely what directs the selection of different heavy chains by a B lymphocyte. Animal studies have shed some light, however, indicating that the presence of certain cytokines during some stages of B cell differentiation biases the heavy chain expressed.

AFFINITY MATURATION

One final major difference between antibodies produced in the primary and those produced in the secondary response is their affinity. IgM antibodies produced in the primary reponse to an antigen tend to be of relatively, low affinity and may rely upon the additional avidity afforded by their pentameric structure to bind antigen efficiently. However, the IgG and other class antibodies produced in the secondary re-

sponse tend to be of much higher affinity. This change in the characteristic of antibody binding to antigen is termed **affinity maturation**. It is assumed that the process is something of a Darwinian evolutionary change. It is probable that in the lymph node during an antigen challenge, many different IgM-expressing B cells are present, binding antigen with relatively low affinity. They receive positive differentiation signals and undergo class switching. It is at this stage that the process of somatic hypermutation also takes place. The product of these manipulations is a range of antibodies with single affinity, available for selection. Only those B cells receiving the necessary signals to continue their expansion (signals provided by lymph node T cells in the main) will proliferate. In the presence of a limited supply of antigen, the law of the 'immunological jungle' will apply, and only the highest affinity antibodies, which compete most effectively, will receive the next selection signal. We will see the cellular basis of this part of B cell maturation in a later chapter (see p. 100).

GENETIC BASIS FOR IMMUNOGLOBULIN GENE REARRANGEMENT AND CLASS SWITCHING

We have talked blithely of combinatorial processes, class switching and hypermutation; but what are the genetic processes that underlie these? The heavy chain genes on one chromosome are assembled first, with a D_H and $\mathcal{J}_H$ segment combining, before a V_H segment is added. If a successful $V_H D_H \mathcal{J}_H$ gene is produced through this rearrangement, it is likely that the other chromosome is inhibited in some way from undergoing the same process (allelic exclusion). The constant heavy chain is then added to the rearranged $V_H D_H \mathcal{J}_H$ segment. Invariably, the C_μ is selected, and it is worth noting that the appearance in the cytoplasm of this protein product (i.e. the IgM heavy chain) is the first indication that a cell is of the B lymphocyte lineage. Next, the light chain gene segments (V_L and $\mathcal{J}_L$) are rearranged and combined with the constant region gene C_L. In human, the C_κ gene is selected first, and only if the rearrangement is unsuccessful on both strands of chromosome 2 is the C_λ gene then sought (the majority of κ chain gene rearrangements must be successful, since the κ:λ ratio of antibodies in the periphery is 2:1). At this point, sufficient genetic material to produce an immunoglobulin molecule has been constructed. When class switching takes place, the IgM heavy chain must be replaced by selection of the C_γ, C_α or C_ε gene. This is achieved by the use of switch regions, 5′ to the C_H genes. The only C_H gene not to have a switch region is the C_δ gene: this may explain why few mature B cells express sIgD, and why very little immunoglobulin of the IgD class is made.

The precise mechanism by which switch regions allow the new C_H gene to be transcribed is not known, although it may involve loops and excisions, or straight deletions, as proposed in the models of VDJ recombination (see box 'Immunoglobulin gene recombination: twists and palindromes' and Fig. 4.15).

Immunoglobulin genes and antibody diversity

- Antibody diversity is achieved through a variety of genetic mechanisms the changes tending to focus on the hypervariable regions.
- Combinatorial diversity is the random recombination of some of a large pool of gene segments for the light and heavy chains.
- Junctional diversity is the random imprecision in the joining of the segments caused by loss or retention of nucleotides or codons, which results in frame-shifts.
- Somatic hypermutation is the occurrence of a single mutational change after the initial gene rearrangements, probably during class switching.
- In class switching in B cells, the early expression of IgM gives way to the mature, activated expression of other classes of immunoglobulin. B cells with the highest affinity will be stimulated to proliferate further — affinity maturation.

T CELL RECEPTORS FOR ANTIGEN

The T lymphocyte receptors for antigen were identified in the mid-1980s. In broad terms, the genomic organisation of T cell receptor (TCR) genes is similar to that of immunoglobulin genes, with each cell type using a similar approach to the generation of receptor diversity. The TCR exists as a heterodimer, of which there are two types. One is composed of an α and β chain (αβ TCR), and the other of γ and δ chains (γδ TCR). The TCR type is often used to denote the T cell: for example, a T cell expressing an αβ TCR is referred to as an αβ T cell.

The chains of each type of TCR are divided into variable and constant domains, each domain being encoded by separate gene pools. Like the B lymphocyte producing a single clone of immunoglobulin molecules, the T cell expresses only one form of TCR once the genes have been rearranged. The γδ TCR appears on the surface of primitive T lymphocytes in the thymus before cells bearing the αβ TCR can be seen, and for this reason the nomenclature TCR1 (γδ) and TCR2 (αβ) is occasionally used. However, the αβ TCR remains the best studied in humans and is present on over 90% of peripheral T cells (compared with 1–10% for the γδ TCR). Much more is known regarding

---

Immunoglobulin gene recombination: twists and palindromes

One of the most intriguing questions for geneticists was how differing gene segments were successfully selected and combined. Careful analysis of the nucleotides flanking each V, D and J gene segment revealed an interesting set of repetitive sequences (Fig. 4.15). Downstream from each V gene segment, for example, is a sequence of seven particular nucleotides (a heptamer), followed by a random set of nucleotides (invariably 12 or 23 in number) and then a further nine defined nucleotides (a nonamer). At the approach to each gene segment (i.e. upstream) is a similar set, but this time running in the sequence nonamer → random 12 or 23 nucleotides → heptamer. Particularly intriguing was the fact that the two heptamers and nonamers were palindromic (remember a palindrome reads the same forwards and backwards: 'madam', for example). In DNA terms, this means that when read in opposite directions the heptamers and nonamers are complementary with each other. In other words, if the gene region were doubled back onto itself, for example by formation of a loop, the heptamers and nonamers

could form a region of double-stranded DNA. This is made easier since the heptamer and nonamer sequences are separated by random sequences of fixed length, 12 or 23 bases, which correspond to one or two complete turns of a DNA helix. Formation of such loops could allow gene segments not actually in sequence to be brought next to each other and be spliced together by a recombinase, with the excision of the redundant loop. There is one final 'twist' in the story, however. Analysis of the sequences reveals that for two gene segments to join, the heptamer and nonamer must be separated by a 12-mer on one side and a 23-mer on the other. This is termed the **12–23 rule**, and although the mechanism through which it works is not known, careful studies on the flanking sequences of immunoglobulin gene segments indicate that the rule is important because it dictates that V_H cannot join J_H directly, because such a recombination would involve two 23-mers. This ensures the addition of the D_H region in-between.

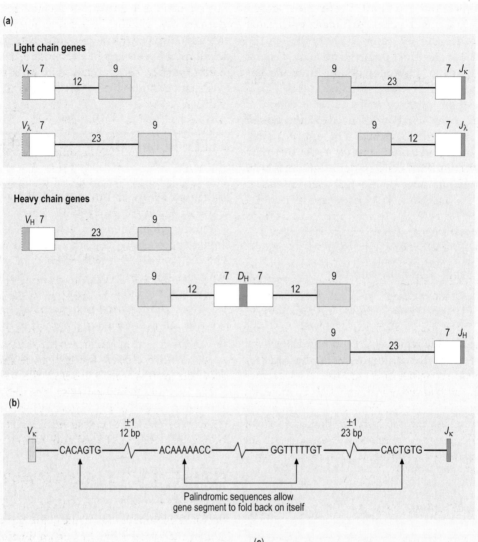

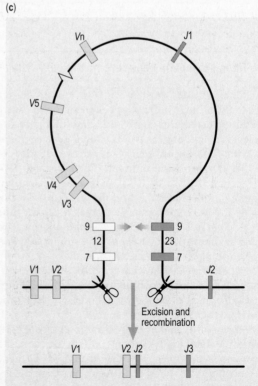

Fig. 4.15 **Mechanisms of gene rearrangements for immunoglobulin segment genes.**
(**a**) Heptamer and nonamer consensus sequences flanking the $V\mathcal{J}$ and $VD\mathcal{J}$ joining sites, showing the 12–23 rule. Note that V–$\mathcal{J}$ joining in the heavy chain is forbidden and that the D segment insertion between V and $\mathcal{J}$ is obligatory. (**b**) Examples of the palindromic heptamer and nonamer sequences flanking the κ light chain segments. (**c**) Probable mechanism of rearrangement of genes within different segments on a chromatid to bring two genes together. Here $V2$ and $\mathcal{J}2$ are brought together by the formation and excision of a loop of redundant DNA.

the antigen responsiveness of αβ T cells; the antigen specificity and functional role of γδ T cells is currently more obscure.

STRUCTURE AND FUNCTION OF THE αβ T CELL RECEPTOR

The αβ TCR is a disulphide-bonded heterodimer comprising an α chain (43–49 kDa) and a β chain (38–44 kDa) (Fig. 4.16). The variable and constant domains follow the nomenclature of the immunoglobulin molecules V_α, V_β, C_α and C_β. Indeed, although structural data on the TCRs are lacking at present because of difficulties in obtaining sufficient purified quantities for X-ray crystallography, the structure of the domains in the TCRs is analogous to that of the immunoglobulin domains, and they form part of the immunoglobulin supergene family. In the absence of clear structural data, modelling of TCR structure on the backbone of what is known about immunoglobulin structure has been very informative. It appears that there are hypervariable regions of the variable domains, forming CDRs 1–3. Remembering that the function of the TCRs is to recognise and bind the shape formed by the peptide embedded within an MHC molecule groove, it is speculated that CDRs 1 and 2 interact with the two α-helices of the α1 and α2 domains of the MHC molecule, as these run along the sides of the antigen-binding groove, whilst CDR3 interacts with the peptide within the groove.

STRUCTURE AND FUNCTION OF THE γδ T CELL RECEPTOR

The γδ TCRs are somewhat distinctive in that their gene rearrangement is an early thymic event. As stated above, γδ T cells in humans are equally represented in peripheral blood and lymphoid organs and appear to function in a similar way to the more numerically dominant αβ T cells. This contrasts with the mouse, in which γδ TCRs have been extensively studied, where it appears that they have a particularly important role in epithelial sites, such as skin, gut and lungs.

Structurally, the γδ TCR shows some important differences from the αβ TCR (Fig. 4.16b). Whilst it does exist as a disulphide-linked heterodimer of γ (50 kDa) and δ (40 kDa) chains, there are two other forms: a non-disulphide-linked heterodimer and a disulphide-linked γγ homodimer. Less is known about the antigen- and MHC-binding characteristics of the γδ TCR, although hypervariable regions within the variable domains do exist.

THE T CELL RECEPTOR GENES

The repertoire of T cell antigen receptors is required to have a similar depth of diversity as that for antibodies. The genes for the TCR were discovered some years after those for immunoglobulin molecules, and as expected, they had a similar genetic organisation. For the α, β, γ and δ chains, the genes are divided into two separate groups, one encoding the variable domains using multiple gene segments, the other for the constant domains. As for immunoglobulin genes, TCR genes must undergo rearrangements from the germline before they are transcribed and translated.

GENES FOR THE α AND β CHAINS

Analogous to the heavy and light chain gene segments of immunoglobulin molecules, the gene encoding the α chain is formed by the recombination of segments from different gene groups, in this case V_α (of which there are 50–100), J_α (50–100) and a single C_α gene segment (Fig. 4.17). The potential diversity achievable for the α chain is, therefore, $100 \times 100 \times 1 = 10\,000$.

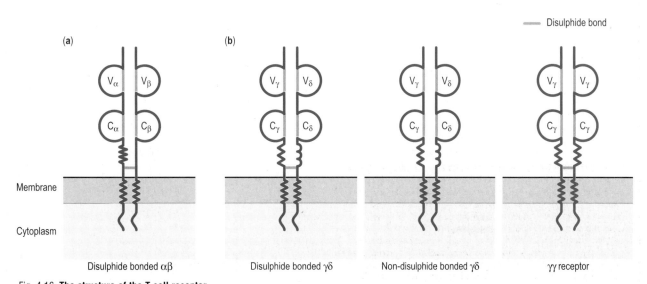

Fig. 4.16 **The structure of the T cell receptor.**
(**a**) The αβ TCR. (**b**) The different types of γδ TCR.

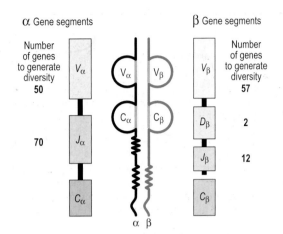

Fig. 4.17 **Numbers of different gene segments used to generate αβ TCR diversity.**

The β chain genes comprise the following different segments: V_β, D_β, J_β and C_β. The V_β genes are divided into some 15–20 families, within which the genes have a very similar structure, with a total of some 50–100 V_β genes all told. The D_β, J_β and C_β segments are clustered together into two pools (one pool arising from a duplication of the other) (Fig. 4.18). Within these are a total of two D_β gene segments, approximately 12 functional J_β segments and two C_β segments. The potential diversity offered by these β chain gene segments is, therefore, $100 \times 2 \times 12 \times 2 = 4800$.

Overall, the diversity achievable from a set of α and β chain genes rearranging and producing two polypeptide chains is $4800 \times 10\,000 = 48$ million.

There are some important differences in the genes and in the genetic processes that give rise to the assembled TCR product compared with immunoglobulin genes. First, the C_α and C_β genes do not appear to encode segments typical of secreted proteins, indicating that secretion of TCRs is not an important functional characteristic. This is borne out in the lack of evidence

for the existence of soluble TCRs. Second, there is no somatic hypermutation in the genes encoding a complete αβ TCR. This is an important difference from immunoglobulins since, as we shall see, it would be dangerous to allow a T lymphocyte, once selected for its antigen receptor and allowed into the periphery in a mature form, to alter subsequently its receptor configuration.

GENES FOR THE γ AND δ CHAINS

The human γ chain gene locus contains three gene segment pools: V_γ (eight genes), J_γ (two genes) and C_γ (two genes) genes. The diversity achievable is, therefore, relatively limited, to $8 \times 2 \times 2 = 32$ different rearranged genes. The δ chain genes are located within the middle of the α chain gene locus, and are arranged in four pools of V_δ (10 genes), D_δ (two genes), J_δ (three genes) and a single C_δ gene segment. The diversity produced is $10 \times 2 \times 3 \times 1 = 60$ possible rearrangements; combined with the γ chain genes the total diversity in the receptor is $32 \times 60 = 1920$.

GENERATION OF T CELL RECEPTOR DIVERSITY

It is likely that the mechanism for bringing different gene components of the TCRs together in order to construct a rearranged TCR gene is the same as that used for the immunoglobulin genes. The major evidence for this is the presence of the nonamer and heptamer sequences as well as the 12 and 23 nucleotide sequences, applying again the '12–23' rule (see the box on immunoglobulin recombination: remember the rule is applied to stop V_H–J_H joining without the insertion of the D_H segment). However, the arrangement of these flanking sequences in the D_β and D_δ gene segments is such that V_β–J_β and V_β–D_β–D_β–J_β configurations could exist, and indeed this has been confirmed at the level of

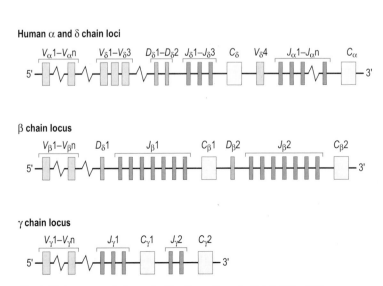

Fig. 4.18 **Arrangement of gene loci for the α, β, γ, δ chains of the TCR.**

rearranged TCR genes in mature T cells. These recombinations are also permitted and have been detected in the δ chain gene segments and could increase the potential diversity of both fully formed TCRs.

Apart from the presence of randomly associating gene segments and the possibility of *V–D–D–J* and *V–J* combinations as well as *V–D–J*, TCR diversity is derived from other mechanisms. In particular, imprecise joining, as for the immunoglobulin gene segments, is common, and the resultant new nucleotide sequences and frame-shift mutations contribute considerably to diversity (Table 4.4). The extent of the total diversity is difficult to estimate, but it is thought to be many orders of magnitude in excess of that indicated in the number of individual gene segments in each of the *V*, *D*, *J* and *C* pools (see Table 4.4).

T cell receptors for antigen

- TCRs have a basic molecule composed of two chains: these may be α/β (90%) or γ/δ. Within the chains are the distinctive motifs which make these molecules members of the immunoglobulin supergene family.
- Like antibodies, TCRs have distinctive regions that are highly variable between different molecules; these regions interact with antigen.
- TCRs vary in structure through the use of a large pool of gene segments for the receptor chains; random recombination of these variable, diversity and joining genes; and highly random imprecision in the joining process.
- TCRs do not mutate somatically after gene rearrangement.
- The function of the TCR is to recognise and bind the complex of a specific antigen with a self MHC molecule, which is formed when the antigenic peptide becomes embedded within the MHC groove.

CHAPTER 5

The human leukocyte antigens

The major histocompatibility complex (MHC) describes a collection of genes that in humans represents about 0.1% of the whole genome and is sited on the short arm of chromosome 6. Many of the genes in the MHC are involved in immune functions. In particular, the MHC contains a group of genes that code for proteins expressed on the surface of a variety of cell types. In humans, these are known as the **human leukocyte antigens**, or HLA system (HLA originally stood for human leukocyte A, the first such molecule to be described). So use of the term MHC refers to this collection of genes in general, while the term HLA refers only to the human MHC. HLA molecules are involved in antigen recognition by T lymphocytes. The T lymphocyte receptor only recognises antigen that is presented as a short peptide embedded within a physical groove created by a HLA molecule.

Knowledge of the physiological role of HLA molecules as presenters of antigenic peptides is relatively new and, aligned with a new nomenclature for the HLA system, it gives the modern student great advantages over pupils past. For many years, our understanding of the role of HLA molecules in immunity was based on three seemingly unconnected facts. First, it has been known for many years that differences in HLA molecules between individuals are responsible for organ graft rejection (hence the name histo- (*tissue*) compatibility; see box: 'MHC genes and organ transplantation'). Second, genetic studies revealed that possession of certain HLA genes was linked to greater susceptibility to particular diseases, such as multiple sclerosis, type 1 diabetes and ankylosing spondylitis (see box: 'MHC loci: disease susceptibility or immune response genes?'). Finally, it had been demonstrated

that differences in the ability of mouse strains to respond to particular antigens could be mapped to genes in the MHC (hence the earlier name of immune response genes). Armed with the knowledge that HLA molecules present antigen, we must now set about accounting for these original observations.

The new HLA nomenclature is based on genotyping (i.e. analysis of DNA sequences; see p. 60) and has been achievable only through the molecular biology revolution. Since many important advances in the field of HLA were made before this, much of our knowledge remains couched in the old terminology; hence it is necessary to have some rudimentary concepts of both.

THE MAJOR HISTOCOMPATIBILITY COMPLEX

THE IMMUNE RESPONSE

In 1974, two scientists called Zinkernagel and Doherty published a series of classic experiments that can be considered as the turning points in our understanding of the physiological role of MHC genes in the immune response (Fig. 5.2), for which they received the 1996 Nobel Prize. The studies demonstrated that in strain A mice infected with lymphocytic choriomeningitis virus (LCMV), cytotoxic T lymphocytes appeared that were capable of killing LCMV-infected cells. However, LCMV-infected target cells obtained from strain B, which differed from strain A at the *H–2* gene loci in the MHC, were not susceptible to killing by cytotoxic T lymphocytes from strain A. LCMV-infected target cells obtained from strains other than A were susceptible to killing by cytotoxic T cells from strain A, as long as they shared identical genes at the *H-2* loci.

It appeared from these studies that recognition of a viral antigen by cytotoxic T cells required the presence on the target cell of molecules encoded by the MHC. More than this, the MHC molecules had to be the same as those present in the animal from which the cytotoxic T cells were obtained. This principle was termed the **law of MHC restriction**: antigen-specific cytotoxic T cell responses are *restricted* to kill only those target cells that bear the correct MHC molecule. Antiviral responses were convenient for these early studies, but, subsequently, the universality of this principle was established for all forms of T lymphocyte response to antigen. Once the law of MHC restriction was established, researchers set about interpreting it. Clearly, it implies that a T lymphocyte is compelled to recognise

MHC genes and organ transplantation

Some of the proteins encoded by genes in the MHC are at the heart of organ graft rejection. Attempts to transplant tissue from one animal to another have been made for over 200 years, with limited success. Early studies on animals revealed that transplanted organs, for example kidneys, did not survive because of a destructive process termed 'rejection', taking place within 1 or 2 weeks of implantation. By the middle part of the current century, surgical techniques had advanced sufficiently for human organ transplantation to be considered viable, and this became a major driving force in the study of rejection. The use of inbreeding in mice to achieve pure strains with complete genetic identity — syngeneity — between individuals demonstrated that skin grafts between such animals were not rejected, while grafts between animals of two genetically different inbred strains were. By careful crossbreeding between different inbred strains, the genes most important in conferring skin graft compatibility between individual mice were soon identified. In mice, the gene complex involved is on chromosome 17, and because of its determinant role in whether tissues are compatible, it was termed the major histocompatibility complex (Table 5.1; Fig. 5.1).

Identification of the human MHC took a little longer for the obvious reason that inbred strains are not readily available. Clues to its existence came from the results of a series of kidney transplants performed in Boston in the early 1950s. Those performed between unrelated individuals were uniformly unsuccessful, but the survival of one of these patients for 6 months encouraged further operations to be undertaken, this time between identical twins. The unqualified success of these grafts was confirmation of the existence of genes determining tissue types in humans, and this was soon followed by the identification of the human MHC. Very much like the ABO blood group system, it was established that the molecules actually involved in determining the 'foreignness' of a graft were present as proteins on the surface of white blood cells, hence the name human leukocyte antigens.

Table 5.1 **Terminology and definitions**

Term	Definition
Major histocompatibility complex (MHC)	Large collection of genes that includes those responsible for determining rejection of transplanted tissue by the immune system; versions of the MHC are possessed by all mammals, and by animals as low as coelenterates (e.g. sea anemones)
Human leukocyte antigens (HLA)	Term for human MHC gene products involved in antigen recognition by T lymphocytes (the term 'antigen' is used rather loosely here, denoting the fact that HLA molecules can elicit immune responses in graft rejection)
Haplotype	A collection of genes (i.e. a section of chromosome) inherited as a whole group
Gene polymorphism	The availability in the gene pool of many different allelic forms of a gene at a particular locus
Linkage disequilibrium	Alleles appearing *together* on the same haplotype more frequently than their single gene frequencies suggest; this implies that meiotic recombination is non-random

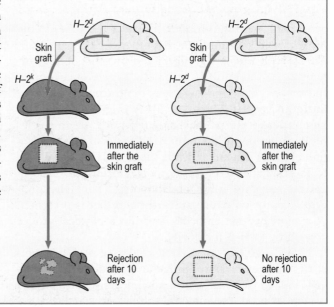

Fig. 5.1 **Influence of MHC genes on skin grafting.**
A graft from a mouse possessing the *d* gene at the *H–2* locus is rejected after 10 days by a mouse possessing the *k* gene at this locus.

a specific antigen (e.g. a virus) *and* MHC molecules simultaneously. It is the molecular basis of this recognition that forms the major subject of this chapter.

STRUCTURE OF THE HLA

The human MHC, or HLA, comprises three major classes (I, II and III) of genes involved in the immune response. The genes are found on the short arm of chromosome 6 (Fig. 5.3). In addition, there are several genes that lie in the HLA region but do not fall into any of the three major categories. These include the genes for 21-hydroxylase (an enzyme important in steroid metabolism), tumour necrosis factor-α, and heat-shock protein 70 (one of a family of proteins produced by cells in response to heat and other injuries).

Genes in the HLA are designated using capital italic letters. The antigen molecules produced by them are designated with capital roman letters and the Greek letters α and β describe the polypeptide chains.

MHC loci: disease susceptibility or immune response genes?

The association between the inheritance of particular genes in the MHC and a higher risk of developing certain diseases was first clearly demonstrated in 1973, when Brewerton showed that over 90% of patients with ankylosing spondylitis, an inflammatory disease of the spine, had *B27* as one of their HLA types. Possible explanations for such associations are discussed in a later chapter (see p. 125), but they serve to underline that this group of genes was known for its relationship with disease and graft rejection before a physiological function could be assigned to it.

First indications of the role of the MHC in the immune response again came from studies using inbred strains of mice. It became possible to characterise certain strains as high or low responders to polypeptide antigens such as insulin on the basis of the amount of anti-insulin antibody produced. Genes determining responsiveness were called immune response genes (Ir) and localised to the *I* region of the mouse major histocompatibility complex, which is termed the *H-2* region.

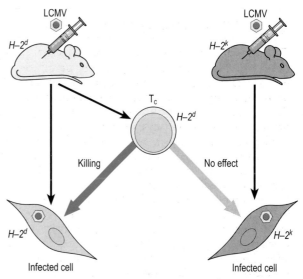

Fig. 5.2 **MHC restriction of immune responses.**
Mice infected with LCMV produced cytotoxic T lymphocytes (T$_c$) capable of killing infected target cells from the same animal. Cells infected with LCMV but possessing different genes at the *H-2* locus to those of the mouse providing the T$_c$ cells are not susceptible to killing.

Class I region

Class I HLA genes are found furthest from the centromere and are designated by capital letters, *HLA-A* to *HLA-J*; of these, *HLA-A*, *HLA-B* and *HLA-C* are the best known. The class I genes in the HLA encode the amino acid sequence of the class I α chains (the *H-2* region is the mouse equivalent). The class I β chain is an invariant molecule (i.e. the same for all the α chains) called **β$_2$-microglobulin**, the gene for which is on chromosome 15. Once α and β chains are assembled,

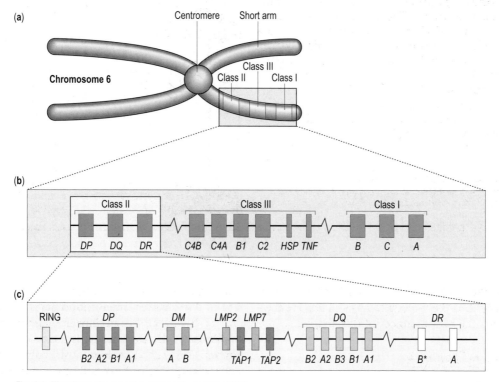

Fig. 5.3 **The three classes of genes in the human MHC.**
(**a**) Site on chromosome 6. (**b**) The major subregions and genes within each of the classes. (**c**) Detailed map of class II region showing the major genes. RING, really interesting new genes; LMP, low molecular mass polypeptide; TAP, transporters associated with processing; HSP, heat-shock protein; TNF, tumour necrosis factor.

the class I molecule has the role of presenting peptide antigens to T lymphocytes.

Class II region

The class II genes have three major subregions, *DP*, *DQ* and *DR* (there are two equivalent regions in the mouse, *I–A* and *I–E*) (see Fig. 5.3). In these subregions are genes encoding molecules that, like those in the class I region, present peptide antigen to T lymphocytes. Molecules encoded in the *HLA-DM* subregion may aid this process.

Two distinct polypeptide chains, termed the α and β chains, combine to form a class II molecule. The *DR* subregion contains only a single α chain gene (*DRA*), and, therefore, all HLA-DR molecules have the same α chain. There exist nine *DRB* genes (*DRB1–9*) of which some are non-functional pseudogenes (*DRB2, 6, 7, 8 and 9*) (Fig. 5.4). Each of the four functional β chain genes (*DRB1, 3, 4 and 5*) encodes a distinct β chain, which can combine with the single invariant α chain to form four distinct DR molecules: DRαβ$_1$, DRαβ$_3$, DRαβ$_4$ and DRαβ$_5$.

However, we do not all express the four distinct DR molecules, DRαβ$_1$, DRαβ$_3$, DRαβ$_4$ and DRαβ$_5$. The number of DRB genes expressed in an individual depends upon the **haplotype** inherited (a haplotype is a group of genes inherited as a unit; Fig. 5.4). In other words, it is possible to inherit a haplotype with, for example, only the *DRB1, DRB5, DRB6* and *DRB9* genes. Possession of this haplotype would result only in formation of DRαβ$_1$ and DRαβ$_5$ heterodimers, since the other *DRB* genes (*DRB6, DRB9*) are non-functional.

The complexity does not end there, however. At each locus of the functional DRB genes, there is the potential for different alleles (i.e. different forms of the same gene). While *DRA* has no allelic forms, and hence the α chain is invariant, each of the different *DRB* genes has a different degree of allelic variability. In some cases, the number of different alleles is considerable, a phenomenon termed **gene polymorphism**. The *DRB1* locus has some 60 different alleles, whereas the *DRB4* locus has only a single allelic form. The result of such gene polymorphism is that there is enormous potential for individuals to differ in the *HLA* genes they possess, and hence the HLA molecules they express. We identify these differences by HLA typing. In the case of HLA-DR molecules, differences are the result of *DRB* gene polymorphisms; hence it is these that determine the particular DR type.

The *DQ* region contains two pairs of genes for the α and β chains. One is a pair of pseudogenes, while the other pair, *DQA1* and *DQB1*, encodes the DQ α and β chains that combine to form the DQ molecule which is expressed on cell surfaces. Both DQ α and β chains are polymorphic (i.e. have numerous possible alleles at the locus) though the DQ β chain bears the majority of the polymorphism.

The *DP* region also contains two sets of α and β chain genes, one of which is a set of non-expressed pseudogenes, while the other, *DPA1* and *DPB1*, encodes the DP α and β chains that form the expressed DP molecule. The DP α chain displays low levels of polymorphism, whereas the DP β chain is highly polymorphic.

Finally, there is the *DM* region, with two genes *DMA* and *DMB*. The product of the *DMA* and *DMB* genes is an αβ heterodimer that, unlike the heterodimers produced by genes in the *DP*, *DQ* and *DR* subregions, is very rarely expressed on the cell surface, if at all. However, in mutant cell lines in which the *DM* region is deleted, peptide presentation on the cell surface by DP, DQ and DR molecules is defective. The consensus view is that the HLA-DM αβ molecule plays a critical role in loading peptide into the other, 'more conventional' class II HLA molecules (see p. 86). The role of the *DN* and *DO* regions remains to be established.

There are three other gene groups of importance in the class II region, of which we shall hear more when the processing of protein antigens for presentation by HLA molecules is discussed in greater depth. *LMP-2* and *LMP-7* encode for two **l**ow **m**olecular **m**ass **p**olypeptides that have peptidase activity. These are contained within a large, multimolecular enzyme complex called the **proteasome**, which can actually be visualised at the electron microscopic level (see p. 90). The role of the LMPs is in the cleavage of proteins into smaller peptides for binding to class I HLA molecules. *TAP-1* and *TAP-2* encode two halves of a peptide transporter. This is reponsible for transporting peptides of the required length into the class I synthesis compartment for loading. The function of the *RING* genes (acronym for really interesting new gene) awaits clarification.

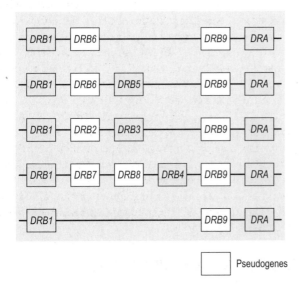

☐ Pseudogenes

Fig. 5.4 **Expression of the HLA-DR locus.**
There are five different haplotypes (groups of genes) and each individual will have one of these on each chromosome. The haplotype will govern the number of DR molecule types produced since some genes are non-functional pseudogenes.

As yet, the identities of the peptidases involved in generating antigenic peptides presented by class II HLA molecules (equivalent to LMP for class I) and the equivalents of the TAP molecules for transporting peptides into the HLA class II assembly site remain unknown.

Class III region

Between the class I and II regions is the class III region, which contains several genes coding for complement components.

The MHC

- The MHC is a collection of genes many of which are involved in immune functions. The human MHC is known as HLA and the genes are found on chromosome 6.
- In some individuals, possession of particular HLA genes confers susceptibility to a disease.
- Molecules encoded by the MHC act as:
  — peptidases to cleave large protein antigens
  — transporters, carrying antigenic peptides to the correct intracellular compartment
  — transporters to load the peptides into the HLA molecules
  — HLA molecules.
- Class I and II HLA molecules are glycoproteins expressed on cell surfaces and bind short processed peptides and present them to the T cell receptor.
- The law of MHC restriction dictates that cytotoxic T cells will only kill target cells that present both a specific antigen and the correct MHC molecule.

INHERITANCE OF THE MHC

Two complementary chromosome strands, one maternal and one paternal, are inherited, each strand providing an MHC haplotype, a string of genes linked together on the same chromosome. For example, in the class I region, an individual might have inherited the *A1* and *B7* genes on a single maternally derived chromosome. The paternal genes at these loci might be *A28* and *B14*. When the genes of maternal and paternal haplotype are transcribed and translated into their protein products, *both* maternally and paternally derived allelic forms are expressed as cell surface proteins, a feature known as **co-dominance**. In our example, A1, A28, B7 and B14 class I molecules are expressed (Fig. 5.5).

Haplotypes encoding class II HLA molecules are inherited in a similar fashion. The major difference is that haplotypes in this region do not necessarily contain a full complement of the *DRB* loci (see Fig. 5.4). Therefore, one haplotype may contain functional alleles of *DRB1* and *DRB5*, another the *DRB1* and *DRB3* genes. Thus, the different haplotypes can contribute genes to make one, two or three DR molecules.

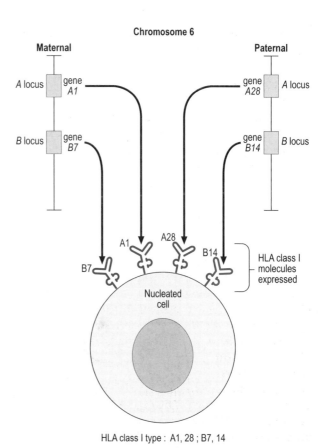

Fig. 5.5 **Inheritance of HLA genes and expression of the gene products, demonstrating co-dominance.**
HLA class I type shown is A1, 28; B7, 14.

Although genes in the MHC follow a Mendelian inheritance pattern, two additional features of this complex serve to set it apart in terms of genetics. One of these is the degree of gene polymorphism and the other is linkage disequilibrium between different loci. **Linkage disequilibrium** describes the fact that certain alleles are found together on the same haplotype with greater frequency than should occur if recombination during meiosis was random. For example, genes for HLA-B8 and HLA-DR3 are found in a Caucasian population with frequencies of 9% and 12%, respectively. Therefore, the expected frequency of a haplotype containing *HLA-B8* and *DR3* is 0.09×0.12, giving 0.0108, or approximately 1%; this haplotype is actually found in over 7% of Caucasians. Linkage disequilibrium results in the inheritance of large portions of the MHC that are intact and have not undergone recombination. It, therefore, gives rise to **extended haplotypes** that incorporate genes from all three MHC classes and are passed on undisturbed from generation to generation.

STUDYING THE MHC: HLA TYPING

Progress in our understanding of the role of the MHC has been enhanced by rapid advances in our ability to analyse its genes and gene products. The speed of this headway has also been a major factor in the difficulty

HLA haplotypes — too much of a good thing?

Selective pressures during the course of evolution may have been the major factor in the survival of certain HLA gene combinations in a haplotype. Inherited together, a collection of class I, II and III genes could offer the optimum protection against a particular infection, providing a positive selection pressure. In contrast, studies since the late 1970s have shown that possession of certain HLA haplotypes is disadvantageous. For example, the extended haplotype of *HLA-A1*, *HLA-B8*, *HLA-DR3* and complement *C4AQ0* alleles present together on a single chromosome is found much more frequently than could occur by chance in patients with a range of diseases that go under the umbrella of 'inflammatory' (e.g. vasculitis) or 'autoimmune' (e.g. the autoimmune form of diabetes) conditions. It has been proposed that these particular gene combinations, which are common in Caucasians, enhanced survival from a viral or bacterial epidemic afflicting northern Europe millennia ago. Those who survived mounted an appropriately vigorous immune response to the infection. It is further speculated that this tendency to aggressive hyper-responsiveness may leave such individuals prone to developing inappropriate immune responses, giving a greater tendency towards chronic inflammatory conditions and responses to self antigens.

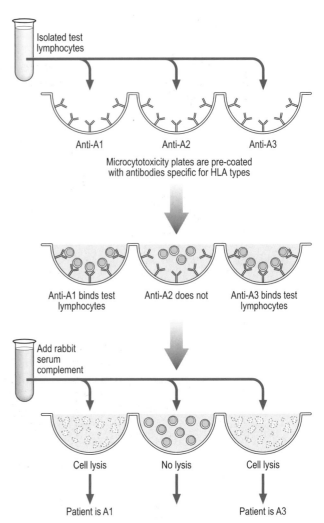

Fig. 5.6 **Microcytotoxicity test to determine HLA class I type.**

many people have in coming to terms with the complexity of the MHC. Understanding how the genes and molecules are identified helps overcome this.

The basic approach is termed **HLA typing**. It is carried out at the phenotypic level (i.e. what types of protein are expressed on the cell surface) and the genotypic level (i.e. what DNA sequence is present in the genes). Originally, HLA typing was carried out almost exclusively at the phenotypic level using antibodies to different HLA molecules. The antibodies are human in origin and are obtained from the serum of individuals who for one reason or another have formed an antibody response to an HLA molecule that they had encountered. For the most part, these are multiparous women (i.e. women who have given birth to several children), making antibody responses to paternally derived HLA molecules. Since it is based on the use of serum-derived antibodies, the approach is known as **serological HLA typing** and uses a technique called **microcytotoxicity** (Fig. 5.6). To antiserum-coated plastic plates are added lymphocytes (a good source of expression of HLA molecules) from the person to be typed. After a period of incubation, rabbit complement is added. Lysis of the cells indicates they bear the HLA molecule(s) defined by that antiserum. Serology remains the main technique for class I HLA typing, although DNA-based approaches are fast being developed.

For class II HLA typing, serological techniques are not as applicable: the antisera available are frequently unable to distinguish between very similar molecules that are actually the products of different alleles at the same locus. Until recently, serological typing was still widely used for HLA-DR typing, for which antisera identifying the major types were available. Serology is unreliable for DQ typing, however, and does not exist for DP typing.

Clearly, the way around the lack of precision of class II serological typing was to analyse the alleles at the genotypic level. Before techniques for large-scale DNA sequencing were available, this was carried out using analysis of **restriction fragment length polymorphisms** (**RFLP**) (Fig. 5.7). Restriction enzymes cut DNA at particular sites. Whether an enzyme cuts a particular stretch of DNA or not depends on the sequence, and by careful selection of the enzymes used, polymorphisms of a gene can be distinguished by the size and number of fragments generated. To reveal the size and number of fragments, the products of the digestion are separated in an electric field and blotted onto nitrocellulose filters. Radiolabelled portions of DNA complementary to the sequences of interest are synthesised in the laboratory; these are termed probes. Several probes can be used, each specific for a particular *DRB* gene, and

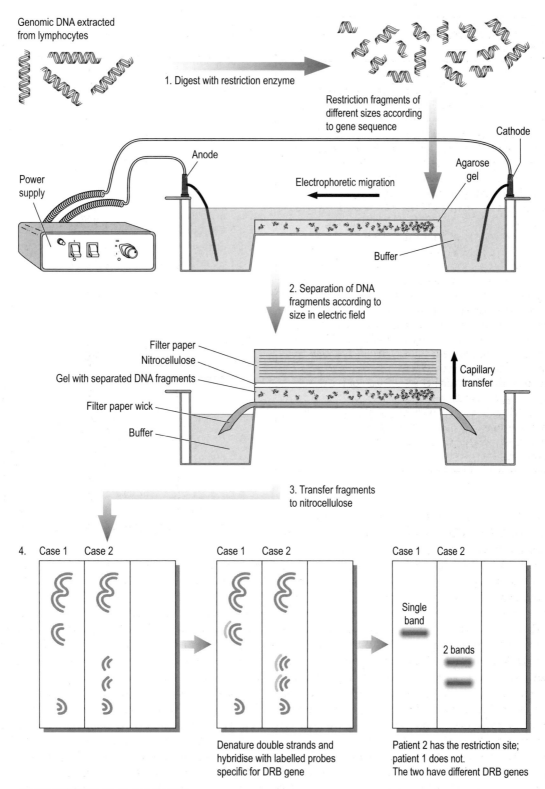

Fig. 5.7 **RFLP analysis of class II genes.**
Genomic DNA is extracted and cut with restriction enzymes. The fragments are separated in an electric field, blotted onto nitrocellulose, denatured into single strands and hybridised to specific probes. After autoradiography, patient 1 shows a single band and has a particular polymorphism of the *DRB* genes; patient 2 had an additional restriction site resulting in two bands and hence has a different *DRB* gene.

these are overlaid onto the cut segments. Differing combinations of bands correspond to different genes. Some alleles, notably in the *DQ* region, share restriction sites and are, therefore, indistinguishable by this technique.

At present, the majority of major HLA typing centres have moved towards identification of the sequences of class II genes. Direct sequencing of a gene locus is expensive and laborious. One of the favoured approaches, therefore, is to amplify the DNA of a

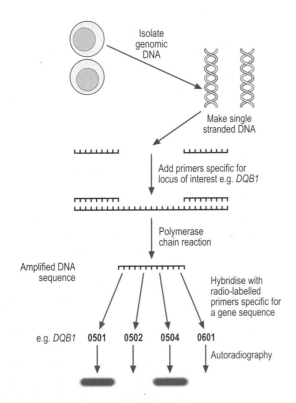

Fig. 5.8 Sequence specific oligonucleotide probe typing.
Single-stranded DNA is amplified using primers that will bind to all polymorphisms of the gene of interest. The amplified sequence is then blotted onto several small nitrocellulose filters. Each filter is hybridised to a different oligonucleotide probe, each designed to be specific for one of the polymorphisms of that gene. One or two filters will indicate a positive reaction (depending on whether the person is homozygous or not).

particular locus using the polymerase chain reaction (PCR) and then to hybridise it with radiolabelled probes designed to be specific for a particular gene sequence (**sequence-specific oligonucleotide (SSO) probe typing**) (Fig. 5.8).

TISSUE DISTRIBUTION OF HLA MOLECULES

Important differences exist in the tissue distribution of HLA molecules that are governed by cell lineage, stage of maturation and state of activation (Table 5.2). Whilst class I molecules are expressed on the surface of virtually all cells except for mature erythrocytes and trophoblast cells, class II molecules are only constitutively expressed on the surface of a small number of cell

Table 5.2 Cells constitutively expressing HLA molecules

Class I	Class II
Virtually all nucleated cells	B lymphocytes Mononuclear phagocytes (macrophages/monocytes) Follicular dendritic cells Tissue representatives of mononuclear phagocytes (e.g. Kupffer cells, mesangial cells) Activated T lymphocytes

types, including macrophages, monocytes, follicular dendritic cells and B lymphocytes, from which class II molecules are progressively lost when these cells differentiate into plasma cells. Most unstimulated T lymphocytes lack detectable class II molecules on their surface but are induced to synthesise and express them after antigen stimulation. In addition, the individual subclasses of class II molecules are differentially expressed. On some cells, such as a subset of macrophages, only DR molecules are expressed, whereas on others, such as B lymphocytes, all three subclasses are present. Even when all three subclasses are expressed, they are present at different densities on the cell surface, such that DR expression is higher than DQ or DP.

Under the influence of cytokines (e.g. interferons-a and g, tumour necrosis factor) a whole range of cells that typically only express class I may be induced to express class II MHC molecules and also to up-regulate the number of surface MHC class I molecules. The ability to regulate MHC expression may be of importance in the eradication of intracellular viral infections and could also be of relevance to the generation of autoimmune disease (see p. 124).

Variation in the MHC

- Inherited maternal and paternal haplotypes are both expressed: co-dominance.
- Haplotypes in the *DRB* locus of class II do not necessarily contain a full complement of the *DRB* genes.
- Gene polymorphism is the occurrence of multiple alleles at some loci, e.g. *DRB1* has around 60 different alleles.
- Linkage disequilibrium occurs where certain alleles remain linked together in a haplotype more often than should occur if recombination during meiosis was random.
- The MHC genes and gene products are typed by DNA sequence identification and serology, respectively: HLA typing.
- HLA polymorphism creates broader protection against potential pathogens but is a barrier to organ transplantation.

STRUCTURE OF HLA MOLECULES

The class I molecules, HLA-A, HLA-B and HLA-C, are formed from polymorphic heavy-chain glycoproteins (44 kDa) that bind non-covalently to β_2-microglobulin, an invariant polypeptide (12 kDa). The class II molecules, HLA-DP, HLA-DQ and HLA-DR, are formed from two glycoproteins, an α chain (34 kDa) and a β chain (29 kDa), both encoded in the HLA region (Fig. 5.9).

The heavy or α chain of class I molecules carries three distinct extracellular regions, or domains, formed

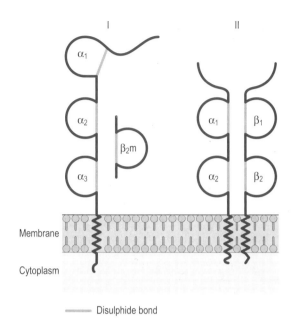

Fig. 5.9 Schematic illustration of the structure of class I and class II molecules.
In class I, the heavy transmembrane α chain is non-covalently bound to β₂-microglobulin. In class II the two chains are both transmembrane and are non-covalently linked.

by disulphide bonding, while the light or β chain is β_2-microglobulin, a much smaller one-domain structure. The class II molecules are heterodimers consisting of two non-covalently linked peptides (α and β), each accommodating two domains formed by disulphide bridging (Fig. 5.9). The domains present in both class I and II molecules can be subdivided into two 'immunoglobulin-like' domains and two 'peptide-binding' domains. For class I MHC molecules, the polymorphic and membrane-anchoring heavy chain contains both

Transcomplementation

To manufacture a class II molecule, the minimum genetic information required is a pair of genes coding for one α and one β chain. The function of HLA molecules is antigen presentation. Antigens come in many different shapes and sizes, so how, with a limited number of functional molecules all of which are invariant (in contrast with the T cell receptor and immunoglobulin, which also bind antigen) can variety of binding be engendered? One strategy is the use of more than one β chain to combine with a single α chain, as occurs in the DR region, giving rise to $DR\alpha\beta_1$, $DR\alpha\beta_3$, $DR\alpha\beta_4$ and $DR\alpha\beta_5$; another mechanism is the use of transcomplementation. This phenomenon was first observed for DQ. The DQ α chain encoded by one chromosome (e.g. maternal) can combine with the DQ β chain encoded by the second chromosome (e.g. paternal) to form a 'hybrid' molecule that is not present in either parent and that bears new epitopes. Transcomplementation may be relevant in HLA-associated predisposition to disease.

peptide-binding domains (α_1 and α_2) and one immunoglobulin domain (α_3), non-covalently bound to the second immunoglobulin domain represented by the invariant β_2-microglobulin. Class II molecules have a symmetrical arrangement in which two transmembrane polypeptides each supplies one peptide-binding (α_1 and β_1) and one immunoglobulin domain (α_2 and β_2) (see also the box 'Transcomplementation').

THREE-DIMENSIONAL STRUCTURE OF HLA MOLECULES

In 1987, sufficient quantities of protein were obtained for X-ray diffraction studies of the HLA-A2 molecule, delineating the first crystal structure of class I MHC glycoproteins. Similar studies on HLA-A68 and HLA-B27 have followed and have revealed many hitherto unknown features of these molecules. Perhaps the most comprehensible view to have of the HLA class I molecule is to take the position of an approaching T cell about to interact with the peptide antigen being presented. The T cell receptor encounters a deep-grooved binding site, 2.5 nm long, 1 nm wide and 1 nm deep, closed at either end and sufficient to accommodate a peptide fragment of around 8 or 9 amino acid residues in length. The groove is situated between two α-helices on top of a floor of eight antiparallel β-pleated sheets (Fig. 5.10). The α-helices contain pockets to accommodate peptide side chains. When HLA-A2 was crystallised, this binding site actually contained electron-dense material that was not continuous with the HLA molecule itself but was so tightly bound that the scientists involved could not remove it; this was interpreted as being a bound peptide. On the basis of these observations, it is now possible to visualise T cell recognition as a T cell receptor clinging to both α-helical sides of the HLA groove and to the peptide lying within it.

Comparisons between the crystallographic structure of HLA-A2 and HLA-A68 show that, with minor perturbations, the polypeptide backbones of the two are extremely similar. The differences between them are primarily owing to the nature of the amino acid side chains at 13 positions of substitution. Ten of these residues are at positions lining the floor and sides of the groove. This means that even a small number of differences between two HLA molecules can have a profound effect on the peptides they could harbour (Fig. 5.11). Analysis of the structure of other class I HLA molecules by sequence alignment with A2 predicts that, in general, the allelic polymorphisms (i.e. the differences between different HLA molecules) are localised predominantly to the sides and floor of the HLA binding groove. This gives a physiological explanation for polymorphism in HLA molecules. Each HLA molecule has a limited repertoire of peptides with which it may bind. Polymorphisms (i.e. slightly altered versions) of HLA molecules, and the fact that we each express several different class I molecules (by having

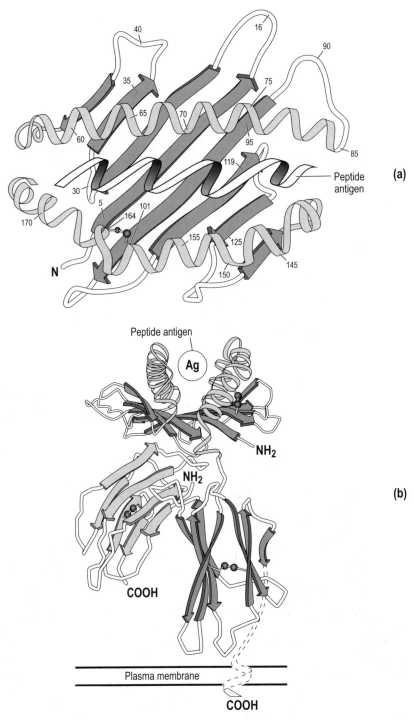

Fig. 5.10 **Structure of the HLA class I molecule.**
(**a**) As seen by an approaching T cell receptor the class I molecule has a deep groove, the antigen-binding site, occupied by a short antigenic peptide. (**b**) Lateral view of the molecule with a peptide in the antigen-binding groove. For amino acid positions refer to Figure 5.11. (Modified with permission from Bjorkman et al 1987 Nature 329: 506–512.)

multiple loci and co-dominance), extend the overall binding repertoire available to an individual. In the context of presenting peptides from infectious agents to T cells, it is not difficult to see that these features are of benefit to the individual, and how extensive polymorphism is of benefit to the species.

The crystallographic structure of a class II molecule, HLA-DR1, was solved in 1993. It has a remarkably similar appearance to that of class I (Fig. 5.12), with some key differences. First, the peptide binding groove is larger and is not closed at either end, allowing the peptide to protrude. This feature is consistent with the finding that class I binding peptides are roughly half the length of those binding class II molecules (see below). Second, there appears to be only a single clearly definable side chain pocket in the class II groove (as opposed to several in class I: see below). This might imply that the binding requirements for class II-

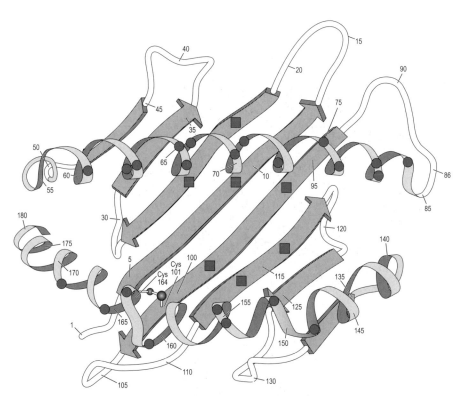

Fig. 5.11 **Sites at which amino acids tend to vary in HLA class I molecules (i.e. polymorphic residues).** Residues shown as circles in the α-helices and as squares in the β-pleated sheets. Note how polymorphism affects antigen binding site. (Modified with permission from Bjorkman et al 1987 Nature 329: 506–512.)

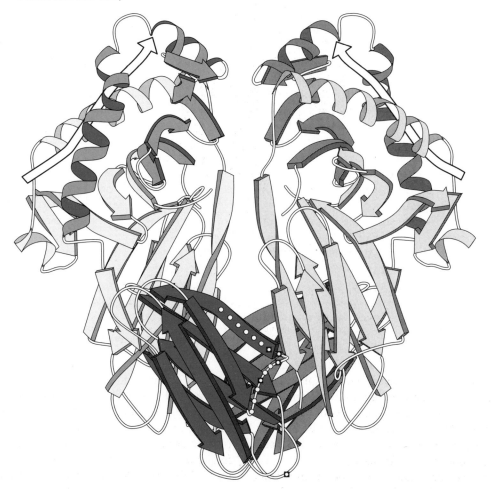

Fig. 5.12 **Structure of HLA class II, following analysis by X-ray crystallography.** The class II αβ heterodimers probably dimerise themselves, to form the 'dimer of dimers'. Peptides can be seen in the class II groove as arrows pointing upwards. (Modified with permission from Brown et al Nature 364: 33–39.)

associated peptides are less stringent than for class I. Finally, all three of the HLA-DR1 crystals made were composed of dimers of the αβ heterodimer. If this is true, and not a crystallographic artefact, it has important implications for the recognition of class II–peptide complexes by the T lymphocyte, a process which will be discussed more fully in a later section (see p. 86).

INTERACTION OF THE HLA MOLECULE AND PEPTIDE

The function of HLA molecules is to bind peptide fragments of antigens degraded inside cells and to present them to the receptors of T cells. As a general rule, the source of the peptide appears to dictate whether it is presented in association with class I or class II molecules. Under physiological conditions, peptides derived from proteins synthesised endogenously, within the cell presenting the antigen, are presented in association with class I HLA molecules. In a viral infection, viral proteins are synthesised endogenously using the host cell's 'machinery'. Hence, viral peptides may also be presented through this **endogenous pathway**, non-covalently bound to class I MHC molecules. In contrast, peptides derived from outside the cell (exogenous antigens) are taken in by endocytosis, processed using proteolytic enzymes (see Ch. 7) and presented following non-covalent association with class II HLA molecules. Antigens presented through this so-called **exogenous pathway** will include a variety of molecules from the external milieu: plasma proteins, for example, as well as proteins located on the surface membranes during endocytosis (e.g. surface receptors). During infection or injury, the nature of the exogenous antigens will change. This is an opportunity for 'foreign' antigens, such as those derived from bacteria, to be processed and presented by class II molecules to T cells. The process of endocytosis and presentation of foreign antigens to T cells is a pivotal event in the initiation of immune responses (see p. 86).

The role of the HLA molecule is the presentation of the peptide antigen fragment in its groove to a responding T lymphocyte. The T lymphocyte, as we shall discuss later, bears a receptor that recognises the HLA molecule–peptide complex. The nature of the T lymphocyte recognition is dictated by another law of MHC restriction: only T cells bearing a surface glycoprotein molecule (termed CD4) that binds to the class II β chain are able to interact with class II-presented peptides. Conversely, only T cells bearing a surface glycoprotein (CD8) that binds to the α chain of the class I molecule are able to recognise peptide presented by class I HLA molecules. With very few exceptions, mature T lymphocytes express either CD4 or CD8, but not both. It seems probable that one of the main functions of these CD4 and CD8 'accessory' molecules is to stabilise the interaction of T cell receptor and the HLA molecule–peptide complex, which is typically of quite low affinity.

Peptide binding to class I molecules

Since the crystallisation of HLA-A2, and the intriguing view of a tightly bound peptide in the groove, extensive studies on the characteristics of this binding have been carried out. One approach has been to use acid dissociation to disrupt the class I molecule and free the bound peptides. From a class I MHC molecule, the eluted peptides are typically nine amino acid residues long and composed from endogenous proteins (Table 5.3). They fit tightly into the groove using non-covalent forces such as hydrogen bonding. In very broad terms, it appears that the class I MHC binding groove can be divided roughly into six pockets, labelled A–F. The peptides appear to 'anchor' at each end of the pocket (A and F; terminal anchor residues). There are then auxiliary anchors along the length of the groove and also pockets that accommodate glycosylated side chains; these vary according to the molecule. In HLA-B27, for example, there is a clear requirement for an arginine residue (R) at position B. It appears that the peptide itself may occasionally be required to bend to fit into the class I groove, which is closed at both ends (Fig. 5.10). This is achieved by making the peptide an integral component of the class I molecule: the α and β chains fold-up around the peptide. This has several important consequences: (1) class I molecules are assembled at a point at which α chain, β_2-microglobulin *and* endogenous peptide are available; (2) there is little or no opportunity for the selected, tightly bound peptide to be replaced during transport to the cell surface; and (3) 'empty' class I molecules will be found only rarely on the surface, since they are unstable. The processes that lead to the formation of the class I molecule–peptide complex will be discussed later (see p. 89).

The binding of peptide to class I molecules is tighter than to class II molecules and can be considered irreversible. This irreversibility correlates with the trap-like geometry of the peptide-binding groove. The kinetics of MHC molecule–peptide interactions can be represented by the dissociation constant, a measurement of the ratio between the rate at which molecules associate and dissociate. This has a value of between 10^{-5} and 10^{-6} M^{-1}, interpreted as indicating a slow association and a very slow dissociation. This dissociation constant is five orders of magnitude higher than interactions

Table 5.3 **Examples of self peptides eluted from the class I molecule HLA-A B27**

Peptide	Source
R **R** I K E I V K **K**	Heat-shock protein 89β
R **R** V K E V V K **K**	Heat-shock protein 89β
G **R** I D K P I L **K**	Ribosomal protein
R **R** S K E I T V **R**	ATP-dependent RNA helicase
F **R** Y N G L I H **R**	60S ribosomal protein
R **R** Y Q K S T E **L**	Histone H3.3
R **R** W L P A G D **A**	Elongation factor 2

Each letter denotes an amino acid (e.g. R = arginine); in bold are some of the terminal anchor residues important in B27 binding; see Appendix 4

between antibody and antigens (i.e. antigen and antibody associate faster and dissociate slower; see page 34). The half-life of the MHC–peptide complex is some 30 hours.

From analysis of the characteristics of peptides eluted from the class I MHC molecule, it has been possible to construct the minimum requirements for peptide binding. These differ for each class I molecule and have been termed **peptide-binding motifs**. Already, such predictions have helped in identifying the critical components of a protein that elicits an antimalarial immune response in individuals with a particular HLA class I molecule (see p. 319) and such knowledge will aid vaccine design.

Peptide binding to class II molecules

The characteristics of peptide binding to class II molecules are marginally less well defined than those associating with class I. Although it would appear that the pathway leading to the generation of class II-binding peptides is designed to present fragments from the external milieu, most studies in this field have taken advantage of class II-expressing cells studied in culture, rather than during an immune response to foreign antigen, which is technically more demanding. Under these conditions, peptides presented include some proteins in the culture fluid acquired into the cell by endocytosis. The majority of the peptides, however, appear to be derived from plasma membrane-associated proteins, suggesting that the process of generating peptides for class II molecules takes place in endosomal or lysosomal compartments near to the cell surface. In particular, many of the plasma membrane-associated self peptides found binding to class II molecules were fragments of MHC molecules themselves (Table 5.4).

On average, the peptides found in class II HLA molecule grooves are between 15 and 18 amino acid residues long (although the range is usually 10–34).

Table 5.4 **Examples of self peptides eluted from the class II molecule HLA-DR4**

Peptide[a]	Source
D T Q F V R F D S D A A S Q R M E P R	HLA-A2
D T Q F V R F D S D A A S P R G E	HLA-Cw9
G S L F V Y N I T T N K Y K A F L D K Q	VLA-4 (a cell activation marker)
G V F Y L Q W G R S T L V S V S	Ig heavy chain
S P E D F V Y Q F K G M C Y F	HLA-DQ 3.2 allele β chain

Each letter denotes an amino acid (e.g. R = arginine); see Appendix 4

Apart from length, there are other important differences between class I- and II-associated peptides (Table 5.5). Class II peptides display 'promiscuity': in other words, the same peptide may bind to several different class II molecules. Binding promiscuity means that predicting class II motifs is also more difficult, though not impossible. In addition, the class II MHC molecule groove is open at both ends, allowing the peptide to 'hang out'; this enables greater variety in length (one eluted peptide described recently was over 70 amino acid residues long). The peptides appear to have a core binding region of 7–10 residues, with at least one aromatic or hydrophobic amino acid as a key component.

HLA POLYMORPHISM

With such a clear vision of the peptide-binding site, it is now possible to visualise the regions of the molecule that are characterised by the extensive polymorphism associated with the MHC. Polymorphism is the phenomenon whereby numerous different alleles — **allotypes** — can occur at a single locus. Gene polymorphism in the HLA region is the most extensive yet described, with the number of known allelic forms of genes increasing constantly with the application of more refined

Table 5.5 **Comparison of major features of class I and class II MHC molecules**

	Class I molecules	Class II molecules
Genetic organisation	Polymorphic α chain genes in MHC (on chromosome 6 in humans) Monomorphic β chain gene (on chromosome 15 in humans)	Polymorphic α and β chain genes in MHC (on chromosome 6 in humans)
Molecular structure	Non-covalently associated αβ dimer	Non-covalently associated αβ dimer; but this may itself form dimers
Binding groove	Two α-helices flanking a floor of β-pleated sheets	Two α-helices flanking a floor of β-pleated sheets
Peptide size	Average 9 (range 8–10) amino acid residues	Average 15 (range 10–34) amino acid residues
Peptide source	Endogenous proteins	Exogenous and endogenous proteins derived from endosomal compartments situated near plasma membrane
Cellular site of peptide binding	Early: during assembly of class I molecule Peptide required for correct folding of dimer	Late: in a specialised endosome Invariant chain (but not peptide) required for folding of dimer
Affinity for peptide	High	Moderate
Role	Presentation of endogenous peptides to the TCR of T lymphocytes bearing the accessory molecule CD8	Presentation of exogenous peptides to the TCR of T lymphocytes bearing the accessory molecule CD4
Tissue distribution	Almost all nucleated cells	Cells of monocyte lineage, dendritic cells, B lymphocytes, activated T lymphocytes

methods of HLA typing. In evolutionary terms, polymorphism has arisen by gene duplication and point mutation to provide a mechanism for increasing the variety of peptides that can be presented to T lymphocytes. The higher the number of different HLA genes possessed by an individual, the wider the range of peptides that can be bound and the broader the ability of T cells to respond. In addition, because MHC genes are co-dominant, heterozygotes will have an advantage over homozygotes by being able to construct a wider range of chain combinations. The groove of a single HLA molecule can accommodate a variety of different peptide antigens, but it cannot bind all peptides against which it would be beneficial to mount an immune response.

Each person is capable of mounting strong responses to some organisms and weaker responses to others. Viewed in evolutionary terms, polymorphism decreases the chance of a population being annihilated by a microorganism against which not all individuals are capable of mounting an effective immune response. Within a species, therefore, the greater the MHC polymorphism, the greater the collective immunity (see the box 'HLA haplotypes', p. 58). Polymorphism of HLA genes has two important consequences for the individual: unrelated individuals have a diverse susceptibility to disease and also promptly reject organ transplants between each other.

The variable regions responsible for HLA polymorphism lie along the α-helices that form the margins of the groove. With one exception (residue 45), all of the positions with high variability in class I molecules have side chains that either point into the binding site and are candidates for contacting bound peptide or are external and candidates for contacting the T cell receptor. Polymorphism, especially on the inner surfaces of the helices and on the floor of the groove, serves to alter binding of peptide fragments and possibly to alter their presentation to the T cell receptor.

NOMENCLATURE

A major revision of the nomenclature of factors in the HLA system has been in progress since 1989. It has been devised in order to assimilate new alleles and gene sequences as easily as possible as they are discovered. Inevitably, the student will be made to suffer for being caught between two systems and yet called upon to recognise both — you have been warned!

Originally, when HLA typing for class I and class II alleles was serologically based, types were assigned according to the antisera with which an individual's cells reacted. As stated above, antisera may recognise epitopes common to more than one molecule. Therefore, molecules shown to be identical by serology may differ at the genotypic and amino acid sequence level.

In the new nomenclature — as previously — an allele is first identified by the letter or letters that designate that locus (e.g. *HLA-A, DR, DP*). For class I alleles, this is followed by an asterisk and then a two digit number (e.g. 01, 02, 03 etc.) defining the HLA type. Where possible, for class I and II alleles, this two digit number is the same as that of the serological equivalent. A further two digits (01, 02, 03 etc.) define the variants of that type (Table 5.6). For class II, the letters defining the locus are followed by *A* or *B* (corresponding to genes coding for α or β chains), a number defining the locus if more than one exists (e.g. DRB1, 3, 4, 5) and an asterisk followed by the types (01, 02, 03 etc.) and their variants (01, 02, 03 etc.) are then defined in an identical fashion to class I. The new system thus allows for novel variants at a locus to be identified at the genetic level and then identified using the next number in sequence. A comprehensive list of HLA types is given in Appendix 3.

Table 5.6 **Examples of the nomenclature for HLA alleles**

General formula for nomenclature		
Locus	Type[a]	Variant
H L A – X*	0 0	0 0

Allele given by new nomenclature	Equivalent serological type
Class I	
H L A – A * 0 1 0 1	HLA-A1
H L A – B * 0 8 0 1	HLA-B8
Class II	
H L A – D R B 1 * 0 1 0 1	HLA-DR1[b]
H L A – D R B 1 * 0 1 0 2	HLA-DR1[b]
H L A – D R B 4 * 0 1 0 1	HLA-DR53

[a]i.e. allele
[b]These are the protein products of alleles with different gene sequences, but they cannot be differentiated by serological techniques

---

HLA structure and peptide binding

- Class I molecules are composed of a three-domain α chain and the invariant β_2-microglobulin and they are expressed on the surface of almost all nucleated cells.
- Class II molecules comprise a pair (α and β) of two-domain chains, and their distribution in health is restricted to cells of the monocyte/macrophage lineage, dendritic cells, B lymphocytes and activated T lymphocytes.
- The binding groove for peptide antigen is formed by a cleft delineated by two flanking α-helices and by a floor of β-pleated sheets. The nature of the groove, and the peptide, differ subtly between class I and II molecules.
- Class I molecules present peptides from endogenous sources; this can include viral proteins if they are made within the cell presenting antigen.
- Class II molecules present exogenous peptides; plasma proteins, cell surface proteins and bacterial proteins.
- The T cell receptor makes contact with the lips of the groove and peptide antigen; only T cells bearing CD4 glycoproteins can bind to class II-presented peptides, while CD8 is required for interaction with those presented by class I.

CHAPTER 6

Cellular immune responses: macrophages, dendritic cells and B lymphocytes

The discussion of cell-mediated immune responses is complex when encountered for the first time. Description of the individual cell types and their functions in isolation is artificial. It is a bit like listening to an orchestra by hearing all of the different sections — woodwind, brass, strings, percussion — on their own one after another. None of it appears to harmonise or relate, and the common themes are lost. Bear in mind, then, that in this chapter and the next we are 'hearing' the monocytes, specialised antigen-presenting cells (APCs), B lymphocytes, T lymphocytes and natural killer cells on their own. In Chapter 8 we will be hearing the full symphony, as these cells combine to regulate one of the most vital but complex systems in mammalian physiology.

Some general principles may help your reading. Phylogenetically and ontogenetically (i.e. in terms of development of the species and development of the individual), macrophages, specialised APCs and natural killer cells are perhaps the most primordial cells, followed by the B, then the T lymphocyte. Macrophages and specialised APCs have none of the cognitive capacities (memory, specificity, amplification) of the acquired immune system on their own. These cells have, however, considerable phagocytic, metabolic and, in the case of macrophages, cytotoxic faculties. The B lymphocyte has specificity in the form of a surface receptor (immunoglobulin) capable of direct binding to antigens of any size in solution or in solid form. The T lymphocyte, in contrast, does not 'see' soluble antigen. As we have learned in our discussions of the function of the MHC system, T lymphocytes require simultaneous interaction with both MHC molecules and antigen. The T lymphocyte is, as it were, completely isolated from the real world of complex, macromolecular antigens. The gulf between the need of a T cell to respond to complex antigens and an inability to 'see' them unmodified is bridged by cells that present antigen (a feature of macrophages, other more specialised APCs, and B lymphocytes) in a way that is 'visible' to the T cell.

CYTOKINES

We have already briefly discussed cytokines, in Chapter 3, as the small, soluble peptides used extensively by the immune system to communicate and influence cellular function. The importance of their role is graphically illustrated by some of the rarest immune defects, which we will encounter later (see Ch. 19). In one of the syndromes described, the molecule responsible for activation of T lymphocytes, interleukin-2 (IL-2), is absent, resulting in a fatal immune deficiency disease. In another, one of the chains of a cytokine receptor is missing, and, again, a severe, fatal (if untreated) immune deficiency disorder follows.

The discussion of cytokines in teaching texts is difficult and frequently results in a sterile list of cells and functions. For this reason, and the fact that cytokines alone are nothing without the cells that release them and the cells that they affect, only a few general principles will be illustrated at this stage. Individual cytokines will be discussed as and when they are relevant. In Appendix 2, a list of cytokines and functions is provided for reference purposes. The important features of cytokines — **pleiotropy**, **autocrine function**, **paracrine function**, **endocrine effects** and **synergism** — are illustrated in Figure 6.1.

CYTOKINE RECEPTORS AND RELATED MOLECULES

Cytokines require specific cell surface receptors through which to mediate their range of actions on different cells. Frequently, the action of a cytokine on a cell will include the up-regulation of surface expression of its receptor, as well as enhanced release of the

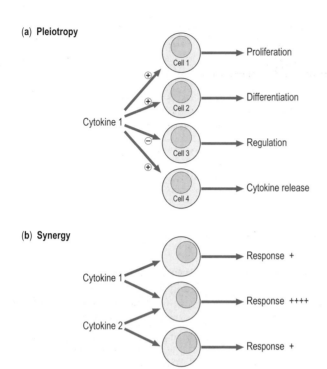

(a) **Pleiotropy**

(b) **Synergy**

(c) **Autocrine, paracrine and endocrine activities**

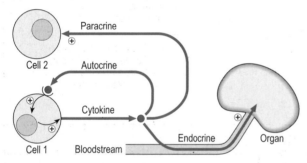

Fig. 6.1 **Important general properties of cytokines.**

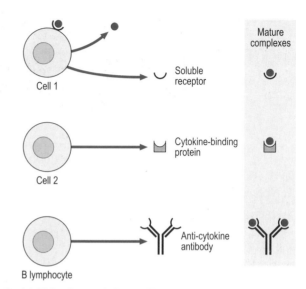

Fig. 6.2 **Molecules regulating cytokine functions.**

molecule itself. Receptors vary in their form, some being single and others multiple chain complexes. Receptors are also frequently found in soluble form in the circulation. The implication of this release of soluble receptors is not yet entirely clear, though the fact that levels tend to increase during inflammatory responses implies that the soluble receptors have a functional role. Some of the soluble receptors are able to bind and functionally inactivate their cytokine ligand, so that one possible function is in the regulation of cytokine effects. Other non-receptor molecules have been identified that bind cytokines and may regulate their responses. Some of these are recently discovered structures and are referred to as binding proteins; these typically have an inhibitory function. Other inhibitory molecules have been identified as antibodies (Fig. 6.2) that bind and inactivate cytokines.

MONONUCLEAR PHAGOCYTES

Cells of the monocyte/macrophage lineage are now frequently referred to as mononuclear phagocytes (MNPs). These cells have for many years been considered as sophisticated phagocytes, with several more complex and refined properties than neutrophils, but possibly no more than that. More recently, however, MNPs have been recognised as an integral part of the cell-mediated, acquired immune response. They form a bridge between the characteristics of cells of the innate immune response, such as neutrophils (i.e. phagocytosis, chemotaxis, killing of organisms), on the one side and, on the other, the requirements of T lymphocyte responses (the need for antigen to be processed and presented to T cells, along with co-signals to achieve activation).

The most important properties of MNPs are:

- antigen processing and presentation
- release of soluble factors (cytokines)
- function specialisation when fixed in the tissues
- cytotoxicity.

MORPHOLOGY, MATURATION AND DISTRIBUTION OF MNPs

Monocytes are the blood form; they are larger than lymphocytes but smaller than neutrophils. They have a large, ovoid nucleus and abundant, clear cytoplasm.

The tissue form of MNPs, known as macrophages or by one of the more specialised names, are distributed throughout the body and, considered as a whole, make up a physiologic system called the **mononuclear-phagocyte system** (MPS, often referred to in the past as the reticuloendothelial system). All MPS cells have common ancestry, morphology and function (Fig. 6.3).

Monocytes migrate in three ways: randomly, into sites of inflammation, or in a tissue-directed way to become specialised cells. Confirmation of the fact that specialised tissue-fixed MNPs (e.g. Kupffer cells in the liver) derive from the bone marrow via the circulation comes from patients after bone marrow transplants

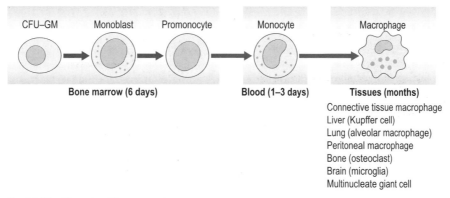

Fig. 6.3 The life cycle of the monocyte.
CFU-GM is a colony forming unit (i.e. stem cell pool) for granulocytes and monocytes.

whose Kupffer cells have the same sex karyotype as the *donor* (e.g. a male recipient of bone marrow from a female donor has 'male' XY karyotype in Kupffer cells). Tissue macrophages may undergo terminal differentiation into **multinucleated giant cells**, typically found at the site of chronic, cell-mediated inflammatory responses such as the **granulomata** characteristic of tuberculosis and other conditions.

Macrophages can be identified by monoclonal antibodies directed against cell-surface molecules. Markers that can be used to identify MNPs include:

- **CD14** (specific marker, function unknown)
- **CD35** complement receptor 1 (CR-1) for C3b
- **CD11b/CD18** leukocyte function-associated antigen 1 (LFA-1)
- **CD4** (but at a considerably lower surface concentration than on CD4$^+$ T cells)
- **CD64** Fc$_\gamma$RI
- **MHC class II** molecules.

Apart from CD14, all the above are expressed on other cell types.

MNP SECRETIONS

MNPs are factories engaged in the production of over 30 secreted products (Table 6.1).

Several cytokines are synthesised by MNPs and influence the function of these cells in antigen presentation and cytotoxicity. (See the boxes on IL-1, IFN and TNF.)

MNP ACTIVATION

Activation of MNPs results in a dramatic up-regulation of a majority of the functions of these cells, increased surface expression of CR1, CR3, the Fc$_\gamma$ receptors, MHC class II molecules and CD4, as well as an increase in the release of secreted products. In particular, increased cytotoxic activity against intracellular organisms (e.g. mycobacteria) and tumour cells is associated with MNP activation. Activated MNPs are bigger, have increased adherence, pseudopod formation and increased numbers of cytoplasmic pinocytotic vesicles.

Table 6.1 Secreted products of mononuclear phagocytes

Product	Function
Lysozyme	Cleaves bacterial cell walls
Collagenase	Enables cell mobility, inflammatory
Elastase	Enables cell mobility, inflammatory
Acid hydrolases	Enable cell mobility, bactericidal
Coagulation factors	Coagulation
Complement (C1, 2, 3, 5, B, D)	Inflammatory, microbicidal
Plasminogen activators	Inflammatory, microbicidal
Superoxides, H$_2$O$_2$	Microbicidal
Leukotrienes, prostaglandins	Inflammatory
Cytokines	
IL-1	T cell activator, inflammatory
IL-6	T cell activator, inflammatory
TNF-α; TNF-β	Cytotoxic, microbicidal
IFN-α; IFN-β	Antiviral, inflammatory

Interleukin 1

Interleukin 1 (IL-1) is a cytokine that is mainly produced by cells of the MPS system, typically in response to such stimuli as bacterial lipopolysaccharide. It is a major mediator of the inflammatory response. There are three related molecules in the IL-1 family: IL-1α and IL-1β (17 kDa), which share little homology but have similar functions and operate through the same receptors; and an IL-1 receptor antagonist protein (IL-1ra), which binds the receptors but has no biological activity. There are two distinct single chain receptors for IL-1 (types I and II), which have slightly differing affinities for the different ligands.

Secreted locally, IL-1 has pro-inflammatory effects: it promotes coagulation and increases endothelial expression of adhesion molecules. It also promotes release of IL-6, a cytokine with similar properties. Secreted systemically, IL-1 has endocrine effects, inducing fever and synthesis of proteins of the acute-phase response in the liver (see p. 19).

Functionally, activated MNPs have increased killing potential, antigen presentation, phagocytosis and secretory capacity. In vivo, the main MNP activators are **interferon-γ** (secreted by T cells), **granulocyte-monocyte colony-stimulating factor** (GM-CSF; see box: 'Colony-stimulating factors') (secreted by T cells) and **tumour necrosis factor-α** (see box: 'Tumour necrosis factor'), which being itself released by MNPs can act in a positive, autocrine feedback loop. MNPs are also activated and show enhanced adherence and chemotaxis in response to complement activation products that typically stimulate neutrophils (see p. 27).

The type I interferons: IFN-α and IFN-β

Interferons were first noticed as part of the innate immune system as natural antiviral agents. Overall, there are two types of interferon: I and II. The type I interferons have antiviral activity and are found in two distinct forms, α and β (the type II interferon, interferon-γ, is discussed later). IFN-α is derived from monocytes and IFN-β is derived from fibroblasts; both act through the type I IFN receptor. These 18 kDa cytokines can act on all cell types in the body in a paracrine protective effect to inhibit virus growth through inhibition of replication of viral RNA and DNA. In addition, these IFNs potentiate the activity of natural killer cells, as well as enhancing MHC class I molecule expression on a range of cell types. In the context of an intracellular infection (e.g. by a virus) increased expression of class I MHC molecules renders a cell more susceptible to killing by cytotoxic T cells (see p. 100). Class II MHC molecule expression is increased on macrophages, enhancing antigen presentation. All in all, these functions greatly enhance the ability of the host defence systems to eradicate viruses, and recombinant IFNs have been used with some considerable success in patients who are chronic carriers of viruses, such as the hepatitis viruses.

Colony-stimulating factors

Numerous cytokines have been identified whose most potent activity is the stimulation of growth and differentiation of bone marrow progenitor cells. Some of the colony-stimulating factors (CSFs) are restricted in their target cell, whilst others are quite broad in their range of actions. IL-3 (20 kDa), released by CD4+ T helper cells has effects on the growth of cells of most lineages and, in mice, is also particularly important in the differentiation of mast cells. IL-7 (25 kDa), released by bone marrow stromal cells, has effects on the development of B cells within the marrow.

Some of the most interesting molecules within this grouping are granulocyte-monocyte-CSF (GM-CSF, 22 kDa), granulocyte CSF (G-CSF, 19 kDa) and monocyte-macrophage CSF (M-CSF, 40 kDa). G-CSF and GM-CSF have already found their way into the clinic, being used extensively in patients whose white blood cells have been ablated temporarily as part of another treatment (e.g. antileukaemic cytotoxic chemotherapy). GM-CSF is made by CD4+ T cells, MPS cells and endothelium. It acts to promote growth of bone marrow cells already committed to the granulocyte and monocyte lineage; it may also activate mature forms of these cells. G-CSF is released by the same cell types as GM-CSF but acts preferentially on cells committed to the granulocyte phenotype. M-CSF is made by MPS and endothelial cells and is primarily produced within the bone marrow to promote MPS cell development.

Tumour necrosis factor

TNF (25 kDa) is a principal mediator in the host inflammatory response, to Gram-negative bacteria in particular, but it may also play a role in other aspects of immune pathology. As for IL-1, with which it shares many similarities, the main cell type secreting TNF is the MNP, and the main stimulus for release is the lipopolysaccharide (LPS) of bacterial cell walls. There are two structurally and functionally similar forms of TNF: α and β. TNFα is secreted by cells of the MPS and TNFβ by T lymphocytes (the β form is occasionally known as lymphotoxin). During an immune response, T cell release of interferon-γ augments TNF release. The name derives from early experimental work that demonstrated the existence of a soluble factor induced by LPS injection in vivo and capable of lysing a range of tumour cell types. T cells and natural killer cells, when activated, may also secrete TNF. TNF has two distinct receptors.

Local release of TNF causes up-regulation of adhesion molecules on vascular endothelium and on neutrophils to enhance cell migration; activation of neutrophils and macrophages to kill microbes; stimulation of cytokine release (IL-1, IL-6, TNF itself) by cells of the MPS; augmentation of expression of class I MHC molecules to enhance presentation of viral peptides in intracellular infections; and induction of expression of class II MHC molecules (this action requires the presence of other cytokines, such as interferon-γ). It can be seen that this range of activities is important in the immune response to bacteria and viruses.

Systemic release of TNF has the same fever-inducing and acute-phase response properties as IL-1. The long-term presence of TNF has an appetite-suppressing effect, giving rise to cachexia (severe weight loss). In addition, systemic TNF contributes to a clinical syndrome similar to shock: low blood pressure, reduced heart muscle contractility and intravascular thrombosis. These are features of the shock associated with Gram-negative bacterial sepsis, malarial and meningococcal infections, in all of which TNF is thought to have a major role.

FUNCTIONAL ACTIVITIES OF MNPS

MNPs are capable of many of the bactericidal activities of neutrophils and have comparable phagocytic, chemotactic, opsonic and cytotoxic activities. In addition, they appear to be particularly important in the ingestion and killing of **intracellular parasites**, such as *Mycobacterium tuberculosis*, hence their involvement in granulomata.

More recently, however, it has become apparent that MNPs have a critical role in activating T lymphocytes in specific immune responses through a process termed **antigen presentation**. This will be described below but the MNP, with its faculties of phagocytosis, class II MHC molecule expression and cytokine secretion, is ideally suited to this function.

During chronic immune responses, particularly related to indigestible materials (e.g. silicon, asbestos) or chronic infections (e.g. tuberculosis, leishmaniasis), MNPs differentiate into an end-stage form, the **multinucleated giant cell**. The function of this stage in the life cycle is not clear. Phagocytosis, killing and cytokine secretion appear to be comparable in these multinucleate cells to that in single-nucleus MNPs. It is possible that they represent a mechanism whereby activated MNP involvement in immune responses is maintained for long periods.

OTHER ANTIGEN-PRESENTING CELLS

There are various types of APC:

- mononuclear phagocytes
- dendritic cells
- B lymphocytes
- Langerhans cells of the skin.

DENDRITIC CELLS

Along with cells of the MPS and B lymphocytes (see below), dendritic cells have a major role as antigen-presenting cells. They are found mainly in the spleen and lymph nodes as well as being present in small numbers in the blood. They are derived from bone marrow and are named after their irregular shape, with numerous dendritic processes (Fig. 6.4). Dendritic cells are particularly important in the presentation of antigen to, and activation of, T cells that have not previously encountered antigen and have not previously been activated (so-called 'naive' or 'virgin' T cells). In other words, dendritic cells are the key cells in establishing the first-time response to an antigen by T lymphocytes (Fig. 6.5). Quite what it is about the dendritic cell that determines this potency is not clear. Dendritic cells permanently express high surface levels of class II MHC molecules (so-called 'constitutive expression'), which will augment antigen presentation. Difficulties in purifying large numbers of dendritic cells have

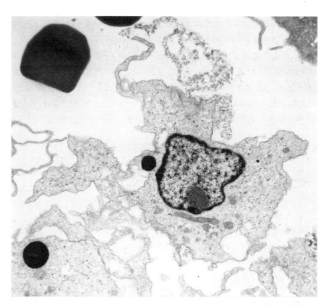

Fig. 6.4 **Dendritic cell.**
Electron micrograph of a mature human dendritic cell showing the distinctive thin cellular processes, × 7500. (Courtesy of Professor S. C. Knight.)

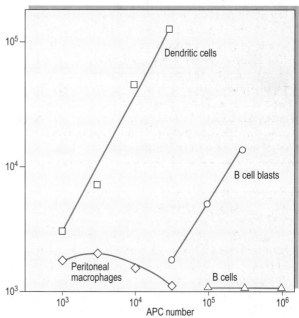

Fig. 6.5 **The ability of different APCs to activate unprimed (virgin) T cells.**
In this experiment the incubation consisted of 3 million virgin T cells, antigen and varying numbers of APCs; proliferation of T cells is measured by the incorporation of [³H] thymidine, see page 86. (With permission from Inaba and Steinman 1984 Journal of Experimental Medicine 160: 1717.)

hampered the study of their surface molecules. Apart from also possessing complement receptors, few other distinctive surface molecules have been defined so far. There are specialised forms of dendritic cells in the lymph nodes (**follicular dendritic cells**) and also in the skin, where the **Langerhans cells** have a morphology highly reminiscent of the dendritic cell.

Research into the functional aspects of antigen presentation by these important cells is hampered by the difficulty in identifying and purifying them, but this is an active area of research given the potential importance of elucidating the mechanism by which primary T cell responses are induced.

Cytokines, MNPs and dendritic cells

- Cytokines are small soluble peptides used by the immune system to communicate and to influence cellular function.
- Cells of the mononuclear–phagocyte system have an important role in innate immune defence, exploiting their characteristic properties of phagocytosis, killing and secretion.
- Equally important is the contribution of these cells to the acquired immune system in the process of antigen presentation to T cells.
- Much of the responsiveness and effector functions of these cells is mediated through the release of two key cytokines in the inflammatory response: IL-1 and TNF.
- Dendritic cells in the blood and lymph nodes, characterised by their distinctive morphology, have a key role in antigen presentation to, and activation of, 'virgin' T lymphocytes.

B LYMPHOCYTES

Source and site

In humans, B lymphocytes develop initially in the fetal liver and transfer to the bone marrow around the 12–16th week of fetal life. From then the marrow is the only site of B lymphocyte generation. B lymphocytes may undergo end-stage differentiation into **plasma cells**. These are non-circulating cells found predominantly in the bone marrow, lymph node medulla and gut and whose role is the production and secretion of antibody.

Apart from the circulation, B lymphocytes reside in lymph nodes, mucosa-associated lymphoid tissue (MALT) and the spleen. In these structures they are found in the middle of germinal centres in lymphoid follicles.

Identification of B lymphocytes

B lymphocytes are indistinguishable from T lymphocytes by light or electron microscopy. They are best identified by surface protein structures, the most obvious being **surface immunoglobulin** (sIg). B lymphocytes produce this special form of immunoglobulin which has a cytoplasmic tail and inserts into the cell membrane.

The surface molecules on B lymphocytes used in identification of these cells include:

- surface immunoglobulin (sIg): specific to B cells

- CD19, CD20, CD21 (the CR-2 complement receptor): specific to B cells
- class II MHC molecules
- CD40, CD23: markers of B cell activation.

B lymphocytes also constitutively express MHC class II molecules on their surface. This attribute endows them, like MNPs, with the ability to interact with T lymphocytes in the process termed antigen presentation.

Plasma cells are identified by their distinctive appearance (eccentric nucleus with a 'clock face') and by their cytoplasmic contents: immunoglobulin heavy and light chains. They do not have the antigen-presentation capacity of B cells.

B lymphocyte functions

B lymphocytes are a component of the **acquired** immune response, which has the two cardinal features of specificity and memory. The major roles of B lymphocytes are:

1. To ensure antibody production against appropriate target antigens, with the help of T cells
2. To present antigen to T lymphocytes and provide signals for T lymphocyte activation.

It is difficult to dissociate these two functions: a B cell presents antigen to a T cell and receives a positive signal for antibody production in return. This is the so-called **cognate interaction** between T and B lymphocytes, which will be dealt with in later sections (see p. 99).

B CELL DIFFERENTIATION AND ACTIVATION

Molecules involved in B cell functions

Several cell surface glycoprotein molecules are uniquely associated with B lymphocyte development and activation. Signalling through the antigen receptor, sIg, involves interaction of several transmembrane molecules, as is also the case for T cells. Molecules of major importance in B cell function form a long list: CD19, CD20, CD22, members of the B7 family (CD80, CD86), CD23, CD40 and CD81. CD23 is the low-affinity IgE receptor (Fc$_\varepsilon$RII), involved in the regulation of IgE production. One other B cell surface molecule, CD5, remains somewhat elusive in terms of ascribing a function to it. The other molecules listed are involved in B cell activation, a complex process discussed below (see p. 76).

B cell receptor complex (BCR). This is analogous to the T cell receptor complex, which comprises the TCR and CD3 molecules. The BCR is composed of (1) sIg as the antigen receptor, and (2) a signal transduction complex comprising the disulphide-bonded heterodimer Ig-α/Ig-β (or CD79a/CD79b). The BCR itself initiates activation signals after antigen binding, through recruitment of protein tyrosine kinases. Ig-α and Ig-β are products of the immunoglobulin supergene family and function through the activation of protein tyrosine kinases of the src family.

CD19, CD21 and CD81. These three B cell surface molecules associate to form a macromolecular complex. The complex is capable of transducing activation signals independent of the BCR. The signalling involves activation of a phosphoinositide (PI) 3-kinase. CD21 is the receptor (CR-2) for complement activation product C3d and provides a co-signal for B cell activation through this complex.

CD20. CD20 is a molecule present on the B cell surface, which is lost on differentiation to plasma cells. It is capable of signal transduction and acts through generation of a Ca^{2+} flux, which is important in the activation of B lymphocytes.

CD22. The function of CD22 is intimately related to that of the BCR. Alone, it is unable to mediate B cell activation, but if it is stimulated simultaneously with the BCR complex this leads to a much enhanced level of activation. CD22 may also function as an adhesion molecule: it has been demonstrated to enhance binding to other B cells and also interacts with the CD45R0 isoform on memory T cells; this is not a surprising finding given that $CD45R0^+$ T cells are potent in enhancing antibody production.

The B7 family. The B7 family of B lymphocyte surface molecules (B7-1, CD80; B7-2, CD86) are important as co-stimulators of T cells. B7 molecules are also found on other APCs. Co-stimulatory molecules provide an extra signal in addition to that provided by contact between antigen presented by the B cell and the T cell receptor. This co-stimulatory function is mediated through interaction with CD28 and a molecule termed CTLA-4 on the T lymphocyte surface. Co-stimulation is essential in the activation of T lymphocytes.

CD40. The interaction between CD40 on B lymphocytes and its ligand (called CD40 ligand, or CD40L) is critical in the development of a B cell response. Stimulation through CD40, accompanied by other signals such as cross-linking of the BCR, promotes B cell proliferation, immunoglobulin production and isotype switching. CD40L is found on activated T cells, and its participation in events within germinal centres of lymph nodes is critical to the generation of B lymphocyte responses.

CD5. CD5 is a marker present on the surface of a small subgroup (10%) of B cells in humans. No specific physiological function has been assigned to these cells with any degree of confidence. The $CD5^+$ B cell subset is well represented at birth, and since it has the capacity to produce copious amounts of poly-specific IgM antibodies (i.e. antibodies that have the capacity to bind with relatively low affinity, but to several different antigens), it may be important in early innate immune defences. Somewhat confusingly, CD5 is also present on most T lymphocytes, for which as yet there is no clear function.

B LYMPHOCYTE LIFE CYCLE

In humans, B cell development takes place in three phases: initially within the bone marrow; in other sites (e.g. lymph nodes, spleen) after export from the marrow; and then within the lymph node germinal centres as responder cells are selected. The nomenclature is carefully chosen to represent these phases:

- **pre-B cells** (bone marrow) do not have fully rearranged antigen receptors
- **immature B cells** (bone marrow) are not ready to respond to antigen
- **virgin B cells** (lymph node, spleen) have fully rearranged immunoglobulin genes but have not encountered antigen
- **mature B cells** (lymph node, spleen) possess antigen specificity in the lymph node
- **memory B cells**, which maintain memory of the encounter with antigen, are resident in the lymphoid system.

In the first phase of B cell development, progenitor cells (pro-B cells) migrate from the periosteal region to the centre of the bone marrow (Fig. 6.6), acquiring markers of maturation and differentiation and rearranging immunoglobulin genes. This process goes on throughout life, and in the adult rodent gives rise to some 2×10^7 cells per day. It is estimated that, during this transition, a single progenitor beginning the journey undergoes six mitotic cycles, giving rise to 64 progeny in 3–4 days. Maturation is supported by marrow stromal cells, with secretion of IL-7 a key signal (see the box on colony-stimulating factors). The first recognisable stage of B cell development (the pre-B cell) is the appearance of cytoplasmic heavy chains of the IgM class. Of the pre-B cells generated in this process, 75% are killed before they leave the marrow. The basis for this selection is not clear: both *positive* (i.e. active selection of a cell for its attributes) and *negative* (i.e. removal of a cell with undesirable attributes) selection processes are involved. The cellular and molecular events taking place during positive and negative selection are not known. One factor known to lead to negative selection is the generation of immunoglobulin gene rearrangements that do not lead to productive expression of heavy and light chains: these cells are deleted.

In the second phase of B cell development, virgin B cells leave the marrow to join the peripheral B cell pool. The blood phase may last as little as 1 hour, before the virgin B cells migrate mainly to the spleen, at this stage expressing surface IgM and IgD. Again, a minority of these virgin B cells survive, deletion occurring predominantly in the spleen. It is presumed that negative

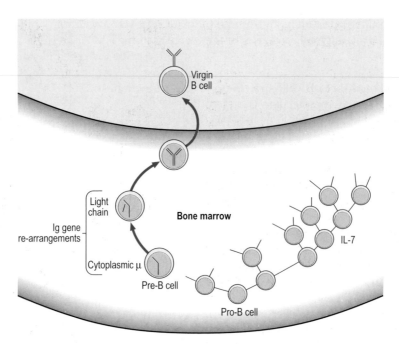

Fig. 6.6 **The first phase of B cell development.**
Pro-B cells are generated in the bone marrow and undergo several rapid rounds
of mitosis under the influence IL-7. They become recognisable as pre-B cells
once cytoplasmic μ chains appear following *VDJ* gene rearrangements. At the
point of export from the marrow into the stable peripheral B cell pool the
uniquely arranged immunoglobulin is expressed on the cell surface.

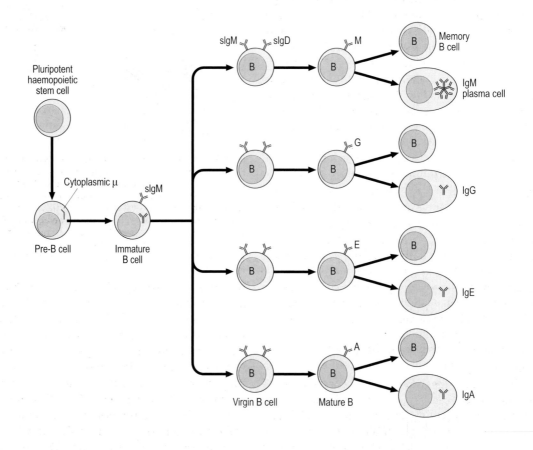

Fig. 6.7 **The life cycle of the B cell in relation to antigen.**
Note how much B cell development is antigen-independent.

selection of 'autoreactive' B cells (i.e. those with dangerous sIg capable of recognising self antigens) takes place in this period. For those B cells remaining in the pool, the length of their life span is a matter of weeks or months, bearing in mind that the pool is being replenished daily. While the majority of the peripheral B cell pool comprises virgin B cells, some members of the pool are memory cells, involved in the process of recirculation.

All of the B cell development described so far is antigen independent (Fig. 6.7). At this stage the B cell typically expresses sIg composed of μ and δ heavy chains. The B cell is ready to encounter specific antigen, and this usually takes place in the lymph node or spleen. Given the correct signals during this meeting, B cell proliferation and diversity generation take place. At this point, diversity generation is restricted to somatic hypermutation; there is no further rearrangement of genes contributing to the variable segments (see p. 46). Alternative heavy chain genes are now selected, in the process of class switching (see p. 45). A single B cell may select any one of the major classes or subclasses of Ig heavy chain. At this point, various different B cells will have been expanded in number in response to the specific antigen. The different clones recognise different parts (epitopes) of the antigen, or the same epitope. The optimum immune response will require selection of the B cells with the highest affinity for antigen. This selection will result naturally from competition for antigen. Those B cells best able to bind and internalise antigen will be able to present the antigen to T cells and receive in return the positive signal for expansion. This is the lymph node version of 'survival of the fittest' (Fig. 6.8) and results in the affinity maturation of antibody responses (see p. 46).

The pool of effector B cells (memory B cells and plasma cells) is constantly being replenished. Cells not receiving appropriate signals within the lymph node germinal centre are lost. Some of the B cells in the peripheral pool are recirculating memory cells, already committed to a specific immune response through a previous encounter with antigen. Memory B cells are more easily primed and can give a swift, specific, high-affinity, class-switched secondary response. If such a response is not needed over a long period (several years), these cells also may die.

Molecular and genetic events in B cell development

During development in the bone marrow, pre-B lymphocytes arise following immunoglobulin gene rearrangements in B lymphocyte precursors (D–J segments first, then a V–DJ recombination; see p. 45). Pre-B lymphocytes can be identified by the presence of cytoplasmic μ chains but no light chains are found. In the next phase, light chain V–J recombinations occur. These genetic recombinations give rise to a unique immunoglobulin gene sequence and, hence, a unique antibody structure. This provides the basis for the

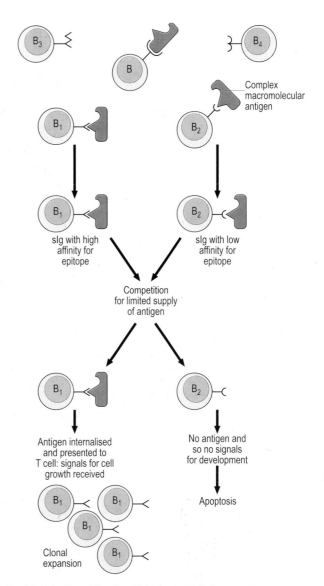

Fig. 6.8 **Selection of B cells with highest affinity for an antigen.**
A complex macromolecular antigen arriving in the lymph node causes expansion of a small number of B cell clones (oligoclonal expansion) Some (e.g. B_1 and B_2) bind the same epitope on the antigen, others (e.g. B_3 and B_4) do not bind antigen and die. In the presence of a limited supply of antigen, the highest affinity sIg (on B_1) is able to compete successfully against lower-affinity sIg (B_2) for its epitope. B_1 internalises antigen and presents it to a T cell, which provides the necessary growth signals for clonal expansion of B_1.

antibody specificity of a given B lymphocyte, which, interestingly, arises long before that cell ever encounters the antigen with which it is capable of binding. Only *one* antigen-binding specificity of immunoglobulin is produced per B lymphocyte, composed of the variable regions of light and heavy chains. The structure of these regions will be maintained without change for the rest of the life cycle of the B lymphocyte (apart from a degree of somatic recombination; see p. 45) while the constant region of the heavy chain, which determines the class (G, A, M, D or E) of antibody, will be changed. The immature B lymphocyte has sIg of the IgM class. This is accompanied by IgD expression, particularly in lymph node germinal centres. Surface IgD is important in the receipt and transduction of activation signals and signifies a virgin B lymphocyte

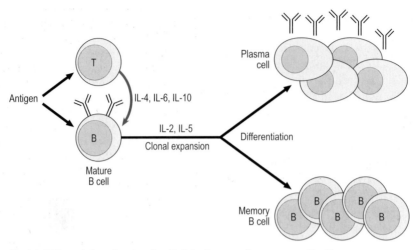

Fig. 6.9 **Differentiation of mature B cells into plasma cells or memory B cells.** See text for detail.

(i.e. one which has not encountered its specific antigen). Surface IgD is lost from the cell after antigenic stimulation. Once activated by encounter with specific antigen under the appropriate conditions during a primary immune response, the B lymphocyte matures. During the activation process, sIg expression is lost temporarily. Following this, when sIg expression returns, the B cell is restricted to display only one isotype of surface immunoglobulin (e.g. a particular G subclass, A subclass, M, D or E) (Fig. 6.7).

B lymphocytes at this stage have two main differentiation pathways. They can become memory B lymphocytes, ready for further rounds of activation and differentiation should the specific antigen be encountered again. Alternatively, they can end-differentiate into a mature plasma cell (Fig. 6.9). Plasma cells have lost all surface immunoglobulin but remain committed to production and *secretion* of a *single* antibody specificity with a *single* light and heavy chain type. Immunoglobulin production and secretion by plasma cells give rise to the IgG, IgA, IgM, IgE (and rarely IgD) found in the circulation and to the IgA secreted across the mucosa. If a plasma cell is committed to the production of neutralising antibody to a pathogen (e.g. poliovirus), immunity is retained in an ever-ready state for as long as that plasma cell continues to secrete antibody. Prolonged or repeated stimulation of antibody production (e.g. by immunisation boosters) will enhance the process of B cell differentiation, more plasma cells will appear, protective antibody levels will be maintained and immunity will be maintained and augmented.

B lymphocyte activation

The majority of B cell activation takes place in the lymph nodes. Primary follicles contain a network of follicular dendritic cells (FDCs), the spaces between the dendrites being filled with B cells (Fig. 6.10). Primary follicles are present in lymph nodes in early fetal life and are also found in animals reared in germ-free environments. This implies that the primary follicle is

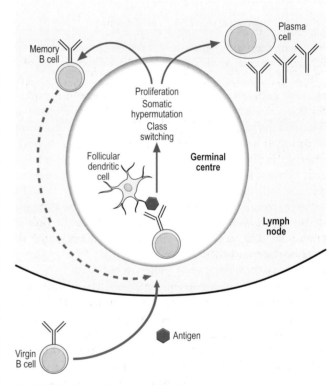

Fig. 6.10 **B cell activation in lymph nodes.**
Virgin B cells from the stable peripheral pool enter lymph node germinal centres. Here, antigen is presented on the processes of follicular dendritic cells. B cells holding sIg recognising the antigen are stimulated into mitosis, during which sIg is lost and there is somatic hypermutation and class switching. B cells with the highest affinity for antigen after this phase are selected as memory B cells or plasma cells, as required. Memory B cells may join the stable peripheral B cell pool.

an architectural site, supplying the cells and structure required for lymphocyte activation in response to antigen. The generation of secondary follicles, which contain activated B cells, is, therefore, clearly dependent on antigenic stimulation. Few secondary follicles are found in congenitally athymic mice, indicating that they are also largely T cell dependent. Secondary follicles consist of a mantle, or corona, of packed resting

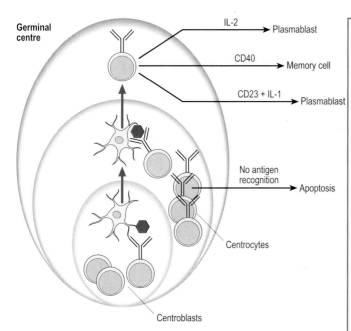

Fig. 6.11 **B cell development within the germinal centre.**
B cells recognising specific antigen are stimulated into an oligoclonal expansion (centroblast stage). These expanded cells migrate further into the germinal centre. There are several possible outcomes of the centrocyte stage. If affinity for antigen is lost after somatic hypermutation, there is no positive signalling and the cells cannot be rescued from apoptosis. Centrocytes remaining highly specific for the antigen may be influenced in three different ways. Interaction with T lymphocytes expressing CD40L stimulates CD40-expressing centrocytes to become memory cells. Either IL-2 or a combination of CD23 and IL-1 influence centrocytes towards the plasmablast and then plasma cell stage.

small B cells (sIgM$^+$ and sIgD$^+$) of the peripheral pool. In the centre of a secondary follicle is the germinal centre, a collection of activated B (mainly) and T lymphocytes and macrophages. Here the B cell activation and maturation process takes place.

The FDCs take up antigen in the form of immune complexes (i.e. antigen–antibody–complement). FDCs have the capacity to preserve and present this antigen to B and T lymphocytes, through mechanisms which are not yet clear. B cells with sIg complementary to the antigen undergo proliferation, and the germinal centre begins to develop. These blasts, termed centroblasts, lose sIg and are typically localised at one pole of the follicle (Fig. 6.11). Centroblasts begin to generate progeny (termed centrocytes) that now express sIg and migrate towards the outer zone of the follicle. During the generation of centroblasts and centrocytes, it has been assumed that somatic hypermutation (see p. 45) takes place. This would coincide with the period during which sIg expression is temporarily lost. However, confirmatory evidence of when hypermutation takes place is lacking. Similarly, it is assumed that class switching, with selection of heavy chains, takes place at this stage. Cell death is a major feature of the generation of centroblasts and centrocytes. Therefore, it seems likely that unless positive centrocyte and centroblast selection take place apoptosis follows (see box: 'Apoptosis: the role of cell death in lymphocyte development').

Apoptosis: the role of cell death in lymphocyte development

As we have seen, cell death is a frequent accompaniment to the process of activation and selection. The term apoptosis has been applied to this process, and it is now clear that at the sites of lymphocyte development (bone marrow and lymph node for B cells, thymus for T cells) apoptosis is an important phenomenon. A considerable body of knowledge about the process of apoptosis has been built up recently. Central to this is a protein termed bcl-2, of molecular mass 26 kDa and found predominantly in the mitochondria and cytoplasm. Whilst the precise function of bcl-2 is not known, it has become clear that B and T lymphocytes undergoing apoptosis have low intracellular bcl-2 levels. Manipulations that increase bcl-2 expression (e.g. transfection of the *bcl-2* gene into the cell) save cells destined for apoptosis. Equally, other manipulations that save cells (e.g. for B cells the signals from T cells or addition of anti-CD40 monoclonal antibody; for T cells the addition of IL-2) also have the associated effect of enhancing intracellular bcl-2 levels.

The importance of apoptosis can be illustrated by recent work on an animal strain, the *lpr* (for lymphoproliferative) mouse. This mouse lacks a key molecule in the process of apoptosis. This molecule, termed Fas (CD95), is present on the surface membrane of many cells, including T lymphocytes. Positive signals received through Fas instruct the cells to die. In the absence of Fas in the *lpr* mice, the instruction for apoptosis is not given. These mice develop a syndrome characterised by massive proliferation of lymphocytes and swelling of lymph nodes, and this is frequently associated with additional complications, such as autoimmune disease. This model serves to underline the important homeostatic role of apoptosis in the immune system. Interestingly, two children were described recently who had a similar syndrome and defective Fas-mediated killing of their lymphocytes.

What then saves germinal centrocytes from apoptosis? First, it appears that they must be capable of successful binding to the antigen currently being expressed in that germinal centre. If this is the case, there are three separate pathways of maturation. First, stimulation of centrocytes through the cell surface molecule CD40 leads to the generation of memory B cells. The ligand for CD40 is a glycoprotein of molecular mass 39 kDa (gp39) expressed on the surface of CD4$^+$ T lymphocytes and known at present as CD40 ligand (CD40L) (see box: 'X-linked hyper IgM syndrome — the importance of CD40–CD40L'). CD40L is expressed on T cells almost exclusively, and its expression is tightly controlled, being inducible by T cell activation within 2–8 hours but being lost again from the surface after 24 hours. The second manoeuvre that saves centrocytes from apoptosis is exposure to soluble CD23 (a surface protein found on B cells and FDCs)

X-linked hyper IgM syndrome: the importance of CD40–CD40L

The identification of the CD40–CD40L interaction in rescuing antigen-specific B cells from apoptosis has elucidated the pathogenesis of a disease characterised by deficiency of antibody production. This immune deficiency is termed X-linked hyper IgM syndrome, since it is found only in males, who typically have high levels of IgM antibodies but no mature B lymphocytes producing the other immunoglobulin classes. The IgM produced tends to be ineffective in protection against bacterial infections, and boys affected with the disease are at risk of serious infections unless treated. It was known for some years that the B cells themselves are not particularly abnormal and could be stimulated effectively using T cells from unaffected donors. It has been recently demonstrated that the genetic basis for this syndrome is the presence of mutations in the *CD40L* gene, which is present on the X-chromosome. In the absence of a CD40L–CD40 interaction, some developing B cells are not rescued from apoptosis, whilst some remain viable but do not receive the correct maturation signals. These latter B cells may escape cell death, but in the absence of T cell help remain only as producers of IgM, hence the high levels of this antibody class seen in this condition.

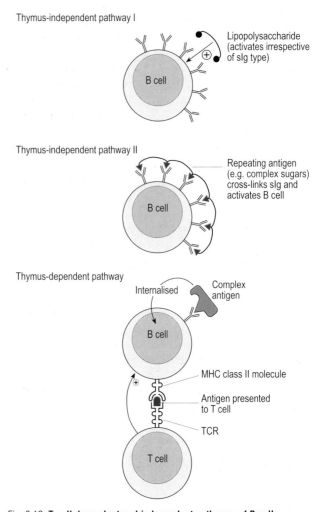

Fig. 6.12 **T cell dependent and independent pathways of B cell activation**.

and IL-1α, inducing differentiation into plasmablasts (i.e. pre-plasma cells). This is followed by migration into the lymph node medullary cords and then out to the gut lamina propria, bone marrow and spleen, which are the main resident sites for plasma cells, the end-stage differentiated B cell. A third mechanism of rescue from apoptosis can be provided by IL-2, which also induces the production of plasmablasts.

THE ROLE OF T CELLS IN B CELL DEVELOPMENT

There are three mechanisms by which immature B lymphocytes may become activated to differentiate. These are termed the thymus-independent pathways I and II and the thymus-dependent pathway (Fig. 6.12). The term 'thymus dependent/independent' denotes whether T lymphocyte help is required or not. This should remind you of the classic experiment described on page 3, when the thymus was removed from birds. They lost the ability for T cell responses and, surprisingly, also to some extent for B lymphocyte responses, indicating the dependence of B cells on the T lymphocyte. The three pathways of B lymphocyte activation are all demonstrable in vitro. It is likely that the dominant pathway in vivo is the thymus-dependent pathway, but that B lymphocytes may also become activated through the thymus-independent pathways.

The thymus-independent pathway I results in activation of *all* B lymphocytes (so-called **polyclonal**

activation) directly. This activation is typical of the action of certain bacterial products, such as lipopolysaccharides. Activation here is not related to the antigen specificity of the B cells and quite to whose benefit the activation is, host or pathogen, is unclear. The type II pathway involves repeating linear antigens, which cross-link several *antigen-specific* surface Ig molecules simultaneously, thus providing a sufficiently strong activation stimulus that T lymphocyte help is not required. T-independent pathways generally give IgM responses and little memory generation.

The thymus-dependent pathway is clearly the most important in that it generates high-affinity, class-switched, specific antibodies. It is this process that has been described in the previous sections: B lymphocytes use their sIg as a receptor for antigen, which is internalised. In the vacuole formed (an **endosome**) enzymes degrade the antigen, and a small peptide fragment of the whole antigen becomes attached to a class II MHC molecule and is exported to the surface (the B lymphocyte acting as an APC). T lymphocytes with a TCR complementary to that of the B lymphocyte (i.e. recognising part of the same antigen) are recruited and activated (the B lymphocyte acting as T lymphocyte activator) and in turn activate the B lymphocyte. This elaborate system ensures that (1) only B lymphocytes and T lymphocytes specific for that antigen are given the activation signal and (2) only antigens against which the immune system is fully committed (i.e. have both T and B lymphocyte recognition for) invoke an immune response. The latter is a protection against developing anti-self reactions. Do not forget that B lymphocytes are designed to produce millions of different specificities, some of which may cross-react with self. This potentially dangerous complication is the price paid for diversity.

Signals in B lymphocyte activation

Several T lymphocyte-derived interleukins are important in B lymphocyte activation, growth, clonal expansion and class (isotype) switching. **IL-4** is the main B lymphocyte activator (Fig. 6.9). It also stimulates B lymphocyte growth. **IL-5** and, to some degree, **IL-2** promote clonal expansion. **IL-6** is a B lymphocyte growth factor that also enhances the switch to IgG production. What influences production of different Ig isotypes is not fully characterised. Control by cytokines undoubtedly exists, but also environmental factors have a role (e.g. IgA production by mucosal B lymphocytes).

SEQUELAE OF B LYMPHOCYTE ACTIVATION

The important results of B lymphocyte activation are **clonal expansion** with the generation of memory B lymphocytes and plasma cells. When a B lymphocyte is activated by antigen, the first response is IgM production, beginning after 5–10 days, followed 2–3 days later by the appearance of IgG in the serum. This constitutes the primary response. When there is a rechallenge with the same antigen, memory cells are already primed and present. Activation of primed cells is quicker and leads to the secondary response. This has several different characteristics: it is quicker (3–5 days), IgG is produced early and it is produced in much greater quantities (see p. 41).

In vitro mechanisms of B cell activation

It is frequently useful to assess B cell function by in vitro studies. Agents that are capable of activating B cells in vitro typically do so by activating all cells through a common pathway. Activation in this polyclonal fashion is termed **mitogenesis**, since the agents inevitably induce mitosis. There is a B cell mitogen called **pokeweed mitogen** (PWM) and B cells may also be activated by antibodies to sIg, which act by mimicking antigen–sIg interaction.

Physiological importance of B lymphocyte responses

The role of B lymphocytes in host protection is exemplified by a rare genetic disease, X-linked agamma-globulinaemia. Children born with the syndrome have no circulating B lymphocytes, although pre-B lymphocytes can be identified in the bone marrow. No B lymphocytes means no antibodies, and patients suffer from repeated life-threatening infections.

In medical practice, we have found ways of manipulating B lymphocytes, especially in **vaccination/ immunisation**. In these processes, a harmless, inactivated form of a pathogen is used to stimulate the primary antibody response, so that when the real pathogen is met, there is pre-existing immunity and the secondary response can be invoked to boost the level of immunity very quickly.

Class and subclass switching, and the production of IgE

Class switching involves the selection during B cell development of different immunoglobulin C_H genes. To what extent this takes place as a spontaneous event and to what extent it is driven remains a moot point in immunological circles. Certain facts relating to the results of in vitro culture studies are pertinent. In particular, the control of IgE production has been quite well studied, for the obvious reason that it may be relevant to the development of allergy (see Ch. 10). For example, co-culture of B cells with a polyclonal activator alone typically results in IgM production in the culture fluid. Addition of IL-4 induces switching to IgE production. In contrast, addition of IFN-γ induces production of IgG class antibodies, and no IgE (Fig. 6.13).

The other factors that clearly must have an effect on class switching are the nature of the antigen, since some antibody responses are skewed to certain isotypes (see Table 4.2), as well as the site of production, since antibodies produced in mucosally associated lymphoid tissue tend to be of the IgA class. It seems likely that the T cells at these sites have an influence: B lymphocytes from other sites co-cultured with mucosally derived T cells can be switched to IgA production.

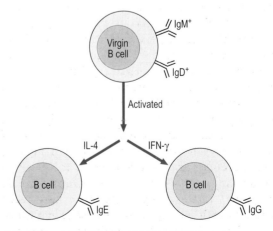

Fig. 6.13 **The control of IgE production by cytokines.** See text for details.

B lymphocytes

- B lymphocytes mature from bone marrow precursors and express surface immunoglobulin molecules unique to each cell.
- B cells are selected for expansion and differentiation by T cells, with the generation of plasma cells to produce circulating protective antibodies, and memory B cells.
- A complex interaction of T and B cells, with the important influence of cytokines, takes place in lymph nodes to achieve B cell activation.
- In this unique position of presenting internalised antigens to T cells, the B cell is also an important source of antigen-presenting function, with consequent T cell activation.

Table 6.2 **The β1 integrins (very late activation molecules)**

Chain composition	Conventional name	CD nomenclature
$\alpha_1\beta_1$	VLA-1	CD49a/CD29
$\alpha_2\beta_1$	VLA-2	CD49b/CD29
$\alpha_3\beta_1$	VLA-3	CD49c/CD29
$\alpha_4\beta_1$	VLA-4	CD49d/CD29
$\alpha_5\beta_1$	VLA-5	CD49e/CD29
$\alpha_6\beta_1$	VLA-6	CD49f/CD29

ADHESION MOLECULES IN LYMPHOCYTE FUNCTIONS

The integrins and selectins are important in T and B cell functions and serve the same purpose as they do for granulocytes, namely directed adherence to endothelium and migration into the tissues (the molecular basis for these has already been discussed). LFA-1 (one of the β_2 integrins) is expressed on virtually all mature resting and activated peripheral T and B cells. LFA-1 is particularly important in migration of lymphocytes into the tissues. In addition, the ligand for LFA-1, ICAM-1, is frequently expressed on other immune cells, as well as on the endothelium. Therefore, when lymphocytes make contact with other lymphocytes or APCs, LFA-1/ICAM-1 adhesion can enhance the interaction and the passage of cell–cell signals. This is illustrated by the fact that anti-LFA-1 monoclonal antibodies can block a range of lymphocyte functions, including antigen presentation to T cells and killing of target cells, as well as adherence to endothelium. L-selectin is also expressed on the majority of T and B lymphocytes.

Another group of integrins are termed the β_1 integrins, and these share expression of a common β chain, CD29. The β_1 integrins are also called the **very late activation** (VLA) molecules. The nomenclature of the VLA molecules is shown in Table 6.2. Three of these, VLA-4, VLA-5 and VLA-6, are particularly strongly expressed by resting T cells and are highly up-regulated on activation. VLA-4 mediates binding of lymphocytes to endothelium at sites of inflammation, where its ligand, VCAM-1, is typically up-regulated.

It seems likely that interactions between the integrins and their ligands provides some accessory signalling for T cell activation.

CD2 is a protein involved in adhesion between lymphoid cells, particularly T cells and natural killer cells. Its principal ligand is LFA-3, expressed on a wide range of haematopoietic cells. Again, although principally involved in cell–cell adhesion, CD2/LFA-3 interaction provides accessory signals for T cell activation.

CHAPTER 7

Cellular immune responses: T lymphocytes, antigen presentation and natural killers

Table 7.1 **Identification of T cells and their subsets**

T cell population	Marker	Typical percentages in blood
T cells	T cell receptor CD3	100% of T cells (70% of lymphocytes)
T helper cells	CD4	66% of T cells
T cytotoxic/suppressor cells	CD8	33% of T cells
Activated T cells	IL-2 receptor Transferrin receptor HLA class II molecules	2–10% of T cells

T LYMPHOCYTES

T LYMPHOCYTE SOURCE AND SUBSETS

Key studies in the 1950s indicated that lymphocytes were the cells responsible for two measurable immune responses: antibody production and graft rejection. Surgical removal of the thymus effectively abolished the ability of a host to reject a tissue graft, and the lymphocytes assumed to derive from the thymus were named T lymphocytes. There is little doubt that these cells have the pivotal role in cellular immune responses. Understanding the complexities of their function is vital for a clear understanding of their role in protective immunity and in disease, whether it be a T cell deficiency disease, or a disease characterised by the immune system attacking self components (autoimmune disease).

Identification of T lymphocytes

The T cell is defined by the presence of its receptor for antigen (T cell receptor, TCR). The genetic basis for this (rearrangement of genes coding for variable and constant chains of the molecule) has been described already (Ch. 4). In concert with expression of the TCR is the constitutive presence of a complex of molecules termed CD3, involved in transduction of antigen-specific activation signals through the TCR.

Subsets of T cells are a key part of the physiology of the cell-mediated immune system. Some two-thirds of T cells express a surface glycoprotein CD4 (CD4+ T

cells), and since these cells were identified many years ago as capable of promoting immune responses such as antibody production, they are termed **T helper** cells. The remaining third of T cells do not express CD4, but express a related glycoprotein, CD8. T cells expressing CD8 (usually called CD8+ T-cells) are associated with functions such as the ability to down-regulate immune responses and kill target cells, hence the term **T suppressor/cytotoxic** cells (Table 7.1).

T cell activation is an important part of any cellular immune response and is much studied. Several cell surface molecules not typically expressed on resting cells are induced following activation by antigen or an artificial stimulus. These include the receptor for interleukin-2 (IL-2R) (see box: 'Interleukin-2'), the transferrin receptor and HLA class II molecules.

T LYMPHOCYTE FUNCTIONS

As the pivotal cell in immune responses, one would expect the T cell to influence most aspects of immunity, and this is not far short of the truth. Much of the functional 'outreach' is done through the secretion of cytokines, although direct cell–cell interaction with B cells is also important in the maturation of antibody responses. Major functions of T cells are as follows:

- Signalling for B cell expansion, inducing them to produce antibody and mature into plasma cells or memory cells.
- Recruitment and activation of cells of the mononuclear phagocyte lineage.
- Recruitment and activation of specialised cytotoxic T cells in antiviral responses.
- Secretion of cytokines responsible for growth and differentiation of a range of cell types, including other T cells, macrophages and eosinophils.
- Regulation of immune reactions.

Interleukin-2

IL-2, originally known as T cell growth factor, is the major cytokine responsible for T lymphocyte activation and proliferation. Its importance in T cell physiology cannot be stressed enough. A major feature of this 15 kDa polypeptide is the auto-crine loop through which it operates: receipt of an appropriate activation signal by a T cell results in massive up-regulation of production of both the cytokine and its receptors, so that IL-2 can feed back activating signals though its receptor. Similarly, local release of IL-2 can lead to activation of nearby T cells in a paracrine fashion. IL-2 also has important growth-promoting functions in relation to B lymphocyte development.

The receptor for IL-2 has three chains: α, β and γ. The minimal receptor configuration for signal transduction is the IL-2Rβγ heterodimer, which binds its ligand with an intermediate affinity (K_d 10^{-9} M), whilst the combination of α, β and γ chains results in high-affinity (K_d 10^{-11} M) binding. The γ chain also appears to be critical for internalisation of the receptor–ligand complex. The α chain alone (also known as CD25) binds IL-2 with a relatively low affinity (K_d 10^{-8} M) and lacks the ability to transduce an activation signal. However, IL-2α chains have a slow turnover rate on the cell surface (> 6 hours compared with 15 minutes

for the IL-2Rαβ heterodimer bound to IL-2) and thus act as a 'trap' for IL-2, which can then be passed to intermediate- or high-affinity receptors, by lateral diffusion, for internalisation (Fig. 7.1). Such a process enhances the overall affinity of a cell for IL-2, increasing the sensitivity of IL-2-mediated activation.

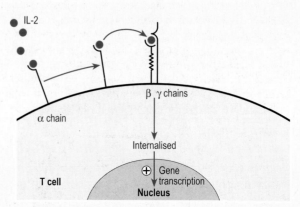

Fig. 7.1 IL-2 receptors.
The T cell growth factor, IL-2, binds the IL-2 receptor α chain which acts as a trap. Transfer of IL-2 to the βγ dimer of the receptor allows internalisation, leading to cell proliferation.

It can be seen from this list that few cells in the immune system remain untouched by the influence of T cells.

Molecules involved in T lymphocyte function

In addition to the TCR, which interacts with specific antigen, there are numerous cell surface molecules critically involved in T lymphocyte functions. Some of the molecules (e.g. the CD3 complex) are an absolute requirement for T cell function. Others have a role in stabilising cell–cell interactions; and yet others provide important additional activation signals; frequently these so-called **accessory molecules** provide adhesion between communicating cells *plus* a signal for T cell activation. As stated earlier, some accessory molecules (e.g. CD4, CD8) are permanently expressed and denote a **functional subset** of T lymphocytes. Other accessory molecules (e.g. CD28, see p. 94) only appear when T cells become activated, and yet others change as the T cell differentiates (e.g. isoforms of the CD45 molecule, p. 95).

In clinical laboratory practice, monoclonal antibodies able to identify the different T cell-associated molecules can be used to subdivide the total T cell population into what are broadly termed **T cell subsets** (see the box). This is of importance in the diagnosis and management of a range of inflammatory diseases, most notably infection with the human immunodeficiency virus (HIV). In this disorder, CD4-expressing T cells are selectively depleted (see p. 279), at a rate which correlates with the progression of the

disease. Measuring numbers of CD4+ T cells is, therefore, a useful tool in managing patients.

The CD3 complex: signal transducer for the T cell receptor

Analogous to the B cell receptor complex, a group of molecules (collectively termed the CD3 complex) have been identified that are closely associated with the T cell receptor. The association is both physical in terms of occupying adjacent locations on the cell membrane and also distributional: cells expressing the TCR also express the CD3 complex. Monoclonal antibodies to CD3 can be used to identify T cells, and CD3 is termed a 'pan-T cell marker'. The major function of the CD3 complex is the transduction of signals coming from the TCR, to initiate cell activation.

The CD3 complex is composed of five different transmembrane protein chains, denoted by Greek letters: γ (25–28 kDa), δ (20 kDa), ε (25 kDa), ζ (zeta, 16 kDa) and η (eta, 22 kDa). One ε chain associates non-covalently with a δ chain and this complex lies adjacent to the α chain of the TCR. An ε–γ complex associates with the β chain, and nearby lies a disulphide-linked ζ–ζ homodimer (90% of T cells) or ζ–η heterodimer (10%) (Fig. 7.3).

CD4 and CD8, accessory molecules in T cell function

CD4 and CD8 are the major accessory molecules in T cell function. CD4 is typically present on about

Identification and counting of immune cells by flow cytofluorimetry

It is often of importance in research and clinical practice to be able to identify and count cell subsets, for example in the peripheral blood. Identification exploits three items: a lineage- or differentiation-specific cell surface molecule (e.g. CD20 for B cells); a monoclonal antibody specific for the molecule; and fluorochromes that fluoresce at a particular wavelength when exposed to an excitatory light source. Fluorochromes typically used are fluorescein, phycoerythrin and Texas red, which fluoresce green, orange and red, respectively, when exposed to an ultraviolet light source. The cell suspension is incubated with a monoclonal antibody conjugated to the fluorochrome of choice. The labelled cells then need to be viewed and counted. Traditionally this has been done by microscopy. Now it is almost entirely done by flow cytofluorimetry, a technique for the study of cells and fluorescence molecules in flow.

The basic skeleton of a flow cytofluorimeter is shown in Figure 7.2. Cells are identified first by the way they scatter light in a forward direction (dependent upon cell size) and at 90° (dependent upon cytoplasmic granularity). The question can then be asked as to whether the cell is also bound by the monoclonal antibody used. Up to four different fluorochromes can be used simultaneously, so that it is possible to ask a lymphocyte are you a T cell (using monoclonal anti-CD3 antibody)? are you a helper cell (anti-CD4)? are you activated (anti-IL-2R)? which TCR are you expressing (anti-αβ)?

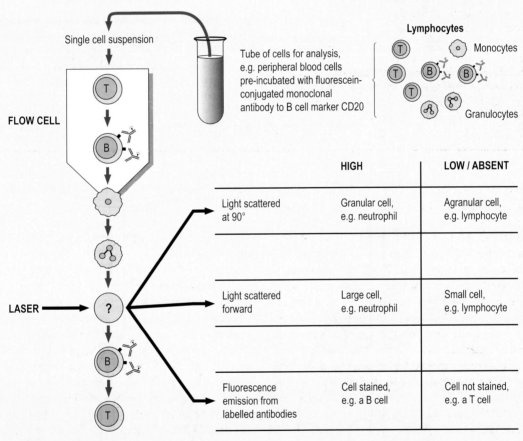

		HIGH	LOW / ABSENT
Light scattered at 90°		Granular cell, e.g. neutrophil	Agranular cell, e.g. lymphocyte
Light scattered forward		Large cell, e.g. neutrophil	Small cell, e.g. lymphocyte
Fluorescence emission from labelled antibodies		Cell stained, e.g. a B cell	Cell not stained, e.g. a T cell

Fig. 7.2 **Flow cytometry.**
The detection of different cellular subsets on the basis of physical characteristics (size, granularity) and binding of fluorochrome-tagged monoclonal antibodies.

two-thirds of mature peripheral blood and lymphoid T cells, and CD8 on the remaining one third.

CD4 is a transmembrane glycoprotein of 55 kDa expressed as a monomer and a member of the immunoglobulin supergene family. As such it has four immunoglobulin-like domains (Fig. 7.4). CD4 is one of the molecules alluded to above that has a dual role in T cell activation: it provides some adhesive forces between interacting cells, and it provides an accessory activation signal (Fig. 7.5). CD4 has specific affinity for the class II MHC molecule. It stabilises the interaction between the T cell and cells presenting antigen through the class II MHC molecule. Without CD4, the TCR–peptide antigen–MHC molecule association, which is of relatively low affinity, is unlikely to be sufficiently secure for T cell activation to take place. The two most external domains of CD4 bind to the β2 domain of the class II MHC molecule.

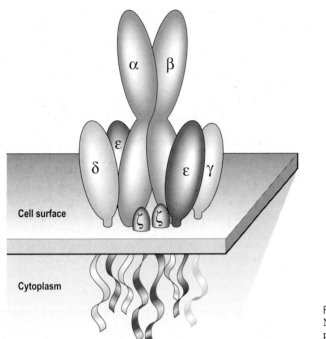

Fig. 7.3 **Schematic representation of the αβ TCR and CD3.**
CD3 chains transduce activation signals emanating from the TCR interaction with presented antigen.

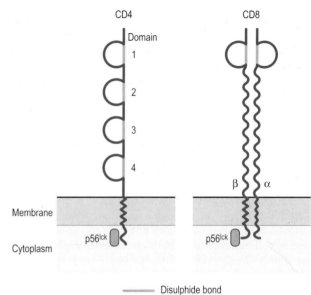

Fig. 7.4 **Schematic representation of CD4 and CD8 accessory molecules.**
Note immunoglobulin-like domain structure and the associated protein tyrosine kinase, p56lck.

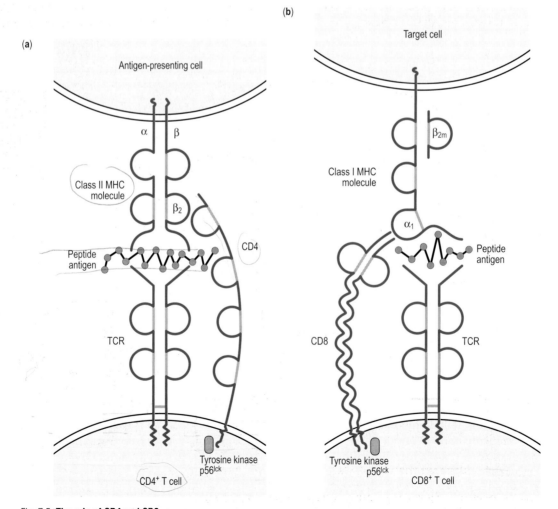

Fig. 7.5 **The role of CD4 and CD8.**
(**a**) Schematic representation of the interaction between TCR and antigenic peptide presented by class II MHC molecules. CD4 stabilises this configuration by binding the class II MHC molecule. (**b**) CD8 has a similar role, but in the interaction with antigen presented by a class I MHC molecule.

That an additional cell activation signal is provided by CD4 is suggested by several facts. First, some anti-CD4 monoclonal antibodies can actually stimulate T cells to become activated and proliferate. Second, a lymphocyte-specific protein tyrosine kinase, called Lck (or p56^{lck}) is physically associated with the cytoplasmic tail of CD4. When T cells become activated, phosphorylation of serine residues in the cytoplasmic tail is an early event. The fact that more than one CD4 molecule may be physically enveloped around a dimeric TCR (see p. 63) is likely to enhance the contribution of p56^{lck} to early events of T cell activation (see p. 97).

Two other important facts about CD4 will become apparent: it has a critical role in thymic development of T cells, and it is the cellular receptor for HIV (see p. 282).

T lymphocyte characteristics

- T lymphocytes arise in the thymus and carry an antigen-specific receptor, the TCR.
- Other key surface molecules acquired in the thymus are CD3 (signal transduction) and accessory molecules (e.g. CD4, CD8).
- CD4 occurs on the surface of two-thirds of T cells; it interacts with class II MHC molecules on cells presenting antigen and increases the affinity of binding. CD4^{+} T cells are termed T helper (T$_{H}$) cells.
- CD8 interacts with class I MHC molecules on cells, stabilising T cell interactions with cells presenting antigen. CD8^{+} T suppressor/cytotoxic (Ts, Tc) cells can down-regulate immune functions and kill target cells.

Separation and testing of lymphocytes for proliferative responses

To examine whether an individual has a T cell response to an antigen, it is conventional to carry out a proliferation assay (Fig. 7.6). First, the lymphocytes must be separated from the whole blood. This is done by exploiting the difference in density between lymphocytes and monocytes, on the one hand, and erythrocytes and granulocytes, on the other. Blood is layered onto a solution of fixed density and then centrifuged. Under these conditions, the denser cells pellet at the bottom of the tube, and the lighter lymphocytes and monocytes remain above the density medium. Selected populations can then be purified using monoclonal

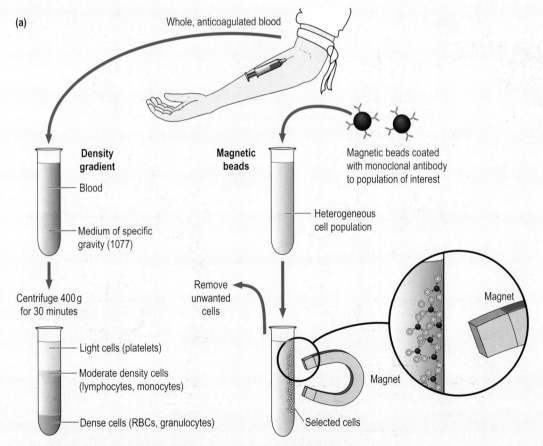

Fig. 7.6 **Purification of leukocyte populations and measuring T cell proliferation.**
(**a**) Separation of blood leukocytes using a density gradient. Purification may also be achieved using specific monoclonal antibodies tagged to magnetic beads.

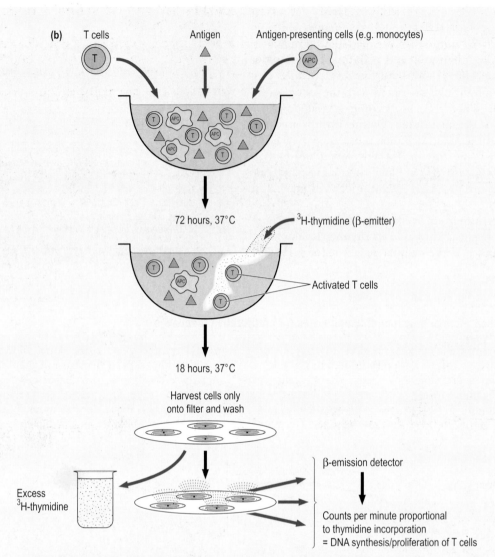

Fig. 7.6 **Purification of leukocyte populations and measuring T cell proliferation.**
(**b**) Proliferation assay to measure T cell response to specific antigen.

antibodies (e.g. anti-CD4, anti-CD8) coated with magnetic beads.

The proliferation assay requires responding T cells and antigen-presenting cells (e.g. monocytes) to be incubated with the antigen for approximately 3–6 days. A radioactive source of the DNA base thymidine is then added and incorporated into the new DNA of dividing cells. The radioactive nuclei of the cells are collected onto a filter and the radioactive emission counted. This provides a measurement of the T cell proliferative response to antigen.

The CD8 molecule differs from CD4 in being a disulphide-linked dimer. The two components may both be α chains, of 32 kDa, or α combined with β, a chain of 34 kDa. Each chain has a single immunoglobulin-like domain (Fig. 7.4). The CD8 molecule is similar in function to CD4. As a cell adhesion molecule it binds through the α chain to the α3 domain of the class I MHC molecule, stabilising T cell interactions with cells presenting antigen through the class I MHC molecule. The cytoplasmic domain of the CD8 molecule becomes phosphorylated and Lck physically associates with this region (Fig. 7.5).

T CELL ACTIVATION: ANTIGEN PROCESSING AND PEPTIDE PRESENTATION

When B cells are incubated in vitro with antigen recognised by the surface immunoglobulin, whole intact antigen can be internalised, providing one of the signals for B cell activation. If purified T cells are incubated with whole intact antigen, there is no TCR recognition event. As stated previously, TCRs do not 'see' native intact antigens. For TCR recognition, the native antigen must be processed intracellularly and presented by MHC molecules. The mechanism by which T cell activation is achieved through antigen processing and presentation is different for CD4$^+$ and CD8$^+$ T cells. The T cell response to presented antigen can be measured as a proliferation of T cells (see box: 'Separation and testing of lymphocytes for proliferative responses').

Antigen presentation to CD4$^+$ T cells: experimental data

Several simple experiments can illustrate these processes (Fig. 7.6). In the first (Fig. 7.7a), the benchmark experiment, CD4$^+$ T cells are incubated with whole native antigen and macrophages from the same donor as

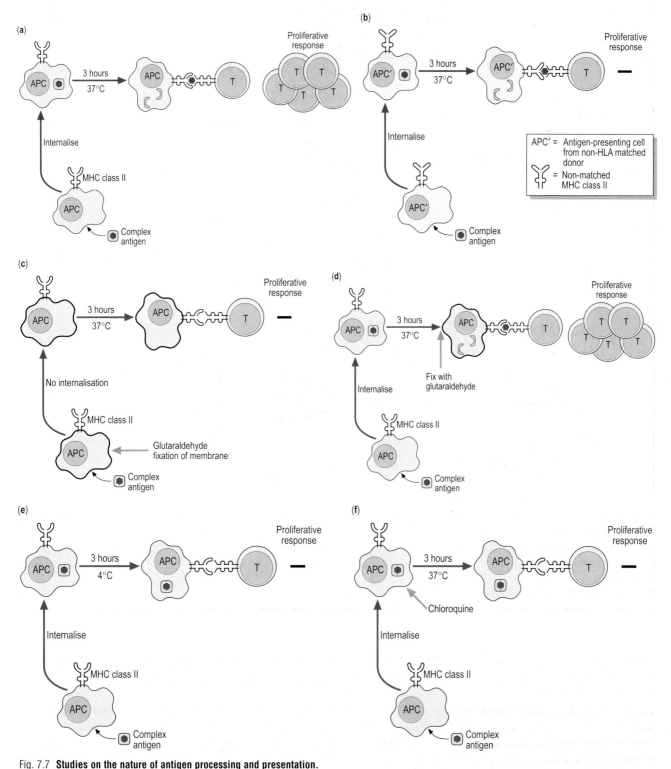

Fig. 7.7 **Studies on the nature of antigen processing and presentation.**
In the model system (**a**), a complex antigen is incubated with the antigen presenting cell (APC) for 3 hours at 37°C. Under these conditions, this APC is capable of inducing proliferation in an antigen-specific T cell (the T cell response takes place over the next 24–48 hours). (**b**) Using an APC from a donor of different class II MHC type gives no T cell response, indicating the need for correct MHC molecules in antigen presentation to T cells. (**c**) Blocking internalisation of the antigen by the APC (by chemical fixation of the membrane) inhibits T cell proliferation, but (**d**) addition of the fixative after the 3 hour incubation does not. (**e**) The processing event requires intact metabolic pathways, since low temperature is inhibitory, and also requires lysosomal activity (**f**) since chloroquine is inhibitory.

the T cells (or macrophages of the same class II HLA type). After 36–48 hours of incubation, using an antigen against which responder T cells are present, T cell proliferation is detectable (see the box). A good example of such an antigen would be tetanus toxoid, with which we are all immunised early in life. Trying to use macrophages from a variety of donors would reveal that only those cells from individuals of similar HLA type to the donor of the responder T cells would work (remember the law of MHC restriction) (Fig. 7.7b).

In a modification of this first experiment (Fig. 7.7c), macrophages are fixed with glutaraldehyde before addition to the culture. Glutaraldehyde permanently cross-links surface membrane proteins such as receptor molecules, disabling them and preventing endocytosis of antigen or antigen presentation. In this case there is no T cell response. In a variation (Fig. 7.7d), macrophages are incubated with native antigen for 3 hours alone and then fixed with glutaraldehyde. Now, there is a detectable T cell response. Clearly, the macrophage needs some time to endocytose and present the antigen. What other requirements are there? The 3-hour pre-incubation of macrophages and whole antigen needs to be at physiological temperatures: at 4°C it is ineffective

(Fig. 7.7e). Evidently, metabolic processes are required. Addition of agents such as chloroquine (Fig. 7.7f) prevents effective processing and presentation: chloroquine is known to interfere with the function of endosomes, the internal cell vacuoles into which complex antigens are taken. Finally, immediate fixation of the macrophages with gluteraldehyde does not completely prevent T cell activation if the antigen is degraded by proteolytic enzymes before addition to the presenting cells. This indicates the need for proteolytic breakdown of the complex antigens before they are able to be presented.

The synthesis of these experimental data is as follows. Alone, T cells cannot respond to antigen. Antigen must be *presented* by a cell bearing the same class II HLA type. Whole antigens are not presented. The macrophage requires time and metabolic activities to *process* the antigen. This, in turn, needs intact endosomal function and proteolytic enzymes. Antigen processing is a specialised active function of cells, which requires internalisation of antigen into an endosomal compartment and proteolytic processing. Presentation by class II HLA molecules can be achieved after fixation of the cell, as long as the appropriate peptide fragment of antigen is made available.

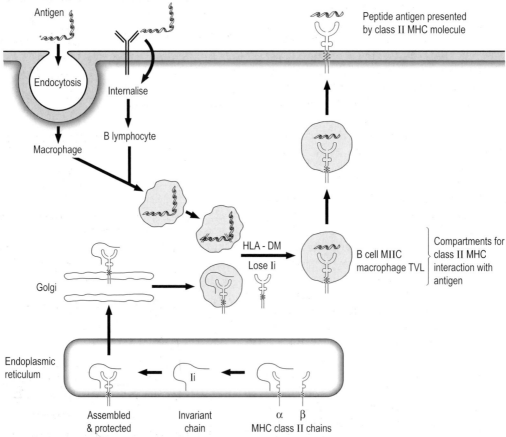

Fig. 7.8 Processing and presentation of exogenous antigen via the MHC class II pathway.
MHC class II molecules are assembled in the endoplasmic reticulum and the peptide-binding groove is protected by the presence of the invariant chain. After modification in the Golgi apparatus, MHC class II molecules migrate to the late endosomal compartments (MIIC in B cells, TVL in macrophages) where they meet antigen that has been internalised and processed by proteolytic enzymes and low pH in late endosomes. The invariant chain is removed and antigenic peptide added to the binding groove, in a process catalysed by the HLA-DM molecule. The MHC–peptide complex now migrates to the cell surface.

Antigen presentation to CD4⁺ T cells: molecules and pathways

Since the process described requires the acquisition of antigens from outside, it is termed the **exogenous pathway** of antigen presentation. The processes involved are described below and in Figure 7.8. Exogenous antigen processing and presentation to CD4⁺ T cells is a function of professional antigen-presenting cells: dendritic cells, macrophages and B lymphocytes. The B–T interaction is particularly easy to envisage: B cells internalise a specific antigen through their sIg molecule and present it only to T cells sharing affinity for a part of the same antigen. The two cells are 'on the same wavelength'.

Antigen is internalised from the external milieu into compartments termed **late endosomes**, because of their proximity to the cell surface (Fig. 7.8). Proteolytic enzymes are added and the pH lowered, and the antigen degrades. In antigen-presenting cells, as part of a continuous process, class II MHC molecules are being generated from gene transcription and translation and assembled in the endoplasmic reticulum (ER). After modifications of the class II molecules in the Golgi apparatus, they are transported in specialised compartments before coming into contact with the late endosomes. The antigen-binding groove of the MHC class II molecule has been protected throughout its journey through the cytoplasm from accepting peptide antigens by the presence of the invariant, Ii, chain. The Ii chain has three major functions in antigen presentation, a result of which has been the coining of the expression **chaperon** for this type of molecule. The Ii chain promotes assembly of new MHC α–β heterodimers; it targets and retains newly synthesised class II MHC molecules into the endosomal pathway, ultimately guiding them to the site at which antigenic peptide binds to the class II dimer; and most importantly it *protects the peptide-binding groove* until the class II MHC molecule has arrived at the appropriate site for peptide loading. The protection of the class II binding groove centres upon a part of the Ii chain called the **CLIP region** (class II-associated invariant chain peptide). It is not yet clear whether the CLIP actually occupies the MHC groove or interferes stoichiometrically with potential peptide binding. However, the importance of CLIP is to exercise control over occupation of the binding groove until the class II molecule arrives at the site at which antigenic peptides are available for binding.

The cellular site at which the CLIP releases and allows interaction between the class II molecule and antigen has yet to be identified categorically, but it is probably localised in a group of vesicles in the late endosomal compartment of B lymphocytes, which have been termed **MIIC** (for MHC class II compartment). The equivalent structures in macrophages are **tubulo-vesicular lysosomes** (TVL). What is known is that these compartments are post-Golgi, acidic and proteolytic. Here, the Ii chain is released and new peptides

from exogenous antigens (15–25 amino acid residues long) are inserted into the MHC molecule groove. This reaction is catalysed by the HLA-DM molecules. The selection process for a particular peptide from a complex molecule is not yet fully characterised. Obviously, to an extent, the ability of the peptide to bind and its ability to compete with other available peptides will determine selection.

Antigen presentation to CD8⁺ T cells

In the **endogenous pathway** of antigen presentation, peptide fragments of endogenous cellular proteins (which would include microbe-derived peptides in the case of an intracellular infection) are loaded into the class I MHC molecule (Fig. 7.9). This takes place at the site of assembly of class I heavy chains with β₂-microglobulin (β₂-m), in the ER. Indeed, there is strong evidence that the assembly of heavy chain and β₂-m is highly inefficient unless peptide (usually 8–10 amino acid residues long) is available to enter the class I binding groove. Analogous to the Ii chain in class II MHC

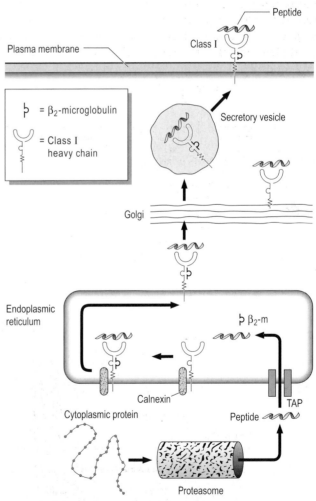

Fig. 7.9 Processing and presentation of endogenous antigen, via the MHC class I pathway.
Cytoplasmic proteins derived endogenously are cleaved into peptides by the action of enzymes in the large proteasome complex. The peptide is transported into the site of class I molecule assembly by specific transporter molecules. Peptide–α chain–β₂-microglobulin (β₂-m) combine and are guided out of the endoplasmic reticulum by the chaperon calnexin, via the secretory vesicle, to the cell surface.

molecule assembly, a molecule termed **calnexin** acts as the molecular chaperon for class I MHC molecules. Calnexin is an ER resident protein that ensures that assembled class I MHC molecules associate with peptide in the correct compartment (in this case peptides derived from the cytoplasm and moved into the ER), and also that any assembled class I molecules with empty peptide-binding grooves are not allowed to leave.

How do the peptides arrive in the ER, and how are they formed? Working backwards, from the site of peptide binding, the first question to address is how the peptides arrive in the MHC class I molecule assembly compartment. Two proteins were identified in the early 1990s that had the characteristics of peptide transporters. These are ATP-dependent molecules termed TAP-1 and TAP-2 (for transporter associated with processing), whose genes lie in the class II MHC region (see p. 55). The TAP transporters act as funnels into the ER and appear to have a selection capability to choose peptides of the correct size (8–10 residues), as well as of an appropriate sequence for class I binding. The supply of appropriate peptides requires a proteolytic machinery. The major known pathway for catalytic turnover of any cytoplasmic protein is a large complex of proteases with multicatalytic capabilities, termed the **proteasome** (Fig. 7.10). A subset of proteasomes contains two components, LMP-2 and LMP-7. The LMP subunits influence proteolysis in such a way as to favour residues suitable for class I binding. There are two other intriguing facts about the LMPs: (1) like the TAPs, they are also encoded in the class II MHC region, indicating a mechanism by which genes in one

region of the MHC can influence those in another; and (2) expression of the LMPs is inducible by IFN-γ, indicating a way of up-regulating antigen presentation during infection.

In vitro mechanisms of T cell activation

As for B cells, in the study of T cell functions it is often desirable to activate the cells non-specifically in vitro. Of the T cell mitogens, the most used are the lectin phytohaemagglutinin (PHA), a phorbol ester, phorbol myristate acetate (PMA) and certain monoclonal anti-CD3 antibodies. As a lectin, PHA is assumed to activate cells by cross-linking cell surface molecules bearing carbohydrate moieties. PMA activates protein kinase C (see p. 97), involved in the intracellular pathway of T cell activation, whilst anti-CD3 antibodies provide a strong activation stimulus through their ability to bind all TCR complexes on the cell surface.

In vivo, there are also molecules that are capable of activating T cells independently of antigen processing and presentation. These molecules bind simultaneously to domains on particular families of V_β chains of the TCR on the T cell surface, and to the β chain of the class II MHC heterodimer on the antigen-presenting cell. In doing so, they activate and expand all T cells bearing this V_β, and they have been termed **super-antigens**. Superantigens are typically derived from retroviruses or as exotoxins of certain bacteria. One of the best studied is staphylococcal enterotoxin B (SEB), which is responsible for expansions of $V_\beta3^+$ and $V_\beta8^+$ T cells in a condition known as **toxic shock syndrome**. A superantigen effect has also been demonstrated recently in Kawasaki's disease, a condition of childhood in which there is blood vessel inflammation. The timing of interaction with superantigen is critical to the outcome: retroviral superantigens encountered during neonatal life cause the deletion, rather than expansion, of certain V_β-expressing T cells.

T LYMPHOCYTE DEVELOPMENT: THYMIC EDUCATION

The bone marrow-derived precursor cells that enter the thymus are not identifiable as T cells. They do not have a T cell receptor rearranged and bear none of the surface molecules typical of T cells. The precursor T cells mature within the thymus, where they are termed **thymocytes**. The process of thymic education for a cell emerging successfully into the periphery takes about 3 weeks. The length of time spent in the thymus by a cell not destined for selection (true of approximately 99% of thymocytes) is about 3.5 days. Any description of the events that take place during the development of thymocytes before release into the periphery must take account of this, and the following facts about a mature T cell:

- in mature T cells, TCR genes are rearranged and the TCR dimer expressed, along with CD3 and one accessory molecule, either CD4 or CD8

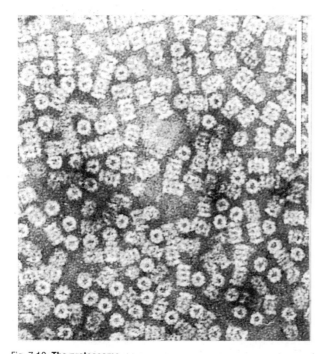

Fig. 7.10 **The proteasome.**
Electron micrograph of a proteasome: the large proteolytic complex responsible for catalytic breakdown of cytoplasmic proteins. Note the cotton reel shape. Proteasomes cleave endogenous peptides for antigen presentation. (Reproduced with permission from Peters J M 1994 Trends in Biochemical Sciences 19: 377–382.)

- CD4$^+$ T cell responses require presentation of peptide antigens by *self* MHC class II molecules
- CD8$^+$ T cell responses require presentation of peptide antigens by *self* MHC class I molecules.

In other words, in the thymus, T cells acquire the 'tools of their trade' (receptors and accessory molecules) and the ability to use them within the laws of MHC restriction described earlier. This process is often referred to as thymic education.

Other facts which must be accounted for in the explanation of thymic development are:

- only 1% of precursor cells entering the thymus leave as mature T cells
- extensive cell apoptosis can be seen in the thymus
- despite the enormously broad repertoire of possible TCR configurations, in health relatively few mature peripheral T cells are able to make responses to self antigens.

Within the thymic events, it seems likely that a process of identification and elimination of strongly self-reactive, and of non-reactive T cells take place. This represents a considerable sacrifice of the potential repertoire, but at the same time offers to the host protection from self-reactivity.

There are two possible types of selection process, positive and negative. Negative selection indicates that thymocytes are excluded on the basis of certain deleterious characteristics; positive selection implies that a thymocyte is selected on the basis of some advantageous attribute. Logic argues for both systems operating in the thymus. First, in view of the ability to make some 10^{16} different αβ TCRs, it is likely that some TCRs will recognise presented self peptide antigens with high affinity, which could be dangerous (see below), and thymocytes bearing these must be deleted by negative selection. Some TCR types are likely to be unable to interact usefully at all with presented peptide antigens, and these will also be deleted. To balance these deletions, there must be a system of positive selection to find those receptors of some use to the individual and avoid redundancy. Experimental data, particularly from transgenic models, support both of these mechanisms being in operation.

Thymic education: lessons from transgenes

Transgenic studies conducted in mice have provided an elegant way of illustrating the processes of thymic selection. In the first such study, a T cell with specificity for a peptide derived from a protein (HY) encoded on the mouse Y (male) chromosome was identified (Fig. 7.11). These T cells were CD8$^+$ and only recognised the HY peptide when it was presented by D^b, a class I molecule in the mouse. (The fact that the T cells were CD8$^+$ is an important fact; see below.) The T cell was induced to proliferate so that sufficient mRNA and then cDNA encoding the α and β chains of the TCR could be obtained. These were introduced transgeni-

cally into mice, with the intention of generating abundant thymocytes expressing this particular αβ TCR. The mice chosen to express the TCR were either: (1) male D^b mice (which would possess the HY peptide and be able to present it on the D^b molecule); (2) female D^b mice (which would not possess the male HY peptide); and (3) D^b-negative male mice (which possess the HY peptide but would be unable to present it on D^b). The outcomes of these manipulations were very revealing about the processes of thymic education, and a number of observations were made.

- In male D^b-positive mice there is negative selection: no T cells expressing the transgenic TCR are present in the periphery, all of them having been deleted in the thymus. The explanation for this result is that the male HY peptide is presented in the thymus by D^b. This is the MHC–peptide complex recognised with exquisite specificity by the TCR transgene. In the thymus, transgene-positive developing T cells would bind with strong affinity to the HY–D^b complex. This would be a potentially dangerous TCR to allow into the periphery. Why? Well, HY peptide will also be widely expressed outside the thymus, in the periphery, and it is likely to be processed and presented in some cells. Therefore, a T cell receptor with high affinity for the HY–D^b complex could inflict damage on host cells: an **autoimmune reaction**. Since this could have disastrous consequences for the host, no transgene-positive cells appear in the periphery.
- In female D^b-positive mice there is positive selection: there were numerous T cells in the periphery that expressed the αβ TCR transgene. By definition, these transgene-positive cells have undergone positive selection. The explanation for this process is that the positive selection of these TCRs has been made on the basis that they are able to recognise *some* peptides presented by D^b. These peptides would not include the HY peptide, which is not available in the females. The peptides must be from other antigens presented in the thymus for which the transgene-positive T cells have an 'acceptable' affinity (i.e. not too high).
- In male D^b-negative mice, transgene-positive TCRs were not found in the periphery. The transgene-expressing TCRs recognise peptides presented by D^b, but not by other class I molecules, and in the absence of D^b, cells bearing transgene TCRs were not selected.

Some aspects of this experiment require further consideration, and it must be said that not all of the answers are currently available. The negative selection of TCRs with high affinity for a peptide to be presented widely in the periphery, as shown in experiment (1), is understandable, from the point of view that such TCRs are potentially dangerous. But why do the female D^b mice in experiment (2) positively select the transgene?

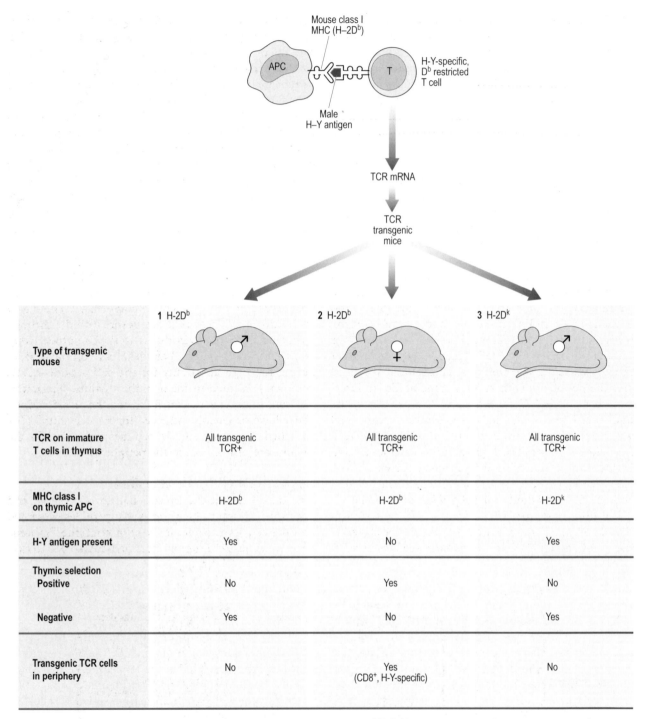

Fig. 7.11 Positive and negative selection of TCRs can be demonstrated in transgenic studies.
See text for details.

First, we know that this selection cannot be on the basis of a high-affinity interaction between TCR and any other peptide–D^b complex, since this results in deletion (see (1)). Second, we know that the selection cannot be based on a lack of recognition of any peptide presented by D^b in the thymus, since experiment (3) shows us that *no recognition* results in *no selection*. The best explanation for the selection of T cells expressing transgene TCRs by female D^b mice is that they recognise peptide antigen presented in the thymus with an acceptable, moderate affinity, not too high to pose a threat in the periphery, not too low to be unselected. This explanation is borne out by one other fact: the transgene-positive TCRs selected in the female mice were all $CD8^+$. If their selection had been a random, or accidental process, equal representation of CD4 and CD8 might be expected. The fact that they are $CD8^+$ shows that the ability to bind the class I molecule D^b is important in the selection process. Exactly what peptide the D^b molecule was expressing during the selection remains unknown, and this is an area of intense research (see below).

Positive and negative selection in the thymus

One of the questions most frequently asked is what do the T cells 'see' during thymic selection? In other words, when a thymocyte is undergoing positive selection for interaction with class II MHC molecules, what is the peptide in the MHC groove? We know that there must be a peptide, since both class I and class II MHC molecules are not assembled and exposed on the cell membrane in the absence of peptide. Equally, we know that a thymocyte that will later mature into a cytotoxic T cell affording protection against influenza virus will not be encountering influenza-derived peptides in the thymus. In other words, positive selection (unlike negative selection) does not require the exogenous peptide antigen that may ultimately be recognised in the periphery to be presented in the thymus.

There is not a good answer yet to the question of what peptides are used to select T cells in the thymus. The best analysis of what takes place in the interaction between TCR, MHC molecule and peptide during positive selection is as follows. The TCR is selected for a moderate affinity for MHC plus 'a peptide'. What this achieves is the selection of a repertoire of T cells to enter the periphery, with at least some ability to interact with a self MHC molecule. In the periphery, the same T cells encounter MHC-presented foreign (e.g. viral, bacterial) peptides in the lymph nodes. Those T cells with a reasonably high affinity for the foreign peptide now receive appropriate signals for expansion. The process of positive selection described ensures that dangerously high affinity for *self peptides* is excluded.

The process of positive selection of T cells sounds (and of course is!) complicated. However, it is based on exactly the same principles as we have seen for B cells, namely to generate as wide a repertoire of antigen receptors as possible, so that every conceivable foreign antigen can be bound. The main difference is that, since T cells are *the* pivotal cell in the immune system, extra care is taken in the final selection process, to insure against self-destruction.

Which cells present the MHC–peptide complexes during thymic selection? The two main candidates are the thymic epithelial cells, which make up the framework of the gland, and bone marrow-derived dendritic cells with specialised antigen-presenting functions. It would appear that positive thymic selection is largely induced by interaction with the thymic epithelium, whilst negative selection may be determined by the dendritic cells.

Negative selection centres upon the unwanted T cell. These T cells make up the majority, and fall into two camps. The easiest to picture is the useless TCR, which fails to bind any MHC–peptide complex presented to it in the thymus. These cells are destined to die through a process of apoptosis in the thymus. The other group of cells negatively selected are dealt with on the basis of having too high an affinity for the self peptide–MHC complex presented to them in the thymus. Numerous different transgenic studies following the one described above have repeatedly indicated the same result: TCRs with high reactivity to self peptides presented in the thymus are unwelcome in the periphery.

An overview of thymic selection

The debate about the precise nature of positive and negative selection in the thymus, the peptides presented and the cells presenting, is likely to continue for some years to come. At this point, it is perhaps as well to take

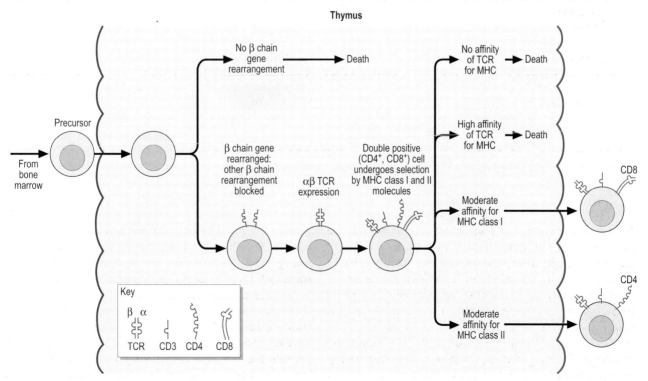

Fig. 7.12 **Model of thymic selection.**
See text for details.

stock of the facts known with certainty and put these into a working schema (Fig. 7.12). It is of some benefit in terms of understanding these principles that many aspects of thymic education parallel the development of B lymphocytes.

The T cell precursor enters the thymus and becomes recognisable as a potential T lymphocyte once the rearranged genes of the β chain give rise to a cytoplasmic form of this part of the receptor. The α chain is subsequently rearranged and expressed, and following this the CD3 complex, and *both* CD4 and CD8 molecules appear on the thymocyte surface. It can be assumed that at this point there is the potential for encounter between these immature thymocytes and peptide antigens presented in the grooves of class II and class I molecules. Having both CD4 and CD8, the thymocyte can potentially interact with whichever presenting molecule is appropriate (see box: 'How does positive selection for CD4 or CD8 lineage take place?'). There are four possible outcomes. (1) No affinity of the rearranged TCR for peptides presented by class I or class II MHC molecules leaves the cell without positive development signals; i.e. death. (2) High affinity for the self peptide–MHC complex is a potentially dangerous characteristic: the same self peptide could be encountered in the periphery by a mature T cell, with disastrous consequences. These thymocytes must also receive the deletional signal. (3) Moderate, but physiologically appropriate, affinity for peptide–class I MHC complex

leads to a positive selection signal and loss of CD4. (4) The reciprocal is true for thymocytes interacting effectively with peptide–class II complexes (i.e. TCR selection and loss of CD8). Virgin T cells leaving the thymus, therefore, express a TCR selected for binding a particular MHC–peptide complex and either CD4 or CD8.

MOLECULES INVOLVED IN T CELL ACTIVATION AND DIFFERENTIATION

Several of the key molecules in T lymphocyte function have already been discussed: the TCR–CD3 complex, CD4 and CD8, the adhesion molecules. Several other molecules also have roles in T cell physiology, many of which are still being elucidated.

The CD45 molecule

CD45 is a cell surface glycoprotein expressed on mature and immature white blood cells, including granulocytes, T and B cells and monocytes. For this reason, it has been known for many years as the **leukocyte common antigen** (LCA) and monoclonal antibodies to it are useful tools as pan-white blood cell markers. The whole CD45 molecule, LCA, has a molecular weight of 200 kDa. The gene encoding the CD45 molecule has a total of 34 exons, some of which can be used variably to generate different isoforms of the molecule. The isoforms are particularly important in T lymphocyte development and differentiation. For example, 'virgin' or unprimed T cells express the **CD45RA** isoform only: after stimulation and activation by antigen, CD45RA is lost from the cell surface and the memory or primed cell now expresses exclusively the **CD45R0** isoform (see box: 'Differential expression of CD45 isoforms: is T cell memory made of this?').

Co-stimulatory molecules in T cell activation

Immunological reactions typically have numerous fail-safe mechanisms, to ensure that the risk of unwarranted activation is minimised. For T cell responses, this means that simple interaction between TCR and antigenic peptide–MHC is insufficient for activation. Indeed, interaction with antigen alone may render the T cell anergic (i.e. unresponsive) (see p. 106). Productive cellular activation can be achieved by the provision of antigen plus **co-signals**. Some of these co-signals are soluble, for example those represented by the release of cytokines, but some of the most powerful involve interactions between surface molecules on the responder cell and their ligands on the antigen-presenting cell. These molecules are termed **co-stimulatory molecules**, and the most important are the CD28/CTLA4 group on T cells and their counterparts, the B7 family on antigen-presenting cells.

Both groups of molecules are members of the immunoglobulin supergene family, and have the familiar domain structure (Fig. 7.14). CTLA-4 is so named because of its initial discovery on cytotoxic T lymphocytes. The B7 group is composed of two main

How does positive selection for CD4 or CD8 lineage take place?

Developing thymocytes have a phase in which both CD4 and CD8 co-receptor molecules are expressed, which is followed by the final selection of one or other of these, but not both. After that selection, the cell is committed for life to interact with either class II or class I MHC molecules and, therefore, to be either a helper or a suppressor/cytotoxic T cell. How is this central decision made? There are currently two models, termed the **instructive** model and the **stochastic** (i.e. randomly selective) model. In the instructive model, it is the interaction between TCR, co-receptor and MHC molecule which is determinant. In other words, a TCR with optimal MHC class I binding characteristics, on interaction with the class I MHC molecule is 'instructed' to cease CD4 expression. Equally, a TCR with MHC class II binding characteristics, through its binding to a class II MHC molecule in the thymus loses CD8 expression. The stochastic model suggests that after the CD4$^+$CD8$^+$ double-positive stage, a thymocyte is randomly programmed to select either CD4 or CD8 expression but not both. Then, the thymocytes are exposed to thymic antigen–presenting cells, and selection on the basis of TCR affinity for MHC–peptide complex takes place. A CD4$^+$ cell that has optimal binding to class II is selected, and so on.

Differential expression of CD45 isoforms: is T cell memory made of this?

The gene complex that gives rise to the CD45 molecule has three particular exons encoding external domains of the molecule (termed A, B and C), which can be alternatively spliced at the RNA level to generate different protein sequences (e.g. A–B–C, A–B, A–C, A, or absent). The different possible forms of the CD45 molecule generated in this process are called CD45 isoforms, denoted CD45R. At present these can be identified at the cell surface by whether they possess the products of the A, B or C exons, or none of these (0), using monoclonal antibodies (see Fig. 7.13). The principal isoforms are called CD45RA, CD45RB, CD45RC and CD45R0. Each CD45R isoform has an importance for different phases of T cell development. Unprimed, virgin T cells leaving the thymus all react with the anti-CD45RA monoclonal antibody; in the peripheral blood of the newborn, almost all T cells are CD45RA⁺. As the individual matures, and the T cells in the periphery mature and become primed to external antigens, the proportion of T cells expressing CD45RA declines, and CD45R0 increases. In an octogenarian, one might expect to see the majority of T cells expressing CD45R0, and indeed this is true, giving this cell population the name primed, or memory, cells. In vitro studies show that CD45RA⁺ unprimed cells are difficult to stimulate with antigen, have low levels of adhesion and activation molecules and fail to support antibody production by B cells. In contrast, the primed cells are easy to stimulate, express high levels of adhesion molecules and activation markers, such as the IL-2 receptor, and avidly assist B cells in making antibody.

It would appear straightforward: unprimed cells become primed, in doing so attain CD45R0 positivity and hold immunological memory, ready for a rapid response to restimulation. Or is it this simple? Studies with tagged cells have shown that the CD45R0 popula-tion is actually relatively short lived (1–2 years). Long-term immunological memory probably resides in the unprimed cells, which are constantly generating short-lived, ready-for-action memory cells, which then die or revert to the unprimed state.

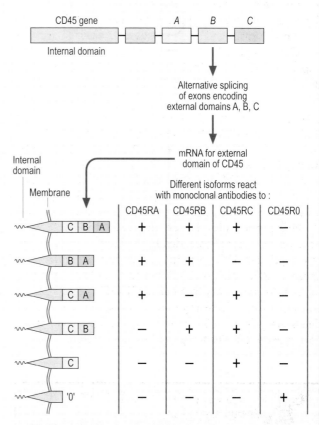

Fig. 7.13 **CD45 and its isoforms.**
Detection by various monoclonal antibodies.

molecules, B7-1 and B7-2. Although both of these will bind with both T cell ligands, B7-1 has a higher affinity for CTLA-4, and B7-2 for CD28 (Table 7.2). CD28 and CTLA-4 may exist as monomers or homodimers.

In functional terms, the interaction between CD28 on a responder T cell and a B7 molecule on the cell presenting antigen leads to a sequence of intracellular events within the T cell that provide a second activation signal. The complexities of T cell signalling are detailed in a later section (see p. 97), but the main intracellular event is the switching on of the gene for IL-2. This is achieved partially by the TCR–antigen–MHC interaction, but stimulation through B7 also up-regulates IL-2 via a different intracellular pathway to that used by the TCR. The activity of CD28 in achieving this relates to its cytoplasmic domain, which binds a phosphoinositide 3-kinase and thus initiates an activation cascade. This co-signal ultimately leads to transcription and translation of the IL-2 and IL-2 receptor genes. As we shall see later, activation of T cells by antigen also leads to up-regulation of synthesis of IL-2 and its receptor, the most important events in T cell proliferation (see p. 97). Therefore, the CD28-mediated co-signal is enhancing the primary T cell activation event, through a different intracellular pathway.

The interaction between B7 and CTLA-4 is intriguing. CTLA-4 takes some time to appear on the activated T cell and actually follows on after T cell activation through B7-2–CD28 interaction. The CTLA-4–B7 interaction is an 'off' signal for the T cell: CTLA-4 has higher affinity than CD28 for both B7 molecules and terminates T cell activation through ligand competition (Fig. 7.15).

LYMPHOCYTE ACTIVATION

INTRACELLULAR PATHWAYS OF ACTIVATION

Binding of antigen to the lymphocyte receptor, accompanied by co-signals supplied through other surface

1. Early generation of enzymes capable of protein tyrosine phosphorylation (e.g. protein tyrosine kinases, PTK).
2. Early activation of the phosphatidylinositol membrane pathway, which leads to generation of high levels of intracellular calcium.
3. Subsequent activation of other cellular protein kinases.
4. Activation of GTP-binding proteins with GTPase activity.
5. Activation of nuclear transcriptional events.

These are the signal transduction events. Additional amplification of the signals is required because the number of surface antigen receptors actually being signalled through in a responding T or B cell is known to be quite small (e.g. only several hundred molecules per cell). Without these additional signals, it is unlikely that the lymphocyte could generate a sufficient head of steam to become activated. Since enzymes are generated in the signal transduction events, there will necessarily be an element of amplification of the signal. However, important amplification is also supplied through enzyme activities in the accessory molecules of T and B cells, notably CD4/CD8 in T cells, and the CD19–CD21–CD81 complex, CD20, CD22 and CD40 molecules in B cells. CD45 appears to supply critical amounts of tyrosine phosphatase activity to both cell types.

Neither the BCR complex (sIg plus Ig-α–Ig-β) nor the TCR complex (TCR plus CD3) have intrinsic PTK activity. However, the Ig-α–Ig-β and CD3 complexes contain numerous distinctive repeating amino acid sequences ('motifs') that are called **antigen rec-ognition activation motifs** (ARAMs) (or may also be called antigen receptor homology (ARH) motifs) (Fig. 7.17). The ARAMs function as substrates for PTKs, thus binding them to the antigen–receptor complex. Some of the important PTKs to be activated are shown in Table 7.3.

The cascade of kinase activities draws nearer to the nucleus. The nuclear events are currently only well characterised for the T cell, mainly because it has been possible to focus on the IL-2 gene as an early and necessary event in T cell activation. One pathway relies upon there being an increase in intracellular Ca^{2+}, generated by membrane events. This activates **calcineurin**, a calcium-dependent protein phosphatase which dephosphorylates a nuclear transcription factor present in the cytoplasm, **NF-AT$_c$** (for nuclear factor of activated T cells$_{cytoplasm}$) which is thus enabled to translocate from the cytoplasm to the nucleus and there to initiate transcription of the IL-2 gene in concert with a similar nuclear transcription factor (**NF-AT$_n$**). Intriguingly, one of the major breakthroughs in clinical trans-

Table 7.3 Protein tyrosine kinases activated in lymphocyte responses

Family of protein tyrosine kinases	Major T cell representatives	Major B cell representatives
Early:		
Src kinases	Lck, Fyn	Lyn, Blk, Fyn
Syk/Zap-70 kinases	Syk, Zap-70	Syk
Late:		
Enzyme groups probably involved	MAP kinases; phospholipase Cγ (PLCγ)	MAP kinases; phospholipase Cγ (PLCγ); phosphoinositide 3-kinase (PI 3-kinase)

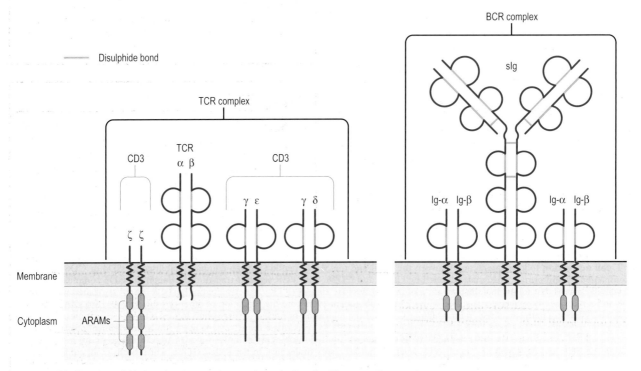

Fig. 7.17 **Binding sites within lymphocyte receptor complexes for tyrosine kinases.** ARAMs, antigen recognition activation motifs.

plantation in the last 10 years has been the introduction of a drug, **cyclosporin**, that interferes with calcineurin function and has a profound inhibitory effect on T cell function (see p. 307).

THE SEQUELAE OF T CELL ACTIVATION: T LYMPHOCYTE-MEDIATED IMMUNE RESPONSES

As T cell physiology became unravelled in the period from the mid-1960s, two distinct labels came to be used for the characters of the immune responses over which these cells presided. On the one hand, T cells promote the responsiveness of other cells. For example, T cells promote activation of macrophages or have a positive influence over B cell production of antibodies. On the other hand, T cells also inhibit such cellular responses. And, in a different type of response altogether, T lymphocytes are capable of killing virally infected cells. These three characters were encapsulated in the terms **helper**, **suppressor**, and **cytotoxic** T cells.

For many years, the populations of cells responsible for these types of response have been delineated by the presence of the glycoproteins CD4 and CD8. Induction (e.g. macrophage activation) and help (e.g. in antibody production) in immune responses are characteristics associated with the CD4$^+$ T cell populations, often called the **helper/inducer subset**. In contrast, suppression and cytotoxicity are the provenance of the CD8$^+$ T cells, hence the term **suppressor/cytotoxic T cells**. These descriptive terms for T cell functions have remained in widespread use for many years and encapsulate the major roles that T cells have in host protection from infection.

T helper lymphocytes

The major areas in which T cells help the functions of other cells are in relation to macrophages, B cells, other helper T cells and cytotoxic T cells. Within recent years, it has become recognised that T helper lymphocytes are not a homogeneous group of cells but can be divided into different subgroups. The subgroups are identifiable by the panel of cytokines they secrete and, thus, the *type* of help they provide. These cytokine profiles subdivide CD4$^+$ T cells into **T helper 1** and **T helper 2** subsets, or T_H1 and T_H2. This subdivision is based on cytokine profiles alone; there are no surface markers or CD numbers that distinguish these two cellular subsets (at present anyway). Not every CD4$^+$ T cell falls into these two categories: some cells have a mixed cytokine secretion pattern and are termed T_H0. The cytokines released by the different T helper subsets are shown in Table 7.4 and the cytokines IL-4, IL-5, IL-6 and IL-10 are described in associated boxes. The T_H subsets arise from a common precursor, and the cytokine influence at a critical point of development determines whether a T_H1 (IL-12 providing the major maturation signal) or T_H2 (IL-4 the main signal) cell is produced.

The mechanism through which T cells provide help to B lymphocytes is illustrated in Figure 7.18. This help is complemented by the cell–cell contact between co-signalling molecules (B7–CD28, CD40–CD40L, adhesion molecules). The net result of this predominantly T_H2-type action is (1) the activation and expansion of B cells and (2) their differentiation along different pathways of antibody production.

The mode of recruitment and activation of macrophages, predominantly mediated by IFN-γ-secreting T cells of the T_H1-type, has been discussed already (see

Table 7.4 **T helper 1 and 2 subsets, their defining cytokine profiles and functions**

Cell	Cytokine profile	Functions of T_H subset
T_H1	IFN-γ, IL-2	Activation of macrophages Activation of cytotoxic cells Antagonism of T_H2 cells
T_H2	IL-2, IL-4, IL-5, IL-6, IL-10	Activation and maturation of B cells Antagonism of T_H1 cells
T_H0	IFN-γ, IL-2, IL-4, IL-5, IL-6, IL-10	Various

Interleukin-4

IL-4 is a 20 kDa polypeptide released predominantly by T_H2 cells, which has important effects in relation to T and especially B cell function. It provides a potent stimulus for B cell switching to production of IgE antibody. As such it is important from a clinical view point in relation to parasitic infections and allergy, in both of which IgE-mediated responses play an important role. IL-4 is an important promoting growth factor for the T_H2 subset of lymphocytes and is an equally important inhibitory cytokine in the growth and differentiation of T_H1 cells. A third major function of IL-4 relates to its inhibitory effects on macrophage function. This effect of IL-4 is shared with IL-10, also secreted by T_H2 cells.

Interleukin-5

This 40 kDa cytokine is released by T_H2 lymphocytes and also by activated mast cells. The major action of IL-5 is in the growth and differentiation of eosinophils and also to activate mature eosinophils to kill helminths. The activities induced by IL-5 are, therefore, a key part of the antiparasitic response and the allergic immune response. It can be envisaged that during a typical response, IgE (promoted by the T_H2 cytokine IL-4) activates mast cells. These in turn recruit, promote the expansion of and activate eosinophils, through release of eosinophil chemotactic factors and IL-5. The T_H2 influence remains as IL-5 is also released by these T cells, strengthening the eosinophil-dominated response. Eosinophils are important in antiparasitic responses; their involvement in allergic responses is an important factor in the tissue damage caused in conditions such as asthma.

Interleukin-6

IL-6 is a cytokine of 26 kDa secreted mainly by the mononuclear-phagocyte system cells, endothelial cells and activated T cells of the T_H2 type. The major stimulus for its secretion is IL-1, with which it shares many actions in common, but TNF-a also induces IL-6 release. IL-6 has a major role in the acute-phase response to inflammatory episodes. It induces the liver to synthesise plasma proteins that are involved in acute-phase reactions, such as clotting and complement factors and C-reactive protein.

IL-6 also has potent effects on B cells. This is graphically illustrated in malignant tumours of plasma cells (called myeloma, see p. 294) when high levels of this factor are released and act as an autonomous growth factor. In non-malignant, physiological responses, IL-6 promotes the growth and differentiation of B cells and has an effect on IgG class switching.

Interleukin-10

CD4$^+$ T cells of the T_H2 subset are the predominant source of IL-10, an 18 kDa peptide, although activated macrophages and B cells may also secrete it. IL-10 inhibits the release of cytokines such as TNF-α and IL-1 by macrophages and also inhibits the accessory cell functions of macrophages in T cell activation. The net result of these actions is to down-regulate T cell immune responses. In contrast, the effect of IL-10 on B cells is stimulatory.

p. 69 and the box: 'Type II interferons: Interferon-γ'): the role of T_H1 cells in the activation of cytotoxic T cell effectors is discussed below.

Cytotoxic T lymphocytes

Cytolytic, or cytotoxic, T lymphocytes (often abbreviated to T_c, or CTL) are important in defence against virally infected cells, in rejection of foreign tissue grafts and possibly also in immune responses to certain tumour types. CTLs are capable of killing targets expressing a specific antigen. They are found predominantly amongst the CD8$^+$ population of T cells. We have already discussed the pathway for antigen presentation to CD8$^+$ T cells: peptide antigen is derived from internally synthesised proteins (the endogenous pathway of antigen presentation) and presented bound to MHC class I molecules. Target peptides for CTLs are fragments of virus, or tumour antigens. CTLs use the same type of TCR, the $\alpha\beta$ heterodimer, as that used by CD4$^+$ T lymphocytes. Recently, CD8$^+$ T cells have been subdivided into two groups on the basis of cytokine production, in much the same way as CD4$^+$ T helper cells have. Although the research is at an early stage, it appears that T_c1 and T_c2 cells, when activated, have similar cytokine profiles to the T_H1 and T_H2 subsets, respectively.

CD8$^+$ T cells, remember, interact with antigen through presentation of peptides in the groove of class I MHC molecules. The induction of a CTL response is dependent upon CD4$^+$ T lymphocytes to provide help, in the form of activation stimuli. The life cycle of a CTL up to the point of killing is as follows. CD8$^+$ T lymphocytes with the potential to become CTLs exit

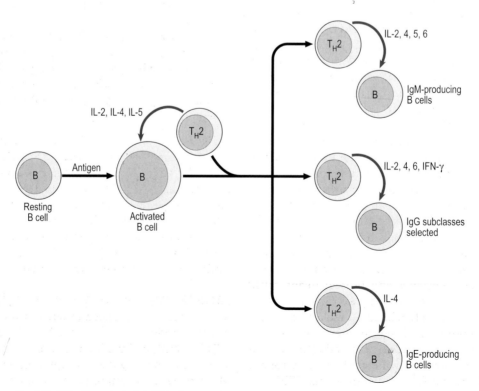

Fig. 7.18 **T_H2 cells promote B cell functions.**

Type II interferons: Interferon-γ

Interferon-γ is a homodimer composed of subunits of approximately 25 kDa. It is released by CD4$^+$ T lymphocytes (both T$_H$1 and T$_H$0) and CD8$^+$ T lymphocytes, as well as by activated natural killer cells. The interferons are known for their antiviral activity, and IFN-γ is no exception. In addition to these innate antiviral effects (similar to the type I interferons, see p. 70), IFN-γ has distinct immunological roles.

First, IFN-γ is a potent activator of macrophages, inducing an increase in metabolic, phagocytic and killing activity (see p. 69). This role is an essential part of the response induced by T$_H$1-like lymphocytes. Second, IFN-γ has the ability to increase MHC class I molecule expression on a range of cell types and induce expression of class II MHC molecules on other cells, either alone or in concert with other cytokines (e.g. TNF). This may be an important component of antiviral protection, since it up-regulates presentation of viral targets by infected cells. Third, as a T$_H$1-cytokine, IFN-γ has profound effects on T cell development (favouring the development of T$_H$1 cells) and B cell differentiation (biasing the production of immunoglobulin in favour of IgG and away from IgE). IFN-γ is also required for the activation of CD8$^+$ cytotoxic T cells (another T$_H$1 function; see this page) and has a role in activating natural killer cells.

the thymus expressing their specific TCR but cannot lyse target cells at this stage. In the periphery, when a cytotoxic response is required, the pre-CTLs are activated by CD4$^+$ T lymphocytes, which are involved in an immune reaction complementary to that of the CTL. For example, a CD4$^+$ T$_H$ lymphocyte is primed to respond to viral peptides after viral particles have been ingested and presented by macrophages at the site of infection. In turn, the activated T$_H$ cells activate virus-specific CTLs (Fig. 7.19). The main cytokine signal is IL-2, but IFN-γ and IL-6 are also stimulators of CTLs. Activation of CTLs requires the typical two-signal activation process of presented antigen and co-signals. The requirement for IL-2 and IFN-γ indicates the importance of T$_H$1 cells in this process.

Following activation, the CTL must prepare the machinery required to lyse target cells. First, membrane-bound granules appear in the cytoplasm. The granules contain a membrane pore-forming protein called **perforin** or **cytolysin** (Fig. 7.19b). In addition, they contain proteolytic enzymes and protein toxins called **lymphotoxins** (note: these lymphotoxins are either identical to, or structurally related to, the cytokine lymphotoxin, or TNF-β, referred to previously; p. 70). Second, there is cytokine production and release: notably IFN-γ, lymphotoxin (which has similar cytotoxic effects to TNF-α) and IL-2. Remember that IFN-γ, as the name implies, also has direct antiviral activity,

which may be of importance when a viral-infected cell is lysed and virions released.

What are the mechanisms of target cell lysis? (See box: 'Detection of cytotoxicity', p. 103.) First, we must define the ground rules. Obviously, killing by CD8$^+$ T cells will be MHC class I restricted. This suggests, and indeed it is the case, that killing requires cell–cell contact. Only those cells to which a CTL becomes attached are killed. There is no 'bystander' death, because the lytic molecules are released only at the site of TCR contact. Finally, CTLs are not themselves damaged during the process.

Lysis involves five steps.

1. **Cell contact** (involves TCR interaction with peptide–MHC class I complex and CD8 interaction with MHC, but other adhesion molecules such as the ICAMs and integrins can be involved).
2. **Activation** of the CTL (activation is first TCR mediated; the second signals necessary come from adhesion molecule interactions).
3. **Delivery of 'lethal hit'**. There are two ways by which target cells are killed. (a) CTLs release perforin, which polymerises in the presence of Ca^{2+} to form a hollow tube, analogous to the membrane attack complex of complement; in fact, C9 and perforin have a high degree of structural homology. If a sufficient number of pores are formed, the cell is killed by osmotic lysis. (b) CTLs release lymphotoxin, which activates enzymes in the target cell to cleave DNA in the nucleus. One of the earliest, characteristic appearances of this form of death is the presence of clumps of nuclear DNA, each of a small, uniform length. This is the consequence of the process of programmed cell death or apoptosis.
4. **Disengagement of CTL**. CTLs are protected from the action of their own granule contents, probably by having a high density of disassembling proteins on their surface (called **protectins**).
5. **Osmotic lysis or programmed cell death of target**.

Recent studies have uncovered an important pair of molecules involved in cell death, namely **Fas** (CD95) and its ligand **FasL**. FasL is expressed on CTLs; Fas is present on a range of different cell types in the immune system. When FasL on CTLs binds Fas on a target cell, apoptosis results. This mechanism of inducing cell death is known to be important in regulating development of immune cells (see p. 77), but it may also have a role in controlling some viral infections.

Immune suppression by T lymphocytes

In any physiological system, there is a key role for negative regulation (i.e. suppression) of the actions of the cells involved, and the immune system is no exception. There are many good examples of experiments in which measurable immune responses by a population of cells are inhibited by a different population. One of

Table 9.2 **The spectrum of autoimmune diseases, from organ-specific to non-organ-specific and the autoantigens typically targeted**

Disease	Main autoantigens targeted
Organ specific	
Myasthenia gravis	Acetylcholine receptor
Graves' disease	Thyroid-stimulating hormone receptor
Hashimoto's thyroiditis	Thyroid peroxidase; thyroglobulin
Type 1 diabetes	Islet cell cytoplasmic targets; insulin; glutamic acid decarboxylase
Pernicious anaemia	H^+K^+ ATPase (gastric proton pump); intrinsic factor
Addison's disease	17α-hydroxylase
Pemphigus	130 kDa member of cadherin adhesion molecules
Bullous pemphigoid	180 kDa hemidesmosomal cell adhesion structure; 230 kDa cell adhesion structure
Vitiligo	Melanocyte cytoplasmic targets
Autoimmune hepatitis	Asialoglycoprotein receptor; cytochrome P4502D6
Autoimmune haemolytic anaemia	Red blood cell surface targets
Overlap between organ- and non-organ-specific diseases	
Primary biliary cirrhosis	Mitochondrial pyruvate dehydrogenase
Goodpasture's syndrome	Non-collagenous domain of type IV collagen in renal and lung basement membrane
Non-organ-specific diseases	
Rheumatoid arthritis	IgG
Systemic lupus erythematosus	Double-stranded DNA; Sm (small nuclear ribonucleoproteins); SS-A (Ro; a 60 kDa ribonucleoprotein); SS-B (La; a 47 kDa ribonucleoprotein); histones
Sjögren's syndrome	SS-A, SS-B
Systemic sclerosis	DNA topoisomerase I; centromere
Mixed connective tissue disease	70 kDa small nuclear ribonucleoprotein
Polymyositis	tRNA synthetase

host as well as foreign antigens. Is this capacity translated into the production of autoreactive T and B lymphocytes?

One approach to answering this question is to generate **clones**. As the name implies, these are the offspring of a single cell, and, therefore, all share the same antigen receptor. This makes it easier to manipulate experimental conditions. The other advantage of cloning techniques is that they generate several million daughter cells, the sort of number required for studying cell function in vitro. Human B cell clones may be derived by fusion of human B cells to a mouse hybridoma (see Ch. 4) or by infection with Epstein–Barr virus. These immortalised B lymphocyte clones produce monoclonal antibodies, up to one third of which have been shown to react with self antigens. This is not simply an in vitro artefact; similar antibodies can be detected in normal human sera. The range of antigens recognised includes actin, DNA, collagen, albumin, IgG, IL-1α, TNF-α, insulin and thyroglobulin.

T cell autoreactivity is a less well-studied phenomenon. Undoubtedly, T lymphocytes reactive with self proteins may be found in the healthy adult human immune system but their frequency is low and T cells that recognise ubiquitous circulatory proteins such as albumin and γ-globulin have not been detected.

These findings suggest that autoreactivity is a feature of a healthy immune system. We could propose that under certain circumstances this provides the background on which clinical autoimmune disease may arise. The physiological role of such autoimmunity is unknown, although it has been suggested that autoantibodies remove the products of tissue breakdown (e.g. collagen by anti-collagen or DNA by anti-DNA antibodies) or that some may have a regulatory role (e.g. anti-cytokine antibodies).

Autoimmune disease could be considered to be one end of a spectrum of autoimmunity stretching from physiology to pathology — in other words a statistical event. However, the fact that autoreactivity does not lead to disease in the vast majority suggests that regulatory mechanisms are critical. This state of balanced, physiological autoimmunity may be described as **tolerance**. On this basis, autoimmune disease may be defined as a pathological process leading to the breakdown of self-tolerance.

IMMUNOLOGICAL TOLERANCE

Tolerance may be defined as the controlled inability to respond to antigens to which an individual has the potential for response. Tolerance is antigen specific and is achieved through deletion of lymphocytes (**clonal deletion**) or their functional inactivation (**clonal anergy**) or through a mechanism of controlling T lymphocyte help, a process which is also termed **suppression**. Although each of these mechanisms operate for T and B lymphocyte tolerance (Fig. 9.1), the main mechanisms for each cell type are probably different. Clonal deletion is predominant in T lymphocyte tolerance whilst anergy is the main mechanism for maintenance of B lymphocyte tolerance.

As we discussed above (see p. 105), tolerance may be induced centrally, in the primary lymphoid organs (thymus for T cell tolerance, bone marrow for B cells) or peripherally.

General features of tolerance include:

- dose dependent: 'large' and 'small' doses of antigen are potent inducers of tolerance

---

Type II interferons: Interferon-γ

Interferon-γ is a homodimer composed of subunits of approximately 25 kDa. It is released by CD4$^+$ T lymphocytes (both T_H1 and T_H0) and CD8$^+$ T lymphocytes, as well as by activated natural killer cells. The interferons are known for their anti-viral activity, and IFN-γ is no exception. In addition to these innate antiviral effects (similar to the type I interferons, see p. 70), IFN-γ has distinct immuno-logical roles.

First, IFN-γ is a potent activator of macrophages, inducing an increase in metabolic, phagocytic and killing activity (see p. 69). This role is an essential part of the response induced by T_H1-like lympho-cytes. Second, IFN-γ has the ability to increase MHC class I molecule expression on a range of cell types and induce expression of class II MHC mol-ecules on other cells, either alone or in concert with other cytokines (e.g. TNF). This may be an impor-tant component of antiviral protection, since it up-regulates presentation of viral targets by infected cells. Third, as a T_H1-cytokine, IFN-γ has profound effects on T cell development (favouring the devel-opment of T_H1 cells) and B cell differentiation (bias-ing the production of immunoglobulin in favour of IgG and away from IgE). IFN-γ is also required for the activation of CD8$^+$ cytotoxic T cells (another T_H1 function; see this page) and has a role in acti-vating natural killer cells.

---

the thymus expressing their specific TCR but cannot lyse target cells at this stage. In the periphery, when a cytotoxic response is required, the pre-CTLs are acti-vated by CD4$^+$ T lymphocytes, which are involved in an immune reaction complementary to that of the CTL. For example, a CD4$^+$ T_H lymphocyte is primed to respond to viral peptides after viral particles have been ingested and presented by macrophages at the site of infection. In turn, the activated T_H cells activate virus-specific CTLs (Fig. 7.19). The main cytokine signal is IL-2, but IFN-γ and IL-6 are also stimulators of CTLs. Activation of CTLs requires the typical two-signal activation process of presented antigen and co-signals. The requirement for IL-2 and IFN-γ indicates the importance of T_H1 cells in this process.

Following activation, the CTL must prepare the machinery required to lyse target cells. First, membrane-bound granules appear in the cytoplasm. The granules contain a membrane pore-forming protein called **perforin** or **cytolysin** (Fig. 7.19b). In addition, they contain proteolytic enzymes and protein toxins called **lymphotoxins** (note: these lymphotoxins are either identical to, or structurally related to, the cytokine lym-photoxin, or TNF-β, referred to previously; p. 70). Second, there is cytokine production and release: nota-bly IFN-γ, lymphotoxin (which has similar cytotoxic effects to TNF-α) and IL-2. Remember that IFN-γ, as the name implies, also has direct antiviral activity,

which may be of importance when a viral-infected cell is lysed and virions released.

What are the mechanisms of target cell lysis? (See box: 'Detection of cytotoxicity', p. 103.) First, we must define the ground rules. Obviously, killing by CD8$^+$ T cells will be MHC class I restricted. This suggests, and indeed it is the case, that killing requires cell–cell con-tact. Only those cells to which a CTL becomes at-tached are killed. There is no 'bystander' death, because the lytic molecules are released only at the site of TCR contact. Finally, CTLs are not themselves damaged during the process.

Lysis involves five steps.

1. **Cell contact** (involves TCR interaction with peptide–MHC class I complex and CD8 interaction with MHC, but other adhesion molecules such as the ICAMs and integrins can be involved).
2. **Activation** of the CTL (activation is first TCR mediated; the second signals necessary come from adhesion molecule interactions).
3. **Delivery of 'lethal hit'**. There are two ways by which target cells are killed. (a) CTLs release perforin, which polymerises in the presence of Ca^{2+} to form a hollow tube, analogous to the membrane attack complex of complement; in fact, C9 and perforin have a high degree of structural homology. If a sufficient number of pores are formed, the cell is killed by osmotic lysis. (b) CTLs release lymphotoxin, which activates enzymes in the target cell to cleave DNA in the nucleus. One of the earliest, characteristic appearances of this form of death is the presence of clumps of nuclear DNA, each of a small, uniform length. This is the consequence of the process of programmed cell death or apoptosis.
4. **Disengagement of CTL**. CTLs are protected from the action of their own granule contents, probably by having a high density of disassembling proteins on their surface (called **protectins**).
5. **Osmotic lysis or programmed cell death of target**.

Recent studies have uncovered an important pair of molecules involved in cell death, namely **Fas** (CD95) and its ligand **FasL**. FasL is expressed on CTLs; Fas is present on a range of different cell types in the immune system. When FasL on CTLs binds Fas on a target cell, apoptosis results. This mechanism of inducing cell death is known to be important in regulating develop-ment of immune cells (see p. 77), but it may also have a role in controlling some viral infections.

Immune suppression by T lymphocytes

In any physiological system, there is a key role for nega-tive regulation (i.e. suppression) of the actions of the cells involved, and the immune system is no exception. There are many good examples of experiments in which measurable immune responses by a population of cells are inhibited by a different population. One of

(a)

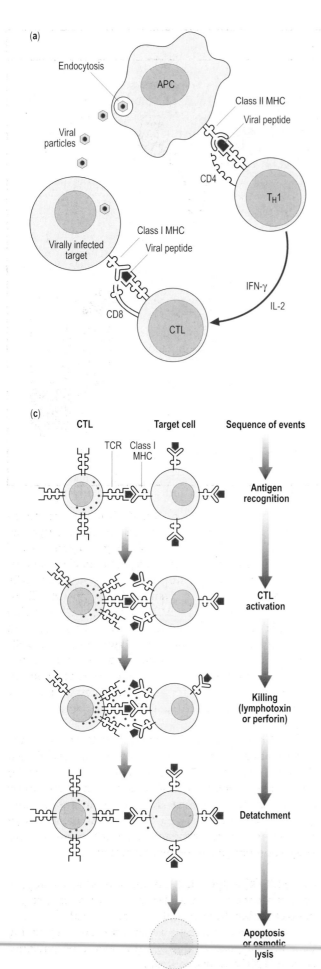

(b)

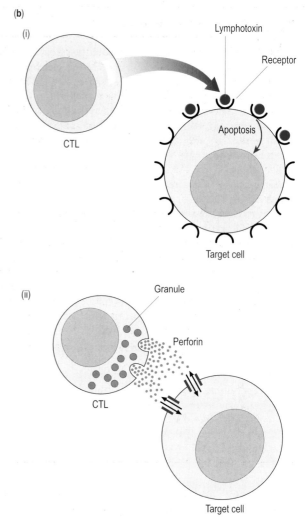

(c)

Fig. 7.19 **Models for activation of CTL responses by CD4+ T lymphocytes.** (**a**) Virus particles excreted from a virally infected cell are endocytosed by APCs and presented to T_H cells. These provide activation signals for CTLs that have TCR specificity for related viral peptides presented by class I MHC molecules on the target cell surface. (**b**) CTLs can kill target cells by (i) inducing suicide (apoptosis) through lymphotoxin release or (ii) forming pores in the target cell through perforin action. (**c**) The cell–cell interactions in CTL killing ensure no bystander cells are killed.

the most elegant ways in which such immune suppression can be demonstrated is by the transfer, from one experimental animal to another, of an inhibitory population of cells (Fig. 7.21, p. 104). In this example, one of the earliest systems to be studied intensively, suppression of antibody production is induced by the delivery of a very large dose of the antigen. The suppressive effect is transferable by whole populations of spleen cells and is clearly a form of cell-mediated regulation of an effector arm of the immune system, namely antibody production. Examples also exist of down-regulation of macrophage functions by the immune system and control of cytotoxicity. The identity of the mediators of suppression (i.e. whether there exists a

Detection of cytotoxicity

Cytotoxicity assays are useful research tools for examining specific lysis by CTLs and also killing by natural killer cells. The assay is based upon incubating together the effector cells and target cells and measuring damage to the targets. In the assessment of CTL activity, the appropriate HLA-matched target cell (e.g. a virus-infected cell from the same donor) must be used. To measure cytotoxicity by natural killer cells, the target used is a cell line known to be highly susceptible to natural killer action (e.g. the erythroleukaemia cell line K562).

Whether performing an assay of cytotoxicity mediated by CTLs or by natural killer cells the appropriate target cells are labelled by incubation with a solution of radioactive sodium chromate (^{51}Cr), which becomes incorporated into the cell cytoplasm (Fig. 7.20). The targets and effectors are then incubated together for 4–5 hours. If target cells are damaged by the effectors, ^{51}Cr is released from the cytoplasm into the culture fluid. Levels of radioactivity in the culture fluid are, therefore, proportional to the degree of target cell lysis.

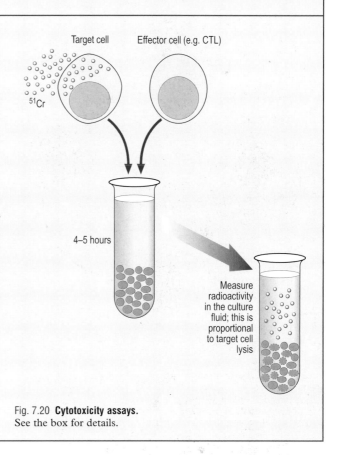

Fig. 7.20 **Cytotoxicity assays.** See the box for details.

---

true subset of 'suppressor' cells) remains an area of controversy and active research. However, in many of the systems studied, the cells responsible for the negative regulation are CD8$^+$ T lymphocytes, frequently relying on CD4$^+$ T cells for their maturation.

The demonstration of the mechanism by which cells of the immune system regulate the functions of other cells, and the nature of the regulatory cells, has proved difficult technically. However, it is possible to identify several ways in which T lymphocytes may suppress the function of another cell. These are: by the release of cytokines; by the release of soluble receptors; by direct cell–cell contact.

1. Soluble inhibitory factors (non-antigen specific). Suppression of certain types of immune response can be mediated by cytokines (Fig. 7.22). Examples of this include: transforming growth factor β (TGF-β; see box: 'Transforming growth factor-β'), which inhibits proliferation of T and B lymphocytes; IL-4 and IL-10, which have a mutually antagonistic relationship with IFN-γ (i.e. when IFN-γ-producing cells are dominant, IL-4 and IL-10 producing cells are down-regulated — see T$_H$1 and T$_H$2 subsets above). In other words, certain subsets of T cells are able to inhibit other populations by the release of cytokines.

2. The 'civil servant' model. A related mechanism of suppression is also proposed. In this, cells absorb T cell activation cytokines, such as IL-2, from the surrounding milieu, dampening down the immune response. This has given rise to the 'civil servant' hypothesis of suppression. In this theory, a rather harsh view is taken of civil servants: that they avidly and enthusiastically take up positions in the running of government offices, obstructing others who are actually trying to get the job done and consuming vital resources in the process. In the same way, these 'civil servant' type suppressor cells become involved in an immune response but do not contribute to the overall immune response and, in fact, obstruct its progress by consuming stimulatory cytokines such as IL-2 (Fig. 7.23).

3. Soluble inhibitory factors (antigen specific). In some experimental systems, it has been demonstrated that the suppressive effects of a population of T cells are (a) mediated by soluble, diffusible factors, and (b) can be antigen specific. This has led to the suggestion that secretion of soluble T cell receptor molecules could be a suppressive mechanism (Fig. 7.24). However, this suggestion remains to be demonstrated.

4. 'Cytotoxic' suppression. As we have seen already, T cells can lethally damage target cells through cell–cell contact. It has been postulated that sublethal damage to activated cells could be a mechanism of suppressing their action, possibly through the release of cytokines such as TNF and lymphotoxin.

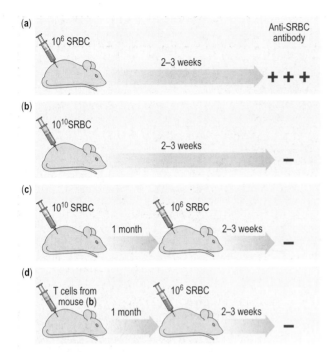

Fig. 7.21 **T lymphocyte-mediated suppression.**
(**a**) A mouse injected with 10^6 sheep red blood cells (SRBC) makes an appropriate antibody response, but a mouse given a much larger dose, 10^{10} SRBC (**b**), makes none. Thus supramaximal doses of antigen are capable of inducing suppression, which is specific for that antigen. (**c**) The suppressed response seen in (b) is maintained despite an additional appropriate stimulating dose of 10^6 SRBC. (**d**) T lymphocytes taken from a 'suppressed' mouse (e.g. the mouse in (b)) adoptively transfer the SRBC-specific suppression to a new recipient, which becomes incapable of responding to a stimulatory dose. This indicates that the suppressive effect is not the result of deletion of a population of T_H cells, but is caused by active suppression by the T lymphocyte population.

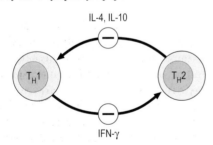

Fig. 7.22 **Soluble T cell suppressor mechanisms.**
Direct suppression by cytokines. T_H1 and T_H2 cytokines are mutually inhibitory.

Transforming growth factor-β

TGF-β is a cytokine with many different actions, and with actions that counter each other depending upon the culture conditions used. Lymphocytes and monocytes secrete predominantly the TGF-β_1 form of the molecule, which is 28 kDa in size, antagonises proliferation of T and B cells and inhibits the mononuclear-phagocyte system cell function. Overall, the effects of TGF-β are down-regulatory, and there has been great interest in harnessing this immunosuppressive effect for therapeutic purposes. Intriguingly, a mouse model in which the TGF-β_1 gene has been 'knocked out' using genetic engineering is characterised by uncontrolled inflammatory reactions.

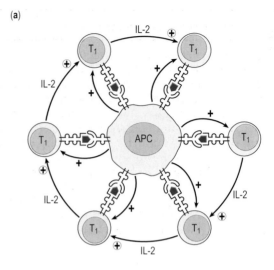

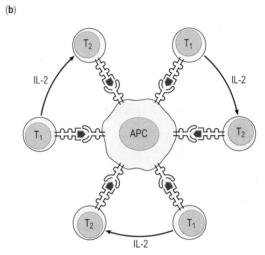

Fig. 7.23 **The 'civil servant' model of antigen-specific immune suppression.**
(**a**) Normal function. (**b**) In the presence of 'suppressing' cells. See text for details.

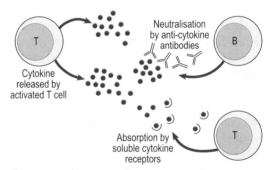

Fig. 7.24 **Suppression of T cells by soluble diffusible factors.**
Indirect suppression may occur through cytokine absorption or via neutralising antibodies. These effects are independent of the antigen inciting the immune response.

5. Idiotype/anti-idiotype-mediated suppression. One explanation for immune suppression is derived from the concept that the immune system exists as a series of networks. The principle relates to the hypothesis that, since each antigen has a unique conformation, the receptor binding to it (e.g. antibody, TCR) also has a

The idiotype/anti-idiotype network

The concept of an idiotype network, dependent upon antibody–anti-antibody interactions has many proponents (and many detractors, this being a controversial area). Experimentally it is possible to observe increases in anti-idiotypes of the type described (Fig. 7.25) after immunisation with antigen. On the basis of this, it has been proposed that the idiotype network could be exploited to generate vaccines. The vaccine (e.g. for a bacterium) would be given in the form of the idiotype that best resembles the bacterial antigen, and the anti-idiotype response would, therefore, also be anti-bacterial. So far, however, results of such research strategies are disappointing.

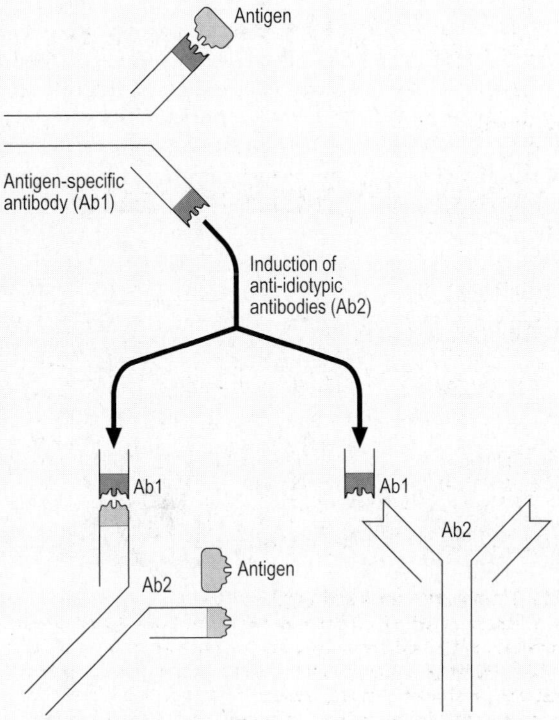

Fig. 7.25 **Production of idiotypes and anti-idiotypic antibodies.** The antigen-specific antibody, Ab1, has a binding site complementary to the shape of the antigen. Anti-idiotypic antibodies (Ab2) directed against Ab1 can either recognise the binding site itself, in which case they can influence antigen responsiveness, or recognise determinants outside the binding site of Ab1.

unique conformation. The antibody or TCR has a structure that is the mirror image of the antigen. If this is so, then the antibody or TCR should itself be immunogenic and capable of eliciting an immune response. This is much easier to view for antibodies than for the TCR. In the case of antibodies, the unique antigen-binding sites (idiotopes) are collectively termed the idiotype. The idiotype becomes the focus of an anti-idiotypic response. The anti-idiotype also has a unique set of idiotopes and can in turn become the target of an anti-anti-idiotype response. Taken to its logical conclusion, the idiotype/anti-idiotype responses form a stable network of interacting receptors (see box: 'The idiotype/anti-idiotype network'). When antigen is added to the network, say in the form of a bacterial toxin, the protective antibody type is expanded to neutralise it (following the general principle of homeostatic mechanisms to restore the equilibrium). This expansion provokes the anti-idiotype to be produced in greater quantities, and so on, until the balanced network is restored.

IMMUNOLOGICAL TOLERANCE

It can be assumed from the life cycles of B and T cells that the potential array of rearranged antigen receptors is vast. The possibility that lymphocytes with receptors

for self proteins do actually arise is a real one, which must be addressed. These receptors for self proteins give rise to the potential for 'autoreactivity': reactivity to self. Lymphocytes with an antigen receptor that could indeed be self-destructive ('*horror autoxicus*' as Ehrlich put it) must be weeded out or tightly controlled.

As we have seen, the immune system is empowered with (1) potentially lethal effector mechanisms and (2) the capacity to develop a sufficient array of receptors to be capable of self-recognition. Yet there is no self-destruction in the vast majority of people! When it does occur, and **autoimmune disease** results, the consequences may be life threatening (it is estimated that 5% of the population have an autoimmune disease during their life). Clearly, the *potential* for response to self is balanced for the most part by an *inability* to respond to self. This state is one of **immunological tolerance** (see box: 'The discovery of immunological tolerance'). It can be likened to living within a community and having a next-door neighbour with a penchant for playing loud rock and roll music every now and then. Rather than make a fuss, which would endanger our relationship with the neighbour, and perhaps on a larger scale damage the community, many of us would tolerate the noise. We have the capacity to respond, but we choose not to. The immune system has the capacity for self-recognition, but for the most part avoids it. How is

The discovery of immunological tolerance

The discovery of the existence of immunological tolerance is credited to Burnet and Medawar, who were awarded the Nobel Prize in 1960 for their contribution. Medawar had become interested in graft rejection during treatment of severe burns in airmen during World War II: skin grafts from distant sites on the same patient usually took, but foreign grafts did not. The key study of Medawar and Burnet was based around the phenomenon of rejection of allogenic (i.e. non-self) skin grafts by mice, which they noted to be associated with heavy lymphocytic infiltration. Injection of allogenic bone marrow cells into the mice at the neonatal stage did not impair general immunity, but when the mice became more mature, they now failed to reject skin grafts from the marrow donors (Fig. 7.26). They had acquired immunological tolerance to the antigens in the skin graft against which the lymphocytic response was raised. The same manoeuvre of bone marrow injection applied to adult mice had no tolerising effect. The importance of the work lay in the demonstration that tolerance to foreign antigens could be achieved, even though the route of neonatal injection was unlikely to become of use in human organ transplantation.

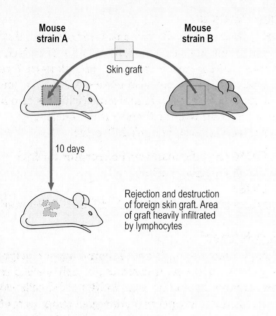

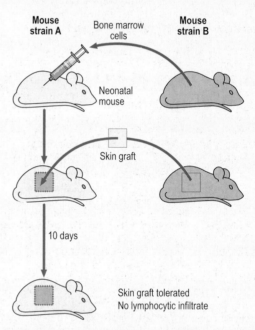

Fig. 7.26 **Induction of immunological tolerance to foreign skin grafts by injection of bone marrow cells into neonates.**

control exercised over individual T and B lymphocytes that may have unwanted specificities for self? There are probably at least three mechanisms for the control of such unwanted clones of cells: **clonal anergy**, or unresponsiveness; **clonal deletion**; and the tight **control of T lymphocyte help**. In clonal anergy, autoreactive lymphocytes remain present but are functionally inactivated and become unresponsive. In clonal deletion, the cells are actually killed. In the control of T cell help, unwanted lymphocyte reactions are held in check by suppressor mechanisms.

Immunological tolerance can be defined as a *specific failure of immune responsiveness, resulting from a prior exposure to antigen*. The term 'specific' relates to the fact that tolerance induced to one antigen does not apply to another. The immune system is essentially intact and healthy, although not responsive to particular antigen(s). The term describing a state of 'immunological tolerance' is generally reserved for the immune system of an organism, rather than a specific cell.

From a clinical viewpoint, there are several disease states in which an understanding of immunological tolerance is of considerable importance. Induction of tolerance to foreign tissue is the goal of the transplant surgeon; reversal of a state of tolerance is desired in some parasitic infections and certain forms of metastatic cancer, when the immune system has become unresponsive to the tumour; in contrast, a return to a state of self-tolerance is the main aim of therapy for autoimmune diseases.

The fact that tolerance induction in a relatively immature lymphoid system is achieved with ease implies that it is dependent upon events in the primary lymphoid organs (the thymus and bone marrow), where the potential responder cells are being generated, and to a large extent this speculation has been borne out for both B and T lymphocytes. This is termed **central tolerance**. The fact that under certain conditions allogenic organ grafts undertaken during adult life can survive for many years is indicative of the fact that a post-thymic form of tolerance also exists, and this is termed **peripheral tolerance**.

The mechanisms of immune tolerance are several and complex. Understanding these processes is particularly important in the investigation of autoimmune diseases. These can be defined as arising from a breakdown of self-tolerance mechanisms, the result of which is often serious and life threatening. Since immunological tolerance is most relevant to these disorders, the mechanisms of tolerance induction, and their breakdown, will be discussed together in Chapter 9.

Lymphocyte activation and sequelae

- Lymphocyte activation requires at least two signals: antigen plus a co-signal. For T cells, CD4, CD8, CD45, adhesion molecules, and co-stimulatory molecules such as CD28 provide the co-signals. For B cells, CD22, CD40, CD19, CD20, and CD45 have the same role.
- To be effective, the signal must be transduced and amplified within the lymphocyte by a series of reactions.
- Once in the periphery, T cells are the pivotal cells in immune responses. Through cell–cell contact and the secretion of a range of powerful cytokines, they activate and promote the growth of other T cells, B cells, monocytes and granulocytes.
- The CD4$^+$ T helper cell subset is divided into T_H1 and T_H2 types, with different functions, according to the cytokines they secrete.
- Cytotoxic T cells (CTLs) kill target cells expressing a specific antigen by inducing cell lysis or apoptosis.
- The potential danger of autoreactive lymphocytes giving rise to autoimmune disease, is avoided: this lack of response to self is termed tolerance, and several mechanisms of tolerance induction exist.

NATURAL KILLER CELLS

Natural killer (NK) cells are the third members (after B and T lymphocytes) of the cell populations typically termed lymphoid, on the basis of their similar morphology, distribution and function. The name is derived from two features. Unlike B and T lymphocytes, NK cells are able to mediate their effector function (i.e. *killing* of target cells) *spontaneously* in the absence of previous known sensitisation to that target. Hence the terms '*killer*' and '*natural*' were coined, without any real understanding of how or why these cells function. NK cells can be identified by incubation with certain types of target cell in a cytotoxicity assay (see box above). The target cells chosen for use in the assay are particularly susceptible to NK-type killing and include certain types of tumour cell.

In morphological terms, NK cells are larger than typical T and B lymphocytes and have azurophilic cytoplasmic granules, leading to the widespread use of the complementary term **large granular lymphocytes**

or LGLs. Much interest recently has focused on how these cells recognise their targets, since none of the conventional antigen receptors typical of T or B lymphocytes are present. Therefore, a current, more acceptable working definition of an NK cell is 'a cytotoxic cell that has the morphology of an LGL but does not express the CD3 complex or any of the known T cell receptor chains'.

In physiological terms, there are two major roles for NK cells: (1) immune surveillance against tumour cells and virus-infected cells; (2) the release of cytokines (mainly IFN-γ) early in infection to activate phagocytic cells and recruit T lymphocytes.

Identification

NK cells carry two distinct surface molecules: the third receptor for the Fc portion of IgG (FcγRIII; also termed CD16) and a molecule of unknown function (CD56). NK cells may also possess CD57, an unusual cell surface carbohydrate molecule (which is also found on some other lymphoid and myeloid cells).

Markers used to identify NK cells:

- **CD16** (specific marker): Fc receptor for IgG
- **CD56** (specific marker)
- **CD57**
- NK cells do *not* carry CD3, the pan-T cell marker.

Development

Commitment to the B and T lymphocyte lineage may be defined as the rearrangement of cell surface receptors (immunoglobulins and TCRs); NK cells do not rearrange these receptors. Although a major part of NK cell development probably takes place in the thymus, NK cells can also undergo maturation under experimental conditions in which the thymus is removed. At present, most of the information on the origin of NK cells is derived from studies in rodents, but some supportive studies have been performed in humans, with the help of cardiothoracic surgeons. For example, a population of lymphoid cells has been identified in the mouse thymus at 15 days of gestation which expresses FcγRIII but not CD4, CD8 or the TCR. When removed from the thymus, such cells are able to differentiate into mature NK cells. In the human studies, thymocytes were obtained during cardiac surgery from children as young as 2 months of age. When cultured with high levels of IL-2 in the absence of any endogenous support cells, the lymphoid cells differentiated into CD16$^+$ NK cells. Similar populations can also be derived from fetal liver.

FUNCTION OF NK CELLS

Activation

Activation of NK cells to kill target cells can be divided into two processes: achievement of an 'activated state' induced by cytokines; and activation for lysis induced by cell–cell contact.

(a)

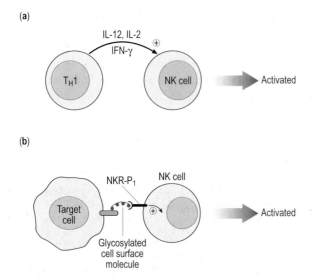

(b)

Fig. 7.27 **Activation of NK cells.**
(**a**) The first stage is mediated by cytokines. (**b**) The second stage is NK–target cell contact. NKR-P1, a lectin that interacts with surface carbohydrate.

(a)

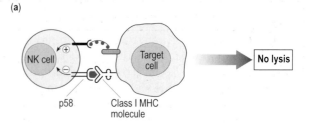

(b)

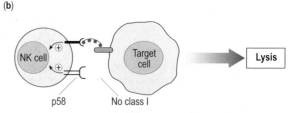

Fig. 7.28 **Target cell recognition by NK cells: the signal to kill.**
(**a**) In this interaction, a positive signal is delivered by the binding of the lectin-like molecule NKR-P1 to a carbohydrate moiety on the potential target cell. The negative signal from the p58–class I MHC molecule interaction over-rides this, and there is no lysis. (**b**) A tumour cell not expressing class I molecules, or expressing abnormal forms of them, is lysed by the NK cell. Certain viruses down-regulate MHC class I molecule expression: this may avoid killing by CTLs, but NK cells can then kill the target cell, providing a 'fail-safe' mechanism.

IFN-γ, IL-2 and IL-12 are the main cytokines responsible for general activation of NK cells, and they may act synergistically. IFN-γ increases adherence of NK cells to targets and increasing the rate of lysis. IL-2 is able clonally to expand NK cells and enhance their cytotoxic activity. IL-12 is a recently described cytokine that has, as a single molecule, the most potent action in activating NK cells, with a strong synergism in the presence of IL-2.

The question of what signals are important to induce NK cells that have bound their target to actually kill is still being examined (Fig. 7.27). Early research in mice indicated that killing by NK cells could be affected by addition of certain carbohydrates, or by addition of a monoclonal antibody to a lectin-like receptor on the NK cell surface, termed NK receptor-P1 (NKR-P1) (remember, lectins bind carbohydrates). These findings are interpreted as indicating that the 'kill' signal for NK cells requires interaction of NKR-P1 with certain carbohydrates on the target cell surface. This is of interest, since cell surface proteins on tumour cells (an example of a cell type targeted by NK cells) are frequently abnormally glycosylated. Once activated, NK cells would appear to lyse target cells using similar mechanisms to those described for cytotoxic T cells (p. 102).

Target cell recognition by NK cells

The NK cell has two major recognition pathways for identifying targets for killing. One form is restricted to NK cells and has a complex mechanism that is still being fully elucidated (Fig. 7.28). One of the early identifiable characteristics of NK cells was their tendency to lyse target cells *not* expressing MHC class I molecules (in direct contrast to CTLs, which require class I MHC molecule expression on target cells). One suggestion was that NK cells might actually be inhib-

ited in the presence of endogenous class I MHC molecules. Recent evidence supports this contention, with the demonstration of NK receptors that bind class I MHC molecules (see box: 'NK cell recognition of MHC molecules'). The absence of class I MHC molecules is a major signal to induce NK cell killing. The opposing requirements for NK cells and CTLs with respect to class I MHC molecule expression could be physiologically important. Viruses can down-regulate class I MHC expression and thus evade recognition by CTLs, but this avoidance would be countered by the activity of NK cells, which would lyse targets not expressing class I MHC molecules, providing a fail-safe system.

The other form of killing of which NK cells are capable can also be carried out by other cell types. Cells to be lysed are targeted by the binding of IgG antibody molecules, and the NK cell is recruited through the binding of the IgG Fc receptor to the FcγRIII (Fig. 7.29). This mechanism is termed **antibody-dependent cellular cytotoxicity** (ADCC), and since the FcγRIII is present on other lymphoid cells (often termed killer (K) cells), it is not restricted as a mechanism to NK cells (it also requires prior sensitisation to produce the specific IgG and is, therefore, not a 'natural' killing process).

The main role of NK cells is lysis of cells such as tumours and virus-infected cells. The NK cell makes use of families of receptors designed to interact with the major types of class I MHC molecule. Recognition that a cell requires killing is achieved in the *absence* of a normal class I MHC molecule. Killing is initiated when a lectin-type surface receptor binds carbohydrate moieties on the target cell surface.

NK cell recognition of MHC molecules

The mechanism described in the main text, by which NK cells recognise whether or not a potential target cell has class I MHC molecules present, requires a receptor molecule capable of recognising class I MHC. Seeking the NK receptor has been a major research goal, with some important recent results. Receptors have been identified, and their genes cloned, that are capable of interacting with class I MHC molecules and inhibiting NK cell lysis (Fig. 7.28). The first family of molecules, at present termed p58 and defined in humans, are typically 55–58 kDa and may function as homo- or heterodimers. The p58 family interacts specifically with HLA-C class I molecules. The p58 molecule binds to a region near the α_1/α_2 domains of the class I MHC molecule, which is actually near the location of the peptide antigen-binding groove. As an example of the experimental evidence, NK cell clones bearing the p58 molecules are typically unable to lyse target tumour cells expressing a particular HLA-C class I molecule, but lysis follows addition of monoclonal antibodies to block p58. Another similar family of receptors, of 70 kDa molecular mass, has been identified more recently, and this interacts in an identical fashion with HLA-B class I molecules. The nomenclature for the NK receptors for class I MHC molecules has yet to be formalised, but will probably describe families of receptors for the different major types of class I MHC molecule (NKB1, NKC1, etc.).

as neutrophils (GM-CSF) and macrophages (IFN-γ) and also providing strong signals to bias T cells towards a T_H1 response. The same cytokines also up-regulate local expression of adhesion molecules and accessory molecules, thus providing the early basis for an effective immune response (Fig. 7.30).

Natural killer cells

- Natural killer cells are a small population of cells that resemble lymphocytes morphologically but form a separate lineage from T and B cells.
- NK cells kill tumour cells and virally infected cells without the need for prior sensitisation.
- NK cells secrete cytokines (mainly IFN-γ), which promote a cellular immune respone, activating phagocytic cells and recruiting T cells.
- NK cells are activated by the cytokines IFN-γ, IL-2 and IL-12, and have two mechanisms of killing targets. In one, target cells are bound by IgG antibody, for which the NK cell has a receptor. In the second, cell–cell contact with the target is required, during which a receptor for class I MHC molecules and one for carbohydrates are involved.

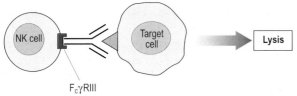

Fig. 7.29 **Antibody-dependent cellular toxicity (ADCC).** Mechanism of killing employed by NK cells and other cell types, such as killer (K) cells, bearing CD16, the FcγRIII. Antibody targets the cell, and cellular cytotoxicity follows after engagement of the CD16$^+$ effector cell.

The immune functions of NK cells

In immune surveillance, NK cells have the ability to identify and lyse a range of target cells that display (by the absence of normal class I MHC molecules) either (1) the presence of an intracellular viral infection, or (2) a neoplastic process. To do so does not require previous activation of the NK cell. During the recognition process, NK cells secrete a number of pro-inflammatory cytokines, mainly IFN-γ and GM-CSF. These cytokines, which have the effect of promoting a cellular immune response, activating phagocytes such

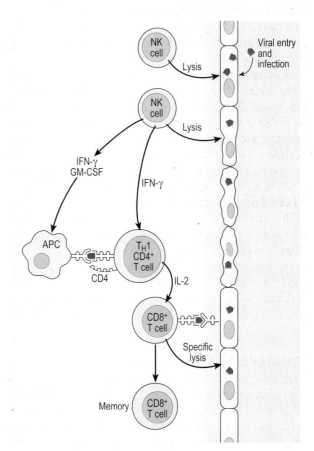

Fig. 7.30 **The role of NK cells in the immune response.**

CHAPTER 8

The immune response to microbes: an overview

The analogy between the players in the immune system and those in an orchestra has already been drawn in an earlier chapter. The orchestra is best appreciated, and the music best understood, when all of the instruments play and are heard together. It is likewise with the components of the immune system. Learning that IL-8 attracts neutrophils, for example, or that LFA-1 interacts with ICAM-1, does not give a full idea of how a pyogenic bacterium is identified and killed.

In this section, the balance of such excessive reductionism is redressed. The immune system is viewed acting in concert, from the moment of entry of a microbe, through to its eradication and the creation of a bank of memory cells equipped for any future encounter. The overview is necessarily general, but each figure panel is accompanied by cross-referencing, so that greater detail can be found if required.

Primary viral infection

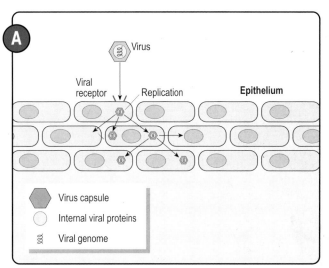

Virus infects epithelial cells and replicates amongst them.

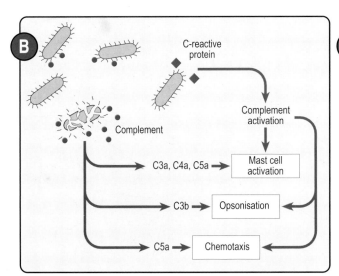

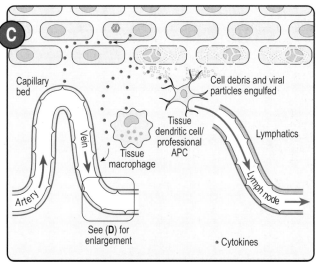

Effect of intracellular viral infection is the activation of cytokine and cytokine-receptor genes (e.g. IFN-α). Secretion of IFN-α involves autocrine feedback loop. Local effects of IFN-α are inhibition of viral gene replication, and upregulation of MHC class I molecules. Viral peptides will appear in the MHC class I peptide-binding groove. See *IFN-α*, p. 70.

Viral infection results in cell death and viral replication. Locally released cytokines activate macrophages and professional antigen-presenting cells (APCs). These engulf and present viral proteins as well as cellular debris. Some professional APCs (e.g. tissue dendritic cells such as Langerhans cells in the skin) transport antigen to local lymph nodes via lymphatics. See *Macrophages*, p. 68; *Dendritic cells*, p. 71; *Antigen presentation*, p. 86.

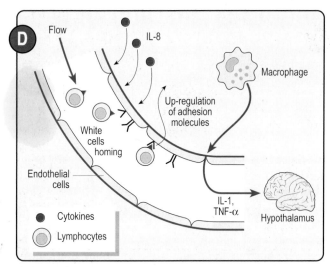

Cytokines up-regulate endothelial cell expression of adhesion molecules such as ICAM-1. Local cytokines with chemotactic activity (e.g. IL-8) are also present. Some locally released cytokines from cells such as macrophages (e.g. IL-1, TNF-α) enter blood-stream and have systemic effects of fever and arthralgia/myalgia. See *Cell adhesion molecules*, p. 24; *IL-1*, p. 69; *TNF-α*, p. 70.

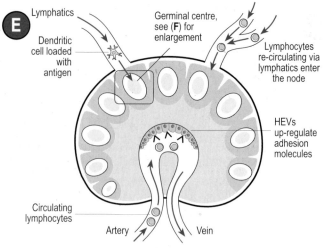

Antigen-presenting cell enters local lymph nodes, and moves to germinal centre. Local inflammation leads to up-regulation of adhesion molecules on high endothelial venules of lymph node, and lymphocytes enter directly from the blood. Circulating lymphocytes in the lymphatics also enter. Many lymphocytes become trapped in the local inflamed node, and the consequent swelling, along with local hyperaemia, leads to the symptom of swollen painful/tender lymph nodes. See *Lymphocyte circulation*, p. 5.

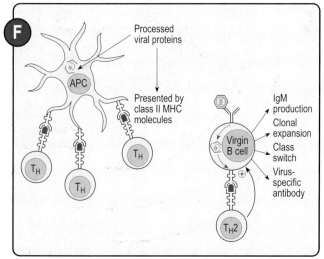

Dendritic cells and other APCs are surrounded in the lymph node germinal centre by T$_H$ cells, where presentation of viral peptides takes place. T$_H$ cells possessing TCRs complementary to the class II MHC molecule/viral peptide complex are activated. Virgin B cells, acquiring viral particles through attachment to surface IgM or IgD, process and present viral peptides to T$_H$2 cells, and in turn receive positive growth and differentiation signals. IgM anti-viral antibody is produced as a result (primary antibody response) whilst some B cells differentiate and class switch, leading later to production of high affinity anti-viral IgG (secondary antibody response). See *Antigen presentation*, p. 86; *B-cell activation*, p. 76.

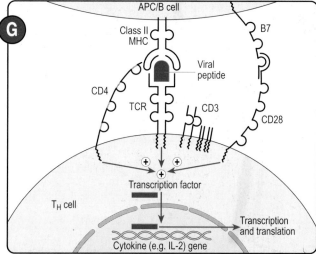

A viral peptide is presented by class II MHC molecules to a complementary TCR on a T$_H$ cell. The interaction is stabilised by CD4/class II MHC and B7/CD28 linkages, which also provide co-stimulatory signals to the T$_H$ cell. See *T-cell activation*, p. 86; *Co-stimulation*, p. 94.

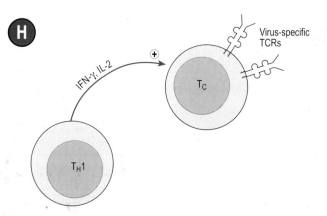

T$_H$1 cells recruit and activate virus-specific T$_C$ cells. See *T activation*, p. 101.

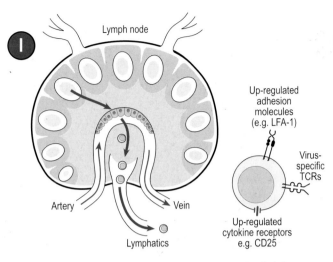

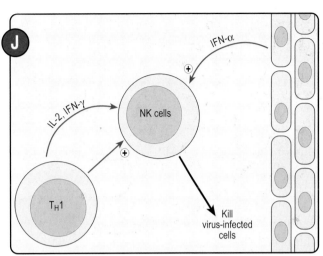

T_H and T_C lymphocytes leave the lymph node via the draining lymphatics towards other lymph nodes, and ultimately enter the blood. At this stage their key attributes are: **1.** virus-specific TCRs; **2.** up-regulated adhesion molecules, to allow migration into the inflamed tissues; **3.** up-regulated cytokine receptors to allow maintenance of cell activation. The up-regulated molecules act as markers of cell activation.

NK cells may be recruited at two points at least during the virus infection. They may have an early, innate anti-viral role following activation by epithelium-derived cytokines. Alternatively, at a later stage they are activated by T_H1 cells specific for the virus. See *NK cells*, p. 107.

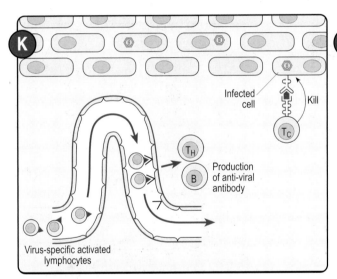

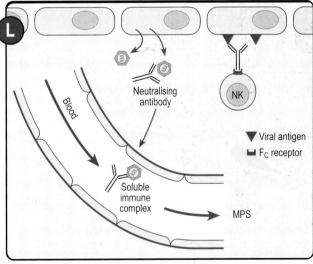

Activated cytotoxic T cells kill virally infected cells. Local T_H1 and T_H2 cells now organise the local anti-viral immune response. See *Cytotoxic reaction*, p. 100.

Virus-infected cells secrete and express viral proteins. These may be neutralised or removed by antibody in the form of immune complexes, which are cleared by the mononuclear phagocyte system (MPS), or antibody may be used to guide Fc receptor-expressing NK cells.

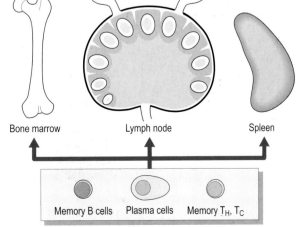

After resolution of the infection, virus-specific memory T and B cells reside long term in lymph nodes, spleen and bone marrow. Plasma cells ensure long-term circulation of protective, virus-neutralising antibody.

Primary bacterial infection

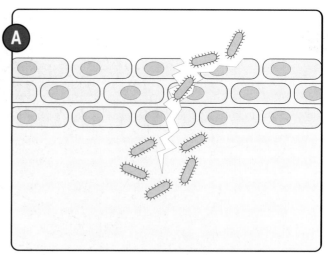

Break in epithelial surface allows bacterial entry and proliferation.

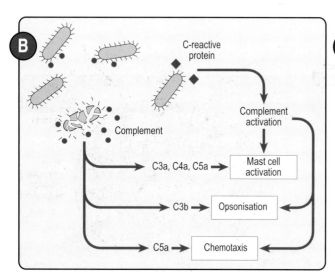

Surface lipopolysaccharide may activate the alternative complement pathway, leading to bacterial lysis. Other complement activators operating at this stage include C-reactive protein, which binds bacterial coat polysaccharides. See *Complement*, p. 10; *Opsonisation*, p. 16; *Chemotaxis*, see p. 18.

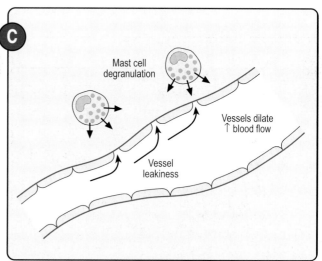

Mast cell degranulation enhances blood flow. The increased blood flow and local oedema are perceived as itchiness and irritation in the inflamed area. See *Mast cell*, pp. 30, 32.

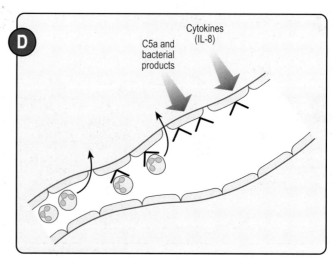

Rolling, marginating neutrophils adhere to the vein wall as locally-released cytokines and bacterial-derived molecules (e.g. endotoxin) activate both the endothelium and the neutrophils, resulting in adhesion between the two. See *Neutrophil adhesion*, pp. 22, 26.

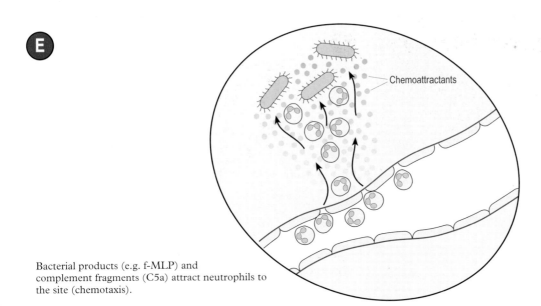

Bacterial products (e.g. f-MLP) and complement fragments (C5a) attract neutrophils to the site (chemotaxis).

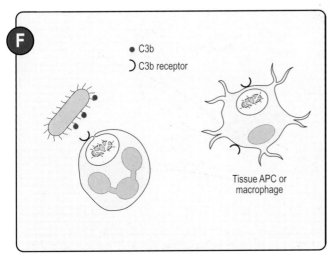

Opsonised bacteria are rapidly engulfed and killed by neutrophils. Tissue APCs also engulf bacteria, for presentation to T cells.

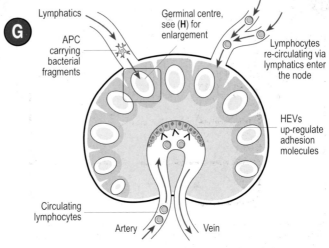

Bacterial antigens are processed and presented in local lymph nodes.

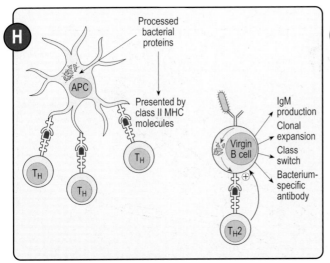

T$_H$ cells are recruited and activated by professional APCs in the lymph node, and by B cells, promoting the production of bacteria-specific antibodies. Initially, IgM class antibody is produced, followed by clonal expansion and switching to other classes. See *B-cell activation*, p. 76.

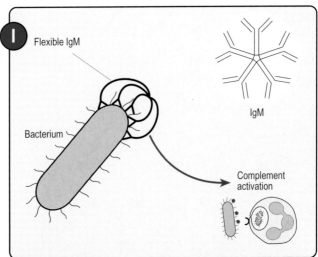

Early antibacterial antibody production is of the IgM class. This relatively low affinity interaction is enhanced by the five adhesion sites on IgM, leading to higher efficiency of binding. IgM is a very potent complement activator and opsonin. Opsonised bacteria are engulfed by phagocytes and lysed by complement. See *IgM*, p. 40.

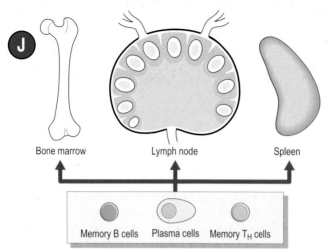

Following the resolution of the bacterial infection, protective mechanisms for future encounters are put in place by the lying down of memory cells.

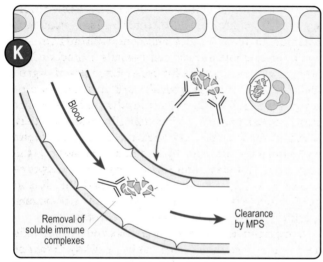

In the resolution of an infection, bacterial debris is removed by local neutrophils, or by antibody as soluble immune complexes, for clearance by the mononuclear phagocyte system (MPS) in the spleen and liver.

CHAPTER 9

Tolerance and mechanisms of autoimmunity

AUTOIMMUNITY

Autoimmune disease, in which an immune response to apparently healthy self components is mounted resulting in morbidity or mortality, is a relatively common occurrence, affecting between 1 and 5% of individuals at some time during their life. Autoimmunity — that is evidence of an immune reaction to self components in the absence of overt disease — is much more common. Indeed, all of us probably have the capacity to mount autoimmune responses, and in some circumstances this may be a healthy, physiological reaction. This spectrum, from autoimmune potential, through physiological autoimmunity to pathological autoreactions holds the key to our understanding of the role of the immune system in many disorders (Table 9.1). Currently, such

Table 9.1 Spectrum of autoimmune responses

Level of response	Characteristics
Autoimmune potential	Ubiquitous; reflects T and B cell receptor diversity; healthy response
Physiological autoimmunity	Sporadic; relates to transient tissue damage; may have homeostatic role
Pathological autoimmunity	Rare (5%); result of complex interactions of genetic and environmental factors

knowledge is being applied to devise immune-based therapies that will cure autoimmune diseases.

Autoimmunity is frequently categorised according to the nature of the target tissues. Some autoimmunity is directed against particular cells in an organ: examples include the insulin-producing β cells of the islets of Langerhans in the pancreas, and the thyroxine-secreting cells in the thyroid. The autoimmune reactions are usually directed against one or more specific cytoplasmic constituents, plasma-membrane structures or secreted products of the cell. This is termed **organ-specific** autoimmunity. In contrast, **non-organ-specific** autoimmunity is directed against structures common to many tissues and found throughout the body: for example nuclear components, mitochondrial proteins or constituents of muscle. Examples of organ-specific and non-organ-specific autoimmune diseases are given in Table 9.2. Some disorders fall in the grey area between the two designations. In primary biliary cirrhosis, for example, although the liver is the organ predominantly affected by autoimmune attack, the ubiquitous mitochondrial enzyme pyruvate dehydrogenase is a target of autoantibodies, and the disease itself often involves manifestations of non-organ-specific disease, notably Sjögren's syndrome.

In organ-specific autoimmune diseases, target cells are frequently damaged irreparably, resulting in loss of endocrine secretions, such as insulin in type 1 diabetes, thyroxine in autoimmune thryoiditis, and adrenocorticosteroid hormones in Addison's disease due to autoimmune adrenocortical insufficiency. In non-organ-specific autoimmune diseases, damage may be widespread, often including the articular joints (rheumatoid arthritis). In other non-organ-specific disorders, small blood vessels may become inflamed (vasculitis) leading to damage to vital organs such as the eyes and kidney.

AUTOREACTIVITY — NORMAL OR ABNORMAL?

Immune recognition of specific antigens is mediated through receptors: immunoglobulin on the B lymphocyte surface and the T cell receptor on T lymphocytes. In order to engender sufficient variety in the immune response to target all possible antigen conformations, both these receptor types are generated in a process ensuring maximum diversity. This is achieved by use of a relatively small number of genes that recombine randomly (see Ch. 4). An obvious consequence of this variety of receptors is the capacity to recognise all

Table 9.2 **The spectrum of autoimmune diseases, from organ-specific to non-organ-specific and the autoantigens typically targeted**

Disease	Main autoantigens targeted
Organ specific	
Myasthenia gravis	Acetylcholine receptor
Graves' disease	Thyroid-stimulating hormone receptor
Hashimoto's thyroiditis	Thyroid peroxidase; thyroglobulin
Type 1 diabetes	Islet cell cytoplasmic targets; insulin; glutamic acid decarboxylase
Pernicious anaemia	H^+K^+ ATPase (gastric proton pump); intrinsic factor
Addison's disease	17α-hydroxylase
Pemphigus	130 kDa member of cadherin adhesion molecules
Bullous pemphigoid	180 kDa hemidesmosomal cell adhesion structure; 230 kDa cell adhesion structure
Vitiligo	Melanocyte cytoplasmic targets
Autoimmune hepatitis	Asialoglycoprotein receptor; cytochrome P4502D6
Autoimmune haemolytic anaemia	Red blood cell surface targets
Overlap between organ- and non-organ-specific diseases	
Primary biliary cirrhosis	Mitochondrial pyruvate dehydrogenase
Goodpasture's syndrome	Non-collagenous domain of type IV collagen in renal and lung basement membrane
Non-organ-specific diseases	
Rheumatoid arthritis	IgG
Systemic lupus erythematosus	Double-stranded DNA; Sm (small nuclear ribonucleoproteins); SS-A (Ro; a 60 kDa ribonucleoprotein); SS-B (La; a 47 kDa ribonucleoprotein); histones
Sjögren's syndrome	SS-A, SS-B
Systemic sclerosis	DNA topoisomerase I; centromere
Mixed connective tissue disease	70 kDa small nuclear ribonucleoprotein
Polymyositis	tRNA synthetase

host as well as foreign antigens. Is this capacity translated into the production of autoreactive T and B lymphocytes?

One approach to answering this question is to generate **clones**. As the name implies, these are the offspring of a single cell, and, therefore, all share the same antigen receptor. This makes it easier to manipulate experimental conditions. The other advantage of cloning techniques is that they generate several million daughter cells, the sort of number required for studying cell function in vitro. Human B cell clones may be derived by fusion of human B cells to a mouse hybridoma (see Ch. 4) or by infection with Epstein–Barr virus. These immortalised B lymphocyte clones produce monoclonal antibodies, up to one third of which have been shown to react with self antigens. This is not simply an in vitro artefact; similar antibodies can be detected in normal human sera. The range of antigens recognised includes actin, DNA, collagen, albumin, IgG, IL-1α, TNF-α, insulin and thyroglobulin.

T cell autoreactivity is a less well-studied phenomenon. Undoubtedly, T lymphocytes reactive with self proteins may be found in the healthy adult human immune system but their frequency is low and T cells that recognise ubiquitous circulatory proteins such as albumin and γ-globulin have not been detected.

These findings suggest that autoreactivity is a feature of a healthy immune system. We could propose that under certain circumstances this provides the background on which clinical autoimmune disease may arise. The physiological role of such autoimmunity is unknown, although it has been suggested that autoantibodies remove the products of tissue breakdown (e.g. collagen by anti-collagen or DNA by anti-DNA antibodies) or that some may have a regulatory role (e.g. anti-cytokine antibodies).

Autoimmune disease could be considered to be one end of a spectrum of autoimmunity stretching from physiology to pathology — in other words a statistical event. However, the fact that autoreactivity does not lead to disease in the vast majority suggests that regulatory mechanisms are critical. This state of balanced, physiological autoimmunity may be described as **tolerance**. On this basis, autoimmune disease may be defined as a pathological process leading to the breakdown of self-tolerance.

IMMUNOLOGICAL TOLERANCE

Tolerance may be defined as the controlled inability to respond to antigens to which an individual has the potential for response. Tolerance is antigen specific and is achieved through deletion of lymphocytes (**clonal deletion**) or their functional inactivation (**clonal anergy**) or through a mechanism of controlling T lymphocyte help, a process which is also termed **suppression**. Although each of these mechanisms operate for T and B lymphocyte tolerance (Fig. 9.1), the main mechanisms for each cell type are probably different. Clonal deletion is predominant in T lymphocyte tolerance whilst anergy is the main mechanism for maintenance of B lymphocyte tolerance.

As we discussed above (see p. 105), tolerance may be induced centrally, in the primary lymphoid organs (thymus for T cell tolerance, bone marrow for B cells) or peripherally.

General features of tolerance include:

- dose dependent: 'large' and 'small' doses of antigen are potent inducers of tolerance

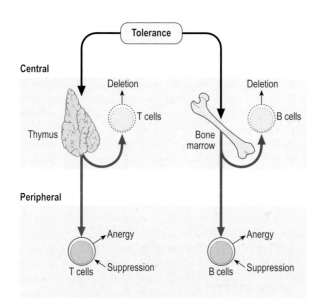

Fig. 9.1 **Sites of lymphocyte tolerance.**

- site dependent: antigens ingested orally are more likely to induce tolerance
- delivery dependent: antigen in the absence of co-signals results in anergy.

MECHANISMS OF CENTRAL TOLERANCE

T lymphocytes

The site for central tolerance induction for T lymphocytes is the thymus. We have already discussed the putative mechanism involved, namely negative thymic selection. During this process, T cells with too high an affinity for the complex of self MHC molecule bearing self peptide are deleted. Such a process is termed clonal deletion, since those clones of T cells with 'dangerous' anti-self T cell receptors are deleted and are not found in the periphery.

Clonal deletion cannot be the full explanation for T cell tolerance to self antigens, since it implies that all self proteins will be present for selection purposes within the thymus, which cannot be the case. Some T lymphocytes, therefore, could be positively selected in the thymus for having a low-affinity interaction with self MHC but arrive in the periphery and encounter a different MHC–self peptide complex for which they actually have a high enough affinity to become activated. There must be a mechanism(s) of maintaining peripheral tolerance (see below), therefore, to control T or B cells with potential autoreactivity.

B lymphocytes

The concept that clonal deletion is important in the control of B lymphocyte tolerance has been prominent for much longer than it has in the T cell arena, since it has been possible to study B cell receptors for longer. One of the earliest experiments, in 1967, remains a convincing example (Fig. 9.2). It involved the radio-iodination of an antigen (to facilitate detection), for example from a common bacterial protein, which was

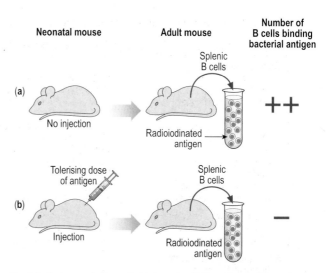

Fig. 9.2 **To demonstrate central tolerance of B lymphocytes through clonal deletion.**
Mouse (**a**) demonstrates that by adulthood, it has acquired a measurable number of B cells with sIg specific for a particular, common bacterial antigen (which has been radioiodinated for detection purposes). Mouse (**b**) is given a large dose of the antigen at an early age, a manoeuvre that typically tolerises the animal to the antigen. The experiment carried out in the adult mouse (**b**) shows that the mechanism of tolerance was clonal deletion of B cells specific for that antigen.

then incubated with splenic B cells from healthy adult mice. A small but measurable number of the B cells were positive for the radioiodine–antigen complex, indicating that they had sIg specific for the antigen. Next, a fresh group of mice, this time only days old, were injected with large, tolerising doses of the antigen. As adults, these mice had virtually no B cells capable of binding the radioiodinated antigen, indicating that they had been removed during the tolerisation process. We have already seen that B cell development involves a considerable amount of apoptotic death in the bone marrow (see p. 77) and it is likely that this is the result of clonal deletion.

In addition to clonal deletion, another mechanism of B cell tolerance exists. In experiments similar to those described above, an antibody to surface IgM is used to mimic the binding of antigen. When this antibody is cultured in large doses in vitro with bone marrow precursor cells (10 µg/ml), clonal deletion appears to be operative, and after 1–2 days when B lymphocytes appear in the culture, none have surface IgM. In contrast, when a smaller dose is used (0.1 µg/ml) surface IgM⁺ B cells appear, but they cannot be induced to proliferate by B cell mitogens (see p. 78). This cellular unresponsiveness is called **anergy**, and the tolerising process it underpins is termed **clonal anergy** (Fig. 9.3). The B cells exist, but through receipt of a particular cellular signal, have been rendered unable to respond.

MECHANISMS OF PERIPHERAL TOLERANCE

Although the dominant sites of tolerance induction are in the primary lymphoid organs, experimental evidence

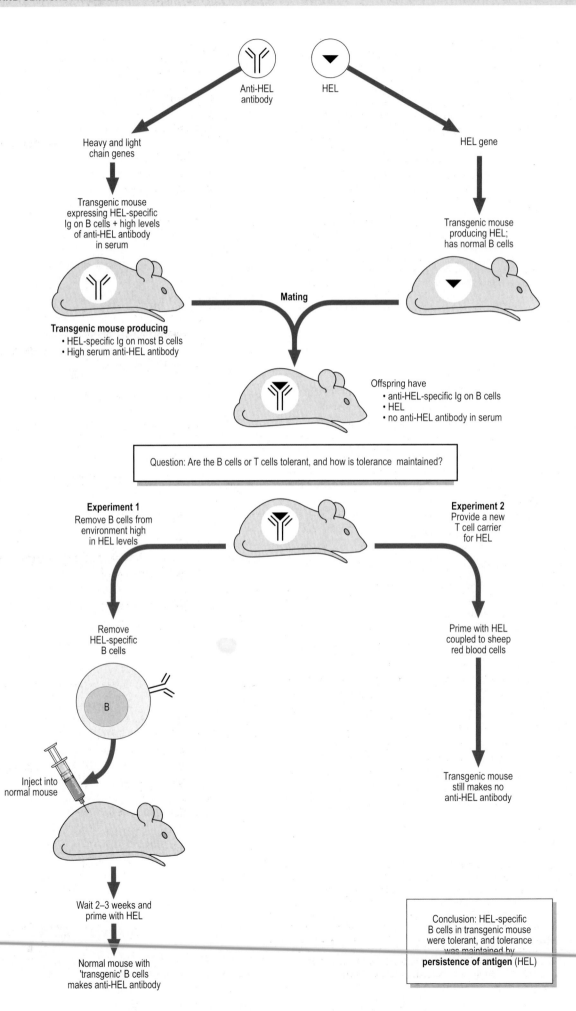

Anti-HEL antibody

HEL

Heavy and light chain genes

HEL gene

Transgenic mouse expressing HEL-specific Ig on B cells + high levels of anti-HEL antibody in serum

Transgenic mouse producing HEL; has normal B cells

Transgenic mouse producing
• HEL-specific Ig on most B cells
• High serum anti-HEL antibody

Mating

Offspring have
• anti-HEL-specific Ig on B cells
• HEL
• no anti-HEL antibody in serum

Question: Are the B cells or T cells tolerant, and how is tolerance maintained?

Experiment 1
Remove B cells from environment high in HEL levels

Experiment 2
Provide a new T cell carrier for HEL

Remove HEL-specific B cells

B

Prime with HEL coupled to sheep red blood cells

Inject into normal mouse

Transgenic mouse still makes no anti-HEL antibody

Wait 2–3 weeks and prime with HEL

Conclusion: HEL-specific B cells in transgenic mouse were tolerant, and tolerance was maintained by **persistence of antigen** (HEL)

Normal mouse with 'transgenic' B cells makes anti-HEL antibody

Fig. 9.3 Induction of B lymphocyte anergy.
A transgenic mouse is produced which expresses the heavy and light chain genes that encode an immunoglobulin molecule specific for the antigen hen egg lysozyme (HEL). The transgenic animal produces B cells expressing surface anti-HEL and anti-HEL antibody in the serum. It is mated with a different transgenic mouse, which has the genes encoding HEL inserted. The offspring from this mating produces cells expressing HEL, B cells expressing anti-HEL, but no circulating anti-HEL antibody. In addition, it does not produce anti-HEL even when boosted with HEL injections. The offspring mouse is tolerant of HEL, an autoantigen present in abundance. This could be the result of B or T cell tolerance to HEL. One way around T cell tolerance to HEL would be to couple the same protein to a new carrier, such as a sheep red blood cell (SRBC), and provide new T helper cells specific for the HEL–SRBC complex. This should generate T cells responsive to SRBC (this is like T cell bypass; see Fig. 9.5). Since HEL and SRBC are coupled, the anti-SRBC T cells should instruct B cells to make antibody to the coupled protein HEL. No anti-HEL antibody is made, however, suggesting that it is the B cells which are tolerised to HEL. This is confirmed by the fact that B cells from this mouse transferred into a normal mouse recover the ability to produce anti-HEL. Presumably in the F1 hybrid, tolerance is maintained by the presence of the antigen HEL.

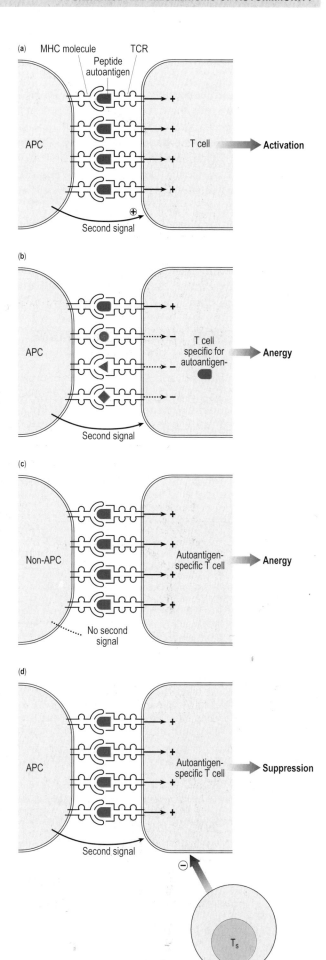

suggests that tolerisation can also be achieved in mature T and B cells. For example, a transgenic mouse model was created by introduction of the gene for a foreign class I MHC molecule, under the influence of a promoter designed such that expression was confined to the liver, kidney and pancreas. As expected, there was no autoimmunity to the transgene protein. When competent spleen cells from a non-transgenic mouse were introduced, a destructive form of liver inflammation appeared, reminiscent of autoimmune hepatitis. This was perhaps to be expected, but, somewhat unexpectedly, the inflammation subsided after 3–6 months, and the aggressive anti-foreign class I MHC T lymphocytes could no longer be detected. The interpretation of these results is that a form of peripheral tolerance arose spontaneously.

Several recent studies have demonstrated that mature T lymphocytes can be rendered non-responsive if specific antigen is presented to them in the absence of the necessary co-signals (e.g. presented by cells other than professional APCs). A similar mechanism can also be demonstrated for B cells, which appear to require large concentrations of antigen to achieve this form of tolerance. T cell anergy can be induced artificially in vitro in several ways, the best described being the use of low-dose antigen and the lack of provision of the second signal for T cell activation. Thus, a peripheral T lymphocyte encountering low levels of autoantigens

Fig. 9.4 Mechanisms of peripheral T cell tolerance.
(**a**) T lymphocytes interact via the TCR with antigen presented at a sufficient density to generate a positive activation signal. The antigen is presented by a 'professional' APC, which gives an appropriate second signal to result in T cell activation. (**b**) The autoantigen recognised by the autoreactive T cell is presented at low density resulting in anergy. (**c**) The cell presenting antigen is incapable of providing a second signal, resulting in anergy. (**d**) As in (a), the signals via the TCR and from the APC are present, but a regulatory T cell (T_S) suppresses the autoreactive T cell.

presented by MHC molecules that it recognises (e.g. peptides from thyroglobulin) becomes inactivated (Fig. 9.4a). Equally, autoreactive T lymphocytes presented autoantigenic peptides by self class II HLA molecules but without the necessary activation signals from the presenting cell may be rendered anergic (Fig. 9.4b). The latter mechanism may be seen in vitro using activated T lymphocytes as the APC. T cells acquire class II molecules when activated but lack the ability to provide secondary signals such as IL-1, typically released by 'professional' APCs (Fig. 9.4c).

Finally, we can assume that tolerance to an antigen can be acquired peripherally through a process of suppression (see p. 101). This form of tolerance lies in the hands of immunoregulatory groups of T lymphocytes, and it is likely that it can control unwanted B and T lymphocyte responses.

ANIMAL MODELS OF CLINICAL AUTOIMMUNE DISEASE

Many of the major advances in the field of autoimmunity have been achieved using animal models. These allow the natural history of a disease to be studied, including the subclinical prodrome; they allow manipulation of breeding and rearing to study genetic and environmental influences; and they allow experimentation with therapies. Several models have been studied extensively and illustrate important concepts (Table 9.3).

BREAKDOWN OF TOLERANCE: MECHANISMS OF AUTOIMMUNITY

These different mechanisms through which T and B cell tolerance operate lead to an obvious conclusion: several different pathological processes could break tolerance and lead to autoimmunity. It has been argued that the multilayered nature of self-tolerance is a failsafe mechanism: all or several control mechanisms must be breached before disease results. This approach would explain several important principles regarding autoimmune disease: (1) it is usually multifactorial, requiring inheritance of at least one gene and exposure to one or more environmental factors; (2) it often progresses much more slowly than immune reactions to pathogenic organisms, suggesting that control mechanisms may continue to work up to a point; (3) it has a tendency to remit and relapse, indicating that control mechanisms may recover and temporarily restore tolerance.

Several immunological processes that lead to autoimmunity have been postulated. Understandably, most are based on in vitro work or animal model studies, since human autoimmune disease can rarely be followed. From this work, it appears that tolerance to self antigens may be broken by (1) defects in immunoregulatory pathways; (2) the presence of antigenic similarities between pathogenic organisms and self proteins; (3) the provision of new T cell epitopes to bypass tolerant T cells; (4) the release of 'hidden' self antigens; (5) the so-called 'aberrant' expression of class II MHC molecules; and (6) the influence of cytokines.

DEFECTIVE IMMUNOREGULATION

Implicit in this theory is the assumption that immunoregulatory pathways — essentially suppressive in nature — control potentially autoaggressive immune responses. CD4 and CD8 T lymphocytes represent the broadest categories of immunoregulatory T cells. One approach

---

Autoimmunity and tolerance

- Autoimmune disease occurs when an immune response arises to apparently healthy self components.
- Autoimmunity can be organ or non-organ specific.
- Tolerance is the controlled ability to refrain from responding to antigens for which the potential to respond exists.
- Tolerance occurs through deletion of lymphocytes, inactivation of lympocytes (anergy) or suppression.
- Tolerance occurs predominantly in T lymphocytes through deletion and in B lymphocytes by anergy.
- Clones are offspring of a single cell that will all have the same characteristics.

Table 9.3 **Animal models of human autoimmune disease**

Animal model	Method of induction	Human equivalent
Non-obese diabetic (NOD) mouse	Diabetes arises spontaneously	Type 1 (insulin-dependent) diabetes
Experimental allergic encephalomyelitis (EAE)	Immunisation with xenogeneic myelin basic protein	Multiple sclerosis
Experimental allergic thyroiditis (EAT)	Immunisation with xenogeneic thyroglobulin	Hashimoto's thyroiditis
Adjuvant arthritis	Immunisation with adjuvant (derived from *Mycobacterium tuberculosis*)	Rheumatoid arthritis
Collagen-induced arthritis	Immunisation with collagen	Rheumatoid arthritis

to the search for immunoregulatory defects in auto-immune disease was to try to quantify suppression. Since it is typically associated with CD8 lymphocytes, these cells were simply counted in peripheral blood. Many studies performed in the 1980s identified reduced numbers of CD8 cells in organ-specific autoimmune diseases, including type 1 diabetes, Graves' disease, Hashimoto's thyroiditis, multiple sclerosis, myasthenia gravis and autoimmune hepatitis.

Immunosuppression, or immunodeficiency, could also interfere with immunoregulation sufficiently to lead to autoimmunity. In human disease, primary immunodeficiency, although rare, is inextricably linked to autoimmunity and autoimmune disease may be the first clinical presentation (see Ch. 19).

Immunoregulatory T cell subsets other than those defined by CD4 and CD8 alone exist and could have a bearing on the development of autoimmune disease. Particular attention has focused on the T_H1 and T_H2 subsets, defined according to their cytokine profile (see p. 99). The current view, in simplistic terms, is that T_H1 cells, generating and activating cytotoxic T cells (through IL-2 secretion) and macrophages (IFN-γ), are tissue damaging and, when dominant, contribute to 'cell-mediated' autoimmune diseases such as type 1 diabetes. By comparison, T_H2 cells provide B cell help (through IL-4, IL-5 and IL-6) and are important in antibody-mediated disease (e.g. Graves' thyroiditis). The evidence of these hypotheses in individual diseases is elaborated in Chapter 13.

MOLECULAR MIMICRY

The term 'molecular mimicry' was first employed in 1968 in a different context to autoimmunity to describe viruses achieving persistent infection by producing antigens similar to self to avoid immune recognition. The concept that pathogenic organisms produce antigens resembling self has been adopted more recently as an explanation for autoimmunity. In this scenario, the immune response to a pathogen capable of mimicking self proteins generates clones of T or B lymphocytes that are simultaneously antimicrobe and antiself (immunological cross-reactivity). These could be in-duced to persist long after the pathogen has dis-appeared by the presence of autoantigens, which drive the autoimmune response. In humans, molecular mimicry could certainly explain the consequences of certain infections, such as rheumatic fever following streptococcal infections, in which autoantibodies to M proteins on the surface of group A streptococci cross-react with cardiac myosin (Table 9.4). However, the evidence for its role in the majority of organ-specific autoimmune diseases is still being weighed in the balance at present. One of the problems is the fact that autoimmune diseases usually have long, often asympto-matic, prodromal periods and associations with viruses as initiating events are, therefore, difficult to find; hence molecular mimicry is often termed the 'hit-and-run' theory.

T CELL BYPASS

As we have seen, potential autoantigen-reactive effector B cell and T cell clones are present in the periphery but are either anergic or kept in check by regulatory lymphocytes. To become activated, they require not simply the recognition of self antigens but also acces-sory signals. One way of bypassing the down-regulatory mechanisms is the provision of a novel T cell epitope associated with the autoantigen (Fig. 9.5). The novel epitope is recognised by a new T_H cell clone that pro-motes responses to associated antigens, which in this case are autoantigens. The key is that the new antigen is sufficiently different from the autoantigen as to provide a different T cell epitope for induction of the immune response but also carries sufficiently similar epitopes to generate some autoreactivity.

The best experimental example of such a bypass is the immunisation of mice with rat erythrocytes. Some of the rat epitopes are perceived as novel, providing new T cell carriers. Other antigens on rat red cells are similar to murine determinants and can be recognised by autoreactive B cells. These B lymphocytes would normally be anergic, but the provision of T cell help leads to anti-red cell antibodies and haemolytic anae-mia. Using the same approach, xenogeneic thyro-globulin or myelin basic protein injected into animals can induce autoimmune disease of the thyroid and central nervous system akin to human autoimmune

Table 9.4 **Examples of viral or bacterial sequences that cross-react with known autoantigens**

Disease	Autoantibody	Autoantigen	Microbial antigen
Chagas' disease	Heart autoantibodies	Laminin	*Trypanosoma cruzi*
Post-streptococcal rheumatic fever	Heart autoantibodies	Myosin; tropomyosin	Group A streptococci
Autoimmune hepatitis	Liver kidney microsomal antibody	Cytochrome P4502D6	Herpes simplex virus-1; hepatitis C virus
Ankylosing spondylitis	Anti-HLA B27	HLA B27	*Klebsiella pneumoniae* nitrogenase
Coeliac disease	Anti-A-gliadin	A-gliadin	Adenovirus 12
Type 1 diabetes	Anti-glutamic acid decarboxylase	Glutamic acid decarboxylase	Coxsackie B4

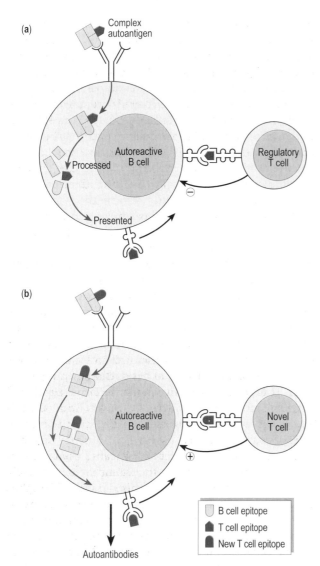

Fig. 9.5 **Mechanism of autoimmunity: T cell bypass.**
(**a**) A complex autoantigen contains a B cell epitope and a T cell epitope. The B cell internalises, processes and presents the autoantigen to a regulatory T cell, which suppresses the B cell from producing autoantibodies. (**b**) The complex autoantigen has been modified (e.g. by a drug or virus), providing a new epitope for a novel T cell, which can then provide the necessary signal(s) for B cell autoantibody production.

thyroiditis and multiple sclerosis (Table 9.3). In both models, T lymphocytes obtained from animals once the disease is established can adoptively transfer it, indicating that autoreactive T cells have been induced.

Examples of human autoimmune disease elicited by a T cell bypass mechanism are generally those induced by drugs or viruses. Methyldopa and *Mycoplasma pneumoniae* infection induce autoimmune haemolytic anaemia by modification of erythrocyte surface proteins to provide a novel, foreign carrier determinant for T cell responses.

RELEASE OR PRESENTATION OF 'HIDDEN' SELF ANTIGENS

It has long been recognised that proteins released from damaged tissues may induce autoantibodies, which could in some instances perpetuate the cellular damage. One of the best examples is the post-myocardial infarction syndrome described by Dressler in 1956. Autoantibodies to cardiac myocytes arise after ischaemic injury to the heart muscle, and tissue damage may be perpetuated, leading to pericarditis and other complications. There are at least three plausible explanations for this breakdown of tolerance, which are not mutually exclusive. First, the production of autoantibodies following tissue damage may be a mechanism for clearing and recycling effete proteins. This is a physiological role for autoimmunity. In this homeostatic model, antibody levels should decline as the antigens are removed, as is indeed the case. Second, it is possible that previously cryptic, intracellular proteins have never been exposed to the immune system and that tolerance is dependent on this state being maintained. Once exposed, autoantigens could incite immune responses. Such a mechanism, following organ damage by a tropic virus for example, is an attractive model for establishing chronic organ-specific autoimmunity, particularly since it allows for the initiating event to become lost in a profusion of autoimmune responses. Third, the appearance of small amounts of an autoantigen to which peripheral tolerance exists may be sufficient to break it, since tolerance is dependent on the concentration of the antigen.

Another mechanism by which autoantigens that are usually 'hidden' may be presented to the immune system is following up-regulation of expression of MHC molecules. Class II expression is the medium for communication between CD4[+] helper T lymphocytes and cells presenting antigen. Since this step is critical in initiating an immune response, class II expression is normally restricted to immune-competent cells, such as B lymphocytes and professional antigen-presenting cells (see Ch. 6). It has been proposed that the appearance of class II MHC molecules on cells that do not typically express them may be sufficient to incite an autoimmune reaction against that cell by CD4[+] T lymphocytes. Indeed, so-called 'aberrant' or 'inappropriate' class II expression has been seen in many autoimmune diseases; on the islet β cells in type 1 diabetes (see box: 'Aberrant expression of class II MHC'), on thyrocytes in Graves' and Hashimoto's thyroiditis and on hepatocytes in autoimmune hepatitis (Fig. 9.6). The hypothesis that this altered state of cell physiology is important in autoimmunity is supported by the demonstration that cytokines such as IFN-γ and tumour necrosis factor, which may have a role in antiviral defence and are likely to be released at sites of inflammation, can induce aberrant class II expression on a range of cell types.

CYTOKINES

Cytokines (see Ch. 3) are soluble factors with pleiotropic effects that act both locally and systemically on cells of the immune system. Their role in the immune

Aberrant expression of class II MHC: primary or secondary?

Since its proposal, the role of aberrant class II expression on target organ cells in autoimmunity has been hotly debated, particularly whether it is a primary, initiating event, or incidental and secondary to local cytokine release by infiltrating lymphocytes and macrophages. Several points remain to be resolved. First if the mechanism is a primary cause of autoimmunity, then endocrine or other cells of epithelial origin must be able to process and present antigens to T lymphocytes. Whether this is indeed the case remains unclear. Second, it must be borne in mind that the exogenous pathway of antigen presentation, involving peptides bound to class II MHC molecules, is designed for proteins derived from the external milieu. It is not known at present whether internally derived, potentially autoantigenic proteins can cross from the endogenous to the exogenous pathways, for what have been speculatively called 'liaisons dangereuses'. Finally, it could also be proposed that presentation of autoantigens to T cells by endocrine cells expressing class II MHC molecules would, in fact, induce peripheral tolerance, not activation, because of the lack of co-signals (see text). Finally, studies on transgenic mice have managed to muddy the waters, rather than clear them. For example, introduction of class I or class II MHC genes under the control of the insulin promoter has ensured hyperexpression of these molecules on the surface of β cells in the islets of Langerhans. Intriguingly, diabetes develops in both sets of transgenic mice, but without the involvement of a single lymphocyte in the islets. In other words, the diabetes in these models is probably not autoimmune in nature. In summary, aberrant expression of class II MHC molecules is an attractive mechanism to explain the development of organ-specific autoimmunity, but its role has yet to be confirmed.

response is the recruitment of immunocompetent cells and modulation of their functions. In these capacities, they will undoubtedly have a role in autoimmune responses. Whether such a role is extraordinary to their physiological functions is the issue in question.

First, as alluded to above, there is the possibility that cytokines induce class II and enhance class I MHC expression on target cells as a primary event in the development of autoimmunity. Other possible mechanisms include cytokine-mediated breakdown of immunological tolerance and a directly cytotoxic effect on target cells (see p. 130).

Anecdotal evidence presents a strong case for cytokines being capable, per se, of inducing the clinical onset of autoimmune disease. IL-2 is a T lymphocyte growth and differentiation factor used therapeutically in some solid-organ tumours to enhance immune-mediated antitumour responses. During such IL-2 treatment, inflammatory lesions involving lymphocytic infiltration have been seen in several organs, including the myocardium, skin and liver, and a thyroiditis resembling Hashimoto's is induced and may progress to hypothyroidism in 10% of cases. Similarly, a patient given IFN-α therapy in an attempt to clear hepatitis C virus infection developed type 1 diabetes, with islet cell antibodies and insulin autoantibodies as evidence of concomitant autoimmunity. In certain mice that rely solely upon peripheral tolerance because thymic tolerance does not take place (for example constitutively athymic or neonatally thymectomised mice), T lymphocyte anergy in the periphery may be overcome by in vivo treatment with IL-2, leading to a systemic autoimmune syndrome. Again, what is unclear about the role of cytokines in the development of autoimmunity is whether they are acting in a primary or secondary capacity, and whether they are inducing autoimmune disease or merely hastening its clinical onset.

It can be envisaged, then, that immune activation associated with large-scale prolonged release of pro-inflammatory cytokines, such as IL-2, IFN-γ or TNF-α might unhinge peripheral tolerance by mechanisms as yet unidentified and precipitate clinical autoimmune disease from a state of smouldering autoimmunity. 'Mild' subclinical autoimmunity may be a common occurrence. Such a process would fit with evidence already discussed, which suggests that T and B cell tolerance is not 'all-or-none', and with the known phenomenon of the diagnosis of autoimmune diseases being associated with recent viral infections and, in some cases, having a seasonal variation, with peaks in the winter months. For example, type 1 diabetes and autoimmune hepatitis have often been described as apparently arising after a 'flu-like' illness.

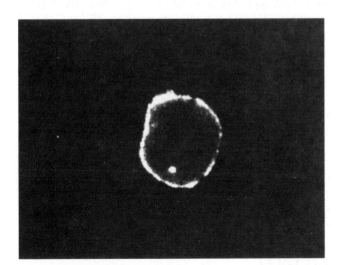

Fig. 9.6 'Aberrant' class II expression.
A hepatocyte from a patient with autoimmune liver disease stained with fluorescent antibody to class II HLA. The hepatocyte expresses surface class II HLA molecules, not normally seen on such cells. (Reproduced with permission from Dr G Senaldi.)

THE ROLE OF HLA IN AUTOIMMUNITY

The role of HLA molecules in antigen presentation

Summary of mechanisms of autoimmunity

	Mechanism	Best examples
Defective immunoregulation	Reduction in suppressor cell number and/or function	Described in thyroid, islet and liver autoimmune diseases
Molecular mimicry	Pathogen has cross-reactive epitopes with autoantigen; anti-pathogen immune response leads to anti-self response	Coxsackie and glutamic acid decarboxylase in type 1 diabetes; adenovirus 12 and gliadin in coeliac disease
T cell bypass	Novel T cell carrier supplied for an associated T or B cell epitope for which tolerance exists; T cell help via new carrier activates tolerised cells	No definite human examples; possible examples include drug- and virus-induced autoimmune cytopenias
'Hidden' self antigens	Tolerance exists to cryptic antigens ('immunological ignorance'); release or presentation of these breaks the tolerance	Sympathetic ophthalmia (see p. 258); post-myocardial complications (Dressler's syndrome)
Cytokines	Cytokines provide additional signals to activate tolerised resting autoreactive cells	Autoimmune thyroid disease following IL-2 therapy

indicates that at a molecular level they are undoubtedly involved in autoimmune responses. Historically, considerable attention has been focused on the place of the MHC in providing a genetic background on which autoimmunity spawns. The first association of HLA and disease in humans was described for Hodgkin's lymphoma in 1967, though this weak linkage has not been consistently confirmed. Several years later, the true avalanche of descriptions of associations had begun with the identification of an association between the class I allele *HLA-B27* and ankylosing spondylitis, an inflammatory process predominantly affecting the synovial and cartilagenous joints of the spine (Table 9.5). Other associations followed, often with class I alleles initially and then, as class II alleles became more easily identified, with these in turn.

A good example of this evolving process is the HLA association with type 1 diabetes, which remains one of the most extensively studied. Early work indicated an association between the class I alleles *HLA-B8* and *HLA-B15* and type 1 diabetes. Subsequently, a stronger association with the serologically defined class II alleles *DR3* and *DR4* was found, with the *DR3/DR4* heterozygous state carrying an even greater risk of developing type 1 diabetes whilst the *DR2* allele confers a degree

of protection. It can be assumed that the class I associations originally described are secondary to the class II associations and arise from linkage disequilibrium (p. 54): in Caucasians, *DR3* is in linkage disequilibrium with *B8*, and *DR4* with *B15*. More recently, as it has become possible to analyse class II *DQ* alleles more precisely with a variety of molecular genetic techniques, attention has focused on the DQ chains (Table 9.6), initially the β but then the α chain. Hugh McDevitt's group drew attention to the 57th amino acid residue position on the DQβ chain, demonstrating in Caucasians that susceptibility to type 1 diabetes was associated most strongly with non-aspartate (Asp) amino acids at this point, whilst resistance was best conferred by having two Asp-57-positive *HLA-DQ*β alleles. It appeared that the association was strongest for Asp-57-negative alleles from *HLA-DR3* or *HLA-DR4* haplotypes, and that between the extremes was a gradation of susceptibility according to the number of Asp-57-negative alleles held. Position 57 is located within the α-helix of the class II peptide-binding groove (Fig. 9.7). Recent attention has focused on the DQα chain (see box: 'Transcomplementation of DQα and β chains').

HLA disease associations bear several interpreta-

Table 9.5 **HLA associations with immune-mediated diseases**

Disease	HLA allele
Ankylosing spondylitis	B27
Type 1 (insulin-dependent) diabetes	B8 DR3 DR4 (susceptibility) B7 DR2 (protection)
Multiple sclerosis	B7 DR2
Rheumatoid arthritis	DR4
Coeliac disease	B8 DR3
Graves' disease	B8 DR3
Autoimmune hepatitis	DR3 (young onset) DR4 (old onset)

Table 9.6 *HLA-DQ* **associations with immune-mediated diseases**

Disease	HLA-DQ alleles
Multiple sclerosis	DQA1* 0102/DQB1* 0602
Pemphigus vulgaris	DQA1* 0101/DQB1* 0503
Type 1 diabetes	DQA1* 0301/DQB1* 0302 (susceptibility) DQA1* 0102/DQB1* 0502 (susceptibility) DQA1* 0102/DQB1* 0602 (protection)
Coeliac disease	DQA1* 0501/DQB1* 0201
Rheumatoid arthritis	DQA1* 0301/DQB1* 0301[a]

[a]Determines severity of disease rather than susceptibility

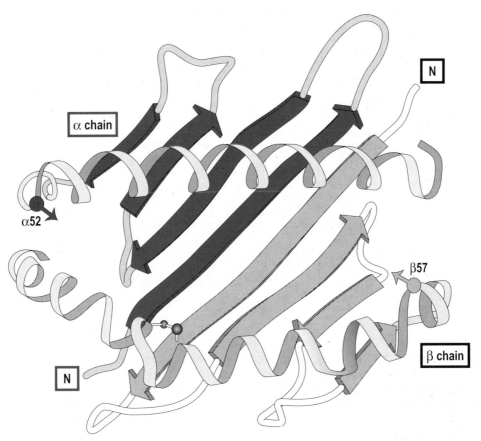

Fig. 9.7 **Susecptibility-determining amino acids on the DQ molecule.**
The probable shape of the class II HLA molecule peptide-binding groove. The amino acid on the DQβ chain 57th position is at one end of the entrance into the peptide-binding groove, and the DQα chain position 52 is at the other. Non-aspartate amino acids and arginine at each of these positions, respectively, confer susceptibility to type 1 diabetes.

Transcomplementation of DQα and β chains

Attention has now turned to the DQα chain. Studies on Caucasian French patients with type 1 diabetes show an association with the presence of arginine (Arg) at position 52 on the DQα chain. In the putative class II molecule structure the residues DQβ57 and DQα52 are at opposite ends of the α-helical side of the antigen-binding groove and, thus, are ideally placed to influence peptide binding (Fig. 9.7). Susceptibility heterodimers composed of Asp-57-negative DQβ and Arg-52-positive DQα heterodimers, occurring *in cis* or *in trans* (i.e. combining an α chain encoded on one chromosome with a β chain from the same or the opposite chromosome, see p. 56), are strongly associated with type 1 diabetes, and there is a gradation of increasing susceptibility with the number of such heterodimers an individual can form. This concept of heterodimers forming between molecules encoded on different chromosomes is called transcomplementation and has been used to account for some anomalies of HLA associations, such as the higher risk for diabetes conferred by the heterozygous *DR3/4* state than for either homozygous state.

tions: some of the mechanisms cited need not necessarily operate independently. In particular, it is worth pointing out that some polymorphisms at some HLA loci are associated with diseases that cannot be described as autoimmune, such as 21-hydroxylase deficiency.

The first possibility, as the evolving process of identifying stronger and stronger correlations as studies of the MHC continue, is that the associations may depend on a true disease-susceptibility gene, which has yet to be identified but which is in linkage disequilibrium with other genes within the MHC. This remains a possible explanation but awaits the identification of all MHC genes and their functions. Three other explanations include molecular mimicry between pathogens and MHC molecules, the molecules themselves acting as receptors for microorganisms, or a mechanism related to the function of MHC molecules in presenting peptide antigen.

Some of the best evidence for molecular mimicry has identified cross-reactivity between HLA-B27 and *Klebsiella pneumoniae* (Table 9.4). Such cross-reactivity could result in an autoimmune disease in *HLA-B27*-positive individuals following infection with *Klebsiella*, but why the inflammation in this disease should then be confined to the vertebral connective tissue and not found at all sites of class I HLA molecule expression remains to be explained. MHC molecules acting as virus receptors have been described, but there remains a gulf between a surface molecule being receptive for a virus and the generation of organ-specific autoimmune reactions.

For many, the role of immunological mechanisms in HLA–disease associations remains the most plausible explanation, given the function of class I and II molecules in presenting peptide antigens to CD8[+] or CD4[+] T lymphocytes. In addition, the demonstration that susceptibility sequences within class II molecules such as the DQα and DQβ chains reside within the antigen-binding groove adds weight to this proposal. A single peptide antigen may bind to many different class II molecules but with varying affinities. One possibility is that a susceptibility class II heterodimer has a particular affinity for an autoantigenic peptide (see box: 'A unified hypothesis for HLA-determined susceptibility'), establishing an idiosyncratically aggressive immune response to target organ damage. However, the mechanism might apply in reverse: a class II molecule may have poor recognition of an epitope of a microorganism, permitting a chronic infection and associated organ damage leading to autoimmune reactions. This explanation could also account for protective alleles and the

---

Mechanisms of autoimmunity

- Autoimmune disease is usually multifactorial, involving at least one gene and environmental factors.
- A number of possible defects that might break tolerance are suggested:
  - regulation, normally suppressive, may be lost, e.g. reduced CD8 cells in thyroid disease
  - antigens of pathogenic organisms might mimic self proteins, e.g. rheumatic fever following streptococcal infections
  - new T cells bypassing tolerant T cells, e.g. in drug/virus-induced disease
  - release of hidden self antigens, e.g. post-myocardial infarction syndrome
  - aberrant class II MHC expression, e.g. on β cells in type 1 diabetes
  - influence of cytokines, e.g. raised levels in virus infections.
- HLA molecules have a key permissive or protective role, relating to presentation of autoantigens.

---

variety of susceptibility alleles in some diseases, such as type 1 diabetes.

A unified hypothesis for HLA-determined susceptibility?

How are we to explain the confusing picture in autoimmune diseases such as diabetes, when some HLA molecules confer susceptibility and some protection? It has been suggested that there is a hierarchy of affinities between class II molecules and a disease-provoking autoantigenic peptide. An individual capable of constructing several class II heterodimers is susceptible to an autoimmune disease only if the susceptibility dimer has the highest affinity for the disease-provoking peptide. In the case of type 1 diabetes, this would involve a diabetogenic peptide binding to the DQ dimer comprising an Asp-57-negative DQβ chain with an Arg-52 DQα chain. Protection could be conferred if the same individual can make another heterodimer, for example DQB1*0602 which is Asp-57-positive and associated with the *DR2* allele and perhaps has a higher affinity for the peptide. What this hypothesis assumes is a single 'diabetogenic' peptide, whilst the available evidence suggests there are several islet β cell and thyroid autoantigens. Nevertheless, the same principle could apply to several different peptides.

Finally, it could be that the critical influence of class II alleles on autoimmune disease takes place in the thymus. Here, the MHC is involved in the selection of the T cell receptor repertoire. A class II molecule that results in selection of potentially autoreactive T cell receptors, or deletion of potentially protective ones, could have a role in predisposing to autoimmunity.

AUTOIMMUNE DISEASE

MECHANISMS OF IMMUNE DAMAGE

The scheme shown in Figure 9.8 is an attempt to distil mechanisms of immune damage in autoimmune disease. For the most part these are pathogenic processes which could apply equally well in physiological immune responses against pathogens.

The central cell in the autoimmune response is likely to be the CD4[+] T_H cell. This will become activated against an autoantigenic peptide displayed within the binding groove of a class II HLA molecule, either on a 'professional' antigen-presenting cell or on the target cell itself aberrantly expressing class II (see p. 125). Whether the target cell can provide the necessary accessory signals (e.g. IL-1) for T cell activation remains unclear. The activated T cell can then recruit other T lymphocytes or other immunocompetent cells. T_H1 cells secreting IL-2 and IFN-γ are likely to promote delayed-type hypersensitivity-like reactions, dominated by other CD4 T cells and macrophages, while T_H2 cells will activate autoantibody production by B lymphocytes. To be damaging, autoantibodies must target surface components and be capable of recruiting effectors such as complement or Fc receptor-bearing killer cells (see p. 109). Macrophages, which are recruited and activated by T_H1 cells, secrete pro-inflammatory and potentially damaging cytokines, such as IL-1 and TNF-α. Direct activation of cytotoxic T cells may result in killing of target cells: such a mechanism requires class I

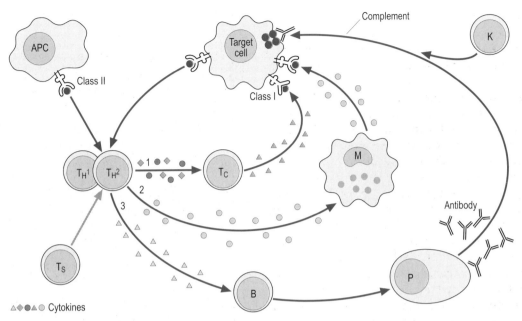

Fig. 9.8 Autoimmune attack on a target organ cell.
A normal component of the cell is presented to helper (T_H1 or T_H2) lymphocytes either directly on the cell's surface or by an APC, in the context of class II HLA molecules. If there is no opposition from T suppressor (T_S) lymphocytes, the T cell differentiates into a T_H1 or T_H2 cell, according to the signals given (IL-12/IFN-γ or IL-4, IL-10 respectively). Then, a variety of effector mechanisms are triggered. Target organ cell destruction could derive from the action of: (1) T cytotoxic (T_C) lymphocytes which react with the self antigen(s) in the context of class I HLA antigens; (2) cytokines produced by T_H1 or T_H2 lymphocytes and recruited macrophages (M) which may be toxic or enhance class I and induce class II MHC molecules; or (3) autoantibodies produced by B lymphocytes (B) or plasma cells (P) with activation of complement and/or engagement of Fc receptor-bearing killer (K) lymphocytes.

expression on the cell surface and presentation of an endogenous autoantigenic peptide.

Evidence for the precise mechanism involved in tissue damage in a range of autoimmune diseases has been sought since the early 1980s. In some autoimmune disorders, antibody-mediated organ dysfunction has been identified. In Graves' disease, for example, hyperthyroidism is mediated by the production of an autoantibody that binds to the receptor for thyrotrophin and provides a stimulatory signal (the autoantibody was originally known as long-acting thyroid stimulator), leading to uncontrolled production and release of thyroid hormones and to thyrotoxicosis. In myasthenia gravis, an autoantibody to the acetylcholine receptor (AChR) acts at the neuromuscular junction to interfere with signal transmission possibly through a complement-mediated mechanism. In other organ-specific autoimmune diseases in which tissue is actually destroyed, such as Hashimoto's thyroiditis (thyrocytes) and type 1 diabetes (insulin-producing β cells), the mechanism of cell death remains elusive. In both disorders, antibody-dependent cell-mediated cytotoxic (ADCC) and complement-dependent lytic reactions have occurred in vitro using endocrine tumour cell lines and autoantibodies from patients, but whether such processes contribute to cell damage in vivo is not known.

Finally, there is the possibility that unwanted damage is caused to target organ cells during an inflammatory response: the so-called 'bystander' phenomenon. This is again well illustrated by type 1 diabetes. In animal models, serial histological studies of pancreata during the period when insulitis is developing demonstrate that macrophages are amongst the earliest cells to appear. Macrophages are potent secretors of IL-1 and TNF-α: IL-1 has been shown to be selectively cytotoxic to β cells in vitro and TNF-α synergises with IFN-γ to damage whole islets (Fig. 9.9). Thus, selective β cell destruction could ensue from a chronic, local inflammatory process which is itself not focused on the β cells.

THERAPIES

Until recently, the mainstays of treatment for autoimmune disorders have either been replacement therapy for loss of endocrine secretions (insulin, thyroxine) or 'blanket' suppression of the immune system. Blanket suppression has been achieved in the main using corticosteroids, which appear to have effects on almost every compartment of the immune system, interfering with cell activation and migration. More recently, drugs such as cyclosporin A and FK506, which inhibit early events in T cell activation and thus inhibit cell-mediated immune responses more selectively, have been used in clinical trials for treatment of type 1 diabetes and rheumatoid arthritis. These approaches, which are described in more detail in Chapter 22, carry risks:

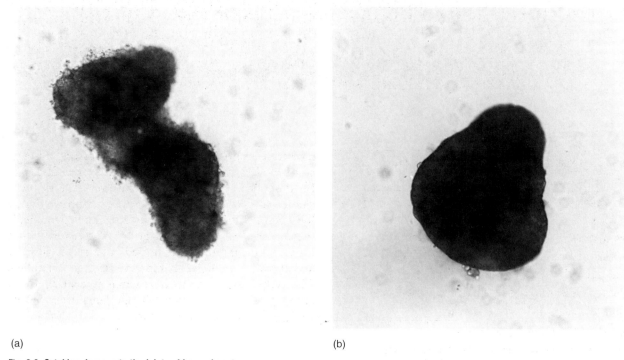

(a)   (b)

Fig. 9.9 **Cytokine damage to the islets of Langerhans.**
Isolated human islets of Langerhans (**a**) incubated with recombinant human IL-1 for 48 hours demonstrate disintegration of islet structure, loss of cell density and death of β cells compared with (**b**) an islet incubated in culture medium alone (×25 original magnification).

corticosteroids have many side effects, and, to be effective, blanket immunosuppression is often used at doses that compromise protective immunity while treating autoimmunity. One approach is to weigh the potential risks and benefits of these therapies: some autoimmune diseases, such as systemic lupus erythematosus, are potentially life threatening, and high-dose steroids plus cytotoxic agents such as azathioprine may be justified. In type 1 diabetes, however, the potential complications of renal damage and secondary cancer associated with cyclosporin A far outweigh the transient remission from insulin dependence that could be achieved.

For these reasons, the search for more specific immune-based therapies has intensified. There is a gradation, from those that will inhibit subsets of T lymphocytes to those specifically designed to disable clones of autoreactive T lymphocytes (see Ch. 22). These approaches make use of monoclonal antibodies to block cell–cell interactions or to neutralise positive signals such as cytokines. A more subtle approach is to compete with the antigenic peptides in an immune response, using peptides that bind but either block or 'switch off' a T cell response.

Autoimmune disease

- Immune attack in autoimmune disease can use the same immune responses that occur physiologically against pathogens.
- Damage can be caused by cytotoxic T cells, cytokines (recruiting macrophages and increasing class I and II MHC expression), B cells or plasma cells producing autoantibodies that activate complement and killer cells.
- Organ dysfunction can occur, e.g. in Graves' disease where the autoantibody binds to the thyrotrophin receptor, stimulating thyroid hormone production.
- Organ cell death can occur, e.g. in type 1 diabetes and Hashimoto's thyroiditis.
- Current therapy involves blanket suppression of the immune response with corticosteroids or selective suppression of T cell activation, e.g. with cyclosporin A.
- Future therapies will be immune based using monoclonal antibodies and 'designer' peptides to block responses.

CHAPTER 10

Hypersensitivity reactions and clinical allergy

For the purpose of host defence, the immune system is charged with damaging and potentially lethal effector mechanisms and molecules. For the most part, these are well controlled. An immune response directed against a pathogen results in clearance of the organism and resolution of any inflammatory process. Under some circumstances, however, resolution does not occur and an exaggerated or persistent immune response results in tissue damage. In other cases, the inciting stimulus is a harmless molecule, ignored by the immune systems of the majority but in some initiating an immune response that leads to tissue damage and even death of the host. These exaggerated, inappropriate reactions come under the umbrella of the term **hypersensitivity reactions**.

Hypersensitivity was originally categorised, according to the effector mechanisms thought to be involved, by Gell and Coombs in the 1970s. At that time, several disorders seemed to fit neatly into one or other of the four categories. In the intervening years, the curtain has slowly been drawn back on the complexity of the immune response in many diseases, and few now fit as well into Gell and Coombs' groups as they once did. However, the classification still serves as a useful guide to the mechanisms whereby immunopathology arises and as such it is an appropriate point at which to start the study of clinical immunology.

Hypersensitivity reaction types II, III and IV describe disease mechanisms but do not usefully define

a discrete group of disorders. For this reason, although some clinical syndromes involving these reactions will be described, the diseases themselves will be considered in depth in their appropriate chapters. Type I hypersensitivity stands alone in defining a pathogenic mechanism that underlies a group of diseases with a similar demographic, genetic and environmental basis and to which a similar therapeutic strategy is applied. The type I hypersensitivity reaction is central to the group of disorders termed 'allergic' and these will be dealt with in full in this chapter.

TYPE I HYPERSENSITIVITY: IgE AND THE MAST CELL

The interaction of antigen, specific IgE, and the high-affinity receptor for IgE on the mast cell surface results in cell degranulation (Fig. 10.1; see also the electron micrographs of mast cell degranulation, Fig. 3.8, p. 31). When this interaction occurs in allergic disease, the antigen is termed an **allergen**. The vasoactive mediators released give rise to vasodilatation and localised oedema. In the skin, where the existence of type I hypersensitivity is usually assessed, this reaction is itchy, has the appearance of a 'wheal and flare' and arises within minutes of the antigen being introduced. The basis for the mast cell reaction and the mediators involved have already been described in Chapter 3. The antigens involved in type I hypersensitivity are usually inert molecules derived from the environment

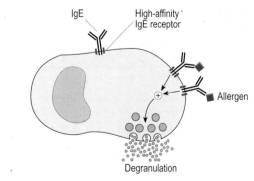

Fig. 10.1 **Mast cell degranulation.**
The mast cell carries high affinity receptors for the Fc portion of IgE. Allergen-specific IgE, occupying these receptors, induces mast cell degranulation when allergens are encountered.

Passive transfer of allergy to fish

In one of the classic medical experiments of this century, the basis for allergic reactions was shown to reside in serum. It is the kind of experiment that would certainly be frowned upon today, but in the early 1920s earned its performers, Carl Prausnitz and Heinz Küstner, the accolade of having an immunological reaction named after them. In the original Prausnitz–Küstner reaction, serum was separated from the blood of Küstner, a professor of obstetrics and gynaecology who was allergic to fish. This was then injected under the skin of the forearm of Prausnitz, a man previously without allergy of any sort. The next day, a fish extract was injected into the same site and for the first time in his life Prausnitz had a positive skin prick test. The factor in serum responsible for this reaction was termed 'reagin'. Finally, in the late 1960s, reagin was identified as a new class of antibody, left undiscovered when IgG, A, M and D were described, because of its very low concentration in normal serum. Two teams identified IgE at almost the same time, one group through studying a patient with high levels caused by allergy, the other following the characterisation of an IgE monoclonal antibody in a patient with a plasma cell tumour (myeloma; see p. 294).

Table 10.1 Common allergens

Allergen source	WHO nomenclature	Molecular weight (kDa)
Perennial rye grass	*Lol p* I	29
(*Lolium perenne*)	*Lol p* II	11
Ragweed	*Amb a* I	35
(*Ambrosia artemisifolia*)	*Amb a* III	11
	Amb a V	5
Cat (*Felis domesticus*)	*Fel d* I	34
House dust mite (*Dermatophagoides pteronyssinus*)	*Der p* I	24

and of no apparent threat to the host organism. The combination of the timing and the innocuous nature of the provoking stimulus has earned this reaction the alternative label of **immediate hypersensitivity**.

THE PATHOGENESIS OF ALLERGIC DISEASE

There are several components to an allergic response: the allergen, the host's state of reactivity and the genetic and environmental influences on this. In addition, it has become clear in recent years that the manifestations of allergic disease do not equate simply with mast cell degranulation and the immediate hypersensitivity reaction. Allergic disorders are also typified by an aftermath, occurring a few hours after exposure and lasting up to several days. These 'late' immune reactions are the indirect result of mast cell degranulation and have important pathogenic and clinical implications.

The allergen

Allergy, derived from the Greek *allos ergos* meaning altered reactivity, is a term much abused. For our purposes it can be defined as a state of heightened reactivity of the immune system to foreign substances. For the sake of clarity, we will also confine the use of the term 'allergic' to those reactions that are initiated when mast cell-bound IgE interacts with its target antigen, known as an allergen. The allergic diseases that cause the greatest morbidity and mortality are **asthma**, a chronic lung disease; **allergic rhinitis** (seasonal allergic rhinitis is 'hay-fever'); **eczema** and **urticaria** (skin disorders); and **generalised anaphylaxis**.

Some of the most intense research into the mechanisms of allergic responses has concentrated on the nature of the allergens. Could these molecules have particular features that give them the power to incite these damaging IgE responses? One result of the interest in this area is that there is now a World Health Organization nomenclature for allergens. The system adopts the first three letters of the name of the genus and the first letter of the species from which the allergen originates, followed by a roman numeral according to the order in which the allergen was identified. Some examples are given in Table 10.1.

Several allergens have now been sequenced, and as yet there appears to be little in their primary structure that sets them apart from non-allergenic proteins. As can be seen from Table 10.1, allergens tend to be of relatively low molecular mass (cf. autoantigens in autoimmune disease; see p. 187), and the carrier particles (e.g. pollen grains, house dust mite faecal material) tend to be of a diameter between 2 and 60 μm. These may be important properties in gaining aerial access to nasal and bronchial mucosa. After all, one of the main functions of the mucosa at these sites, particularly in the nose, is to filter inhaled air. Other common features of aeroallergens are that their source may be dominant (e.g. grass pollen is the most prevalent pollen in the air in the UK, and allergy to it is the main cause of hay fever) and that within a pollen the allergen may be a large proportion of the soluble protein. It is estimated that the total exposure to most allergens is low in comparison with an artificial immunisation, for example against tetanus toxin. Pollen allergen exposure may amount to only 1 μg per season (10 ng/day) and house dust mite 20 ng/day. This low-dose exposure may be important in determining the isotype of antibody produced and, hence, the development of type I hypersensitivity.

Inheritance

The tendency to allergic reactions has a strong heritability, and this tendency has been termed **atopy**. Atopy is most easily defined as the presence of a type I hypersensitivity reaction to an allergen, usually demonstrated in the skin-prick test (see p. 136); this potentially allergic state need not result in disease. Two, one

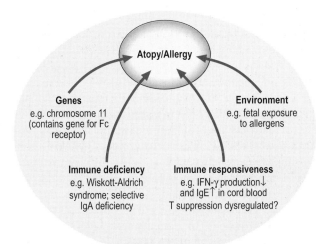

Fig. 10.2 Multifactorial susceptibility to atopy and allergy.
The manifestation of atopy or clinical allergy in an individual is the
end result of numerous different influences. There are genetic
components such as the proposed linkage to chromosome 11, the
effects of subtle or frank immune deficiencies, the nature of the
immune response in an individual and the balance of IFN-γ
production. There are also environmental factors capable of making
atopy and allergy more or less likely.

or no atopic parents pass on the atopic trait to their
children with a risk of 75, 50 and 15%, respectively,
and between 20 and 30% of the population is atopic.

The nature of what exactly is inherited by atopic
individuals and, therefore, what predisposes to allergy
is complex (Fig. 10.2). One research group has shown
an association between increased IgE responses and
gene(s) on the long arm of chromosome 11; others find
no such link. Intriguingly, the gene for the β subunit
of the high-affinity IgE Fc receptor is located in this
region. Allergic disease is also a feature of immune-
deficiency states such as Wiskott–Aldrich syndrome
(eczema) and selective IgA deficiency (eczema and
asthma), and attention has focused on inheritance of
'immune responsiveness'. It has been demonstrated,
for example, that high levels of IgE in the cord blood of
infants predicts future development of atopy. Moreover, stimulated cord blood T cells from infants who
subsequently developed allergic disease produce less
IFN-γ than normal; this is one of the cytokines that
down-regulate IgE production (see p. 79). Obviously,
such features need not be genetically determined; they
could also result from the influence of the environment
(e.g. allergen exposure) during gestation. Intensive
investigation of the HLA types of atopic individuals,
in search of susceptibility loci related to the 'immune-
response' genes, has not been particularly revealing.
The most convincing study has provided evidence that
in a North American population IgE and IgG hyperresponsiveness to one of the ragweed antigens *Amb a* V
is associated with HLA-DR2 in patients with ragweed
pollen allergy. There is no firm evidence as yet, however, that the atopic state is predisposed to by inheritance of particular HLA genes.

Environment

Despite the fact that the familial risks defined above
give the appearance of an autosomal dominant inheritance with variable penetrance, in monozygotic identical
twins (i.e. twins with identical genes) concordance for
asthma (i.e. both twins having the disease) is only 20%.
Environmental factors clearly have a role. The prevalence of asthma, eczema and allergic rhinitis doubled
in 12-year-olds in a South Wales community between
1973 and 1988 without any fundamental change in the
genetic stock of the inhabitants. Asthma is more common in second-generation West Indian immigrants
born in the UK than in their parents raised overseas. As
discussed, the environment could start to have an effect
as early as during fetal life.

A long-running question has been the role of infant
breast-feeding in predisposition to allergy, and eczema
in particular. Early studies indicated a protective effect
of breast-feeding over the use of formula feeds based
on cow's milk. This effect was assigned to the secretory
IgA contained in breast milk, which could protect the
infant gut from undue exposure to potential allergens
in the environment. An alternative explanation was that
cow's milk contained allergenic proteins. More recent
research has failed to show protection resulting from
breast milk. There is no easy interpretation of these
results: modern infant feeds containing cow's milk are
heat treated and hydrolysed and the proteins may be
less allergenic than those used previously. In addition,
it is now clear that antigens from cow's milk proteins
can appear unaltered in breast milk and may even cross
the human placenta. Trials in which mothers have used
low-allergen diets during pregnancy and early infant
life whilst breast-feeding (avoiding cow's milk, egg,
peanuts, wheat) and in which the same foods have been
introduced only slowly to the infant have, at best, only
produced a marginal and transient (6 months) benefit
in controlling childhood eczema.

Other studies have looked at exposure to aeroallergens during infant life in relation to the development of allergic rhinitis and asthma. Individuals raised
at high altitude, where exposure to house dust mite is
comparatively low, have a significantly lower incidence
of asthma. The peak incidence of allergic rhinitis caused
by birch pollen allergy, which is particularly common
in Scandinavia, is found amongst children born during
the months of birch pollen release (February to April).
The recent increase in asthma incidence in the developed countries has provoked considerable discussion.
Some of the favoured explanations are that our use of
central heating and double glazing provides the optimal
conditions — warmth and humidity — under which the
house dust mite (a major allergen in asthma) flourishes,
or that air pollution has a role.

Allergy is a sufficiently common and emotive afflic-
tion that as more predisposing environmental factors
are identified or proposed so families at risk modify
their behaviour. It is important, therefore, that there is
continued research to examine these associations.

The late responses in allergic disease: more than IgE and mast cells

In an attempt to tease out the cells and mediators that result in the symptoms and signs of clinical allergic diseases, models have been developed, mainly in asthma and allergic rhinitis, in which patients are exposed to allergens under controlled conditions. In asthma, for example, allergen is inhaled and then measurements are made of lung function and cells are collected from the fluid bathing the mucosa by bronchoalveolar lavage (BAL). Another approach is to perform skin testing on allergic individuals. Biopsies to examine the cellular infiltrate can be taken from the bronchi and this is also particularly useful in the skin test. In these models, the effects of proved or novel pharmacological therapies can also be assessed.

Some important findings, common to all models, have been made since the mid-1980s and reveal clinical allergy to be much more than the sum of allergen, IgE and mast cell. Taking asthma as one of the best studied models, approximately 15 minutes after endobronchial challenge with allergen there is a fall in the 1-second forced expiratory volume (FEV_1) (Fig. 10.3). This 'early' response recovers spontaneously after 1–2 hours and may be suppressed by pre-treatment with antihistamines. Similarly, in hay fever sufferers, sneezing, increased secretions and nasal congestion occur minutes after nasal challenge with allergen and then subside over the next 2 hours. Again this is sensitive to antihistamines. Further evidence that mast cell products are important in this response comes from the identification of histamine and the leukotrienes B_4, C_4 and D_4 in the nasal secretions. Therefore, it would appear that in immediate hypersensitivity reactions, mast cell activation by allergen-specific IgE is the key pathogenetic event.

However, in over 50% of patients challenged, symptoms recur some 4–6 hours later, the so-called **late-phase response** (LPR). In the asthmatic model, there is the development of a **hyperresponsiveness** in the bronchi to challenge with allergen or histamine, the FEV_1 falls and over the next days there may be recurring episodes of airways limitation. Hyperresponsiveness is one of the key clinical features of allergy, and this constellation of symptoms and signs most closely resembles the clinical picture seen in many asthmatics. These features are not responsive to antihistamines but are suppressed by corticosteroids, again reflecting the clinical experience that steroids give considerable benefit in controlling moderate to severe asthma (see below). Therefore, it appears that, in asthma, the LPR may be of great clinical and pathogenetic importance. In the nasal model, in patients with allergic rhinitis, congestion is the main complaint 4–6 hours after challenge and the nasal mucosa also shows hyperresponsiveness to allergen or histamine exposure.

For these reasons, the LPR has been studied extensively since it appears to hold the key to some of the most debilitating aspects of clinical allergy. Whilst most would admit that it is by no means solved, some important findings, with implications for pharmacotherapy, have been made (Fig. 10.4). First, the cells involved have been identified. In studies on skin biopsies after intradermal challenge, neutrophils are prominent in the first 18 hours of the LPR, but numbers have dwindled by 48 hours. Eosinophils are also prominent and may persist for 2–3 days. T lymphocytes, predominantly $CD4^+$, accumulate around small blood vessels and persist for 1–2 days. Some of these are activated (show

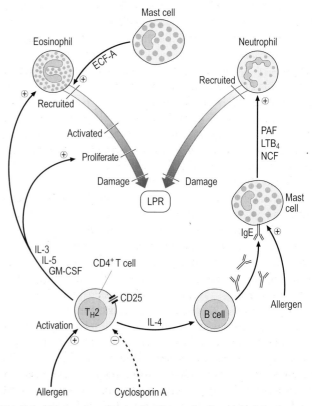

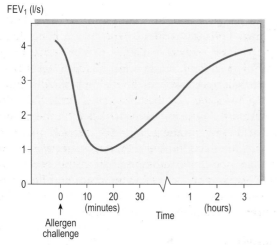

Fig. 10.3 **A patient with allergic asthma is given an endobronchial challenge with allergen and the 1-second forced expiratory volume (FEV_1) is measured.**

Fig. 10.4 **Advances in understanding the mechanism of the late-phase response (LPR) in type I hypersensitivity.** See text for details.

increased surface expression of CD25, the IL-2 receptor). Analysis of BAL fluid in patients with an LPR following endobronchial challenge has revealed similar results. Eosinophils appear in BAL after 6 hours and there is also an expansion of neutrophils and lymphocytes, again of the CD4$^+$ phenotype. Cells are likely to be recruited by release of specific chemotactic factors at the site of allergen-induced inflammation. Platelet activating factor (PAF) and leukotriene B$_4$ attract eosinophils and neutrophils, respectively. These and other mediators are probably also responsible for the activation of neutrophils and eosinophils. One of the features of cellular responses in allergy is that, relative to their proportions in the circulation, eosinophils are recruited in preference to neutrophils. This has been attributed to the actions of IL-5, and eosinophil persistence at these sites is thought to be the result of a combination of IL-3, IL-5 and GM-CSF.

Having arrived at the scene of inflammation, what is the contribution of these cells to the pathogenesis of the LPR? The role of neutrophils is not yet clear, though their phagocytic ability and tendency to release proteolytic enzymes on activation could have a role in tissue damage. Eosinophils are currently amongst the most studied cells in allergic inflammation. A feature of allergic disease known for many years is the associated tissue and blood eosinophilia. Eosinophilia was initially considered a beneficial response, since their granules carry histaminase, which was thought to be an important control mechanism of type I hypersensitivity. The consensus now is that their role is likely to be detrimental. The magnitude of the eosinophil expansion in BAL fluid correlates well with the degree of bronchial constriction in the asthmatic LPR. Several eosinophil cationic granule proteins are damaging to the respiratory epithelium, and eosinophils may also release leukotriene C$_4$ and platelet-activating factor. The current rapid expansion in knowledge about the cell biology of the eosinophil (Ch. 3) promises further surprises. There is certainly evidence at present that eosinophils, long thought to be exclusively derived from bone marrow, may be expanded in the tissues, as T lymphocytes release growth and differentiation factors such as IL-3, IL-5 and GM-CSF.

The unexpected findings in allergic immunopathology have not been confined to the eosinophil. The role of the T lymphocyte has also come into sharp focus recently, such that clinical trials of cyclosporin A, an immunosuppressive drug that targets activated T cells and is more commonly associated with preventing graft rejection, are in progress in asthma. The T cell is clearly involved in allergy: the regulation of IgE production is under the control of T lymphocyte cytokines. But is there any role subsequent to this early step in the development of atopy? Obviously, CD4$^+$ T cells at sites of allergic inflammation may be involved in maintaining the IgE response to an allergen. Several studies using T cell clones (p. 198) generated from patients with allergic disease have described CD4$^+$ T

cells that proliferate in response to incubation with appropriate allergens (e.g. *Der p* I in asthmatics with house dust mite allergy). During this proliferation, responding T cells release IL-4 and, in the presence of B lymphocytes from the same patient, IgE production is stimulated by these T$_H$2 cells. T lymphocytes could also make a significant contribution to the pathogenesis of allergic disease through the recruitment, activation and expansion of eosinophils at sites of allergen exposure (see above). mRNA for IL-5 has been demonstrated in cells in the bronchial mucosa of asthmatics, and cells in the BAL fluid have elevated expression of IL-4 and IL-5 compared with healthy controls. This predominance of T$_H$2 over T$_H$1 responses in relation to type I hypersensitivity is a new theme in allergy research and is likely to be a focus of interest in future studies of immune-based therapies in allergy (see below).

Mechanism of hypersensitivity

- Hypersensitivity is the term used to describe exaggerated or inappropriate immune responses that result in tissue damage.
- Hypersensitivity reaction types I–IV is a useful and simple classification.
- Allergy (type I hypersensitivity) results from the activation of mast cells by allergen-specific IgE.
- An allergen is a small protein which, for reasons unknown, in some individuals induces a persistent IgE response.
- The tendency to allergic reactions (atopy) has both inherited and environmental components.
- T cells, eosinophils and neutrophils are involved in the pathology of clinical allergies such as asthma.

CLINICAL ALLERGY

Approximately two thirds of atopic individuals, defined by a positive allergen skin test (Fig. 10.5), have clinical allergic disease, which itself has a prevalence of between 15 and 20%; males and females are equally affected. Allergic reactions range from being a minor irritation to being life threatening. Occasionally they result in death, usually in association with the chronic lung disease asthma and more rarely through wasp and bee stings or allergy to foods. Allergic disease accounts for up to one third of school absences because of chronic illness, and it is estimated that one of the most common forms, asthma, kills 2000 people in the UK each year, of which 40–45 are children.

Diagnosis

The diagnosis of allergic disease is usually made when the history is taken, and at the same time a good guess

(a)

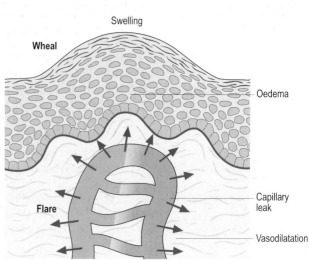

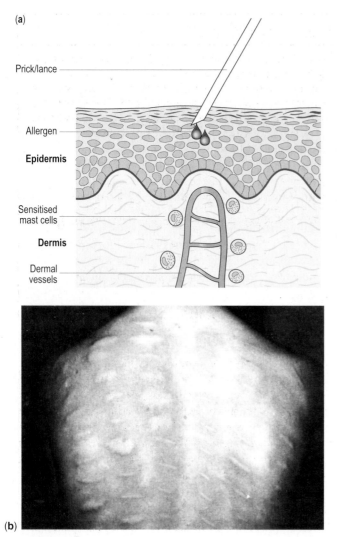

(b)

Fig. 10.5 **The allergen skin test (skin prick test).**
(**a**) Method of testing. (**b**) Back of an atopic individual
demonstrating wheal and flare responses to skin prick tests
administered by subcutaneous scratching with the test allergen.

can be made regarding the nature of the allergens. The timing of the episodes of illness may relate to a seasonal allergy or to exposure to house dust. There is likely to be a family history, and exposure to pets at home or at other people's homes is a frequently recognised trigger.

Skin testing against a wide panel of antigens is usually performed and is almost always positive. Skin tests occasionally reveal sensitisation to allergens not recognised by the patient, and this can help in avoidance. The size of the wheal and flare response, relative to the histamine control or other allergens gives some idea of the importance of each agent. Total IgE levels are raised in the majority of patients. Although the RAST (radioallergosorbent test), which detects serum levels of allergen-specific IgE (see box: 'Detection of allergen-specific IgE by radioallergosorbent test (RAST)'), is often used, it is not a 'diagnose-all'. RAST is expensive to perform and provides little information that a skin test cannot give. In preference, it should be reserved for a few clear indications: when the history and skin test results are at variance; if skin testing cannot be performed because of the continuous use of antihistamines, which suppress the reaction, or a co-existing severe eczema; and when desensitisation is being considered (see below).

A blood eosinophilia (between 0.4×10^9 and 1.0×10^9/l) is often observed in allergic disease. Rarely, a provocation test, exposing the patient to the putative allergen, may be required. These are particularly important in the diagnosis of occupational asthma and should be performed under careful supervision.

Treatment: general principles

Although specific therapies tailored to the disease, particularly with regard to asthma, are important, there are some general principles that can be stated. The first line of therapy is allergen avoidance, followed by drugs. In some allergic disease, the final option may be desensitisation (also termed hyposensitisation or immunotherapy). Avoidance measures may be as obvious as refraining from cycling through the local park in the hay-fever months, or it may be as painful as removing the family pets. Bedding and other furniture is an important source of house dust mites. Mattresses can be encased in plastic, bedding hot-washed regularly and synthetic rather than natural fibres used where possible. Regular vacuuming and damp-dusting helps maintain areas mite-free, and acaricides (mite-killing compounds) are under development. Drug therapy and the use of desensitisation are discussed below.

Detection of allergen-specific IgE by the radioallergosorbent test (RAST)

When skin testing cannot be performed, or desensitisation is being contemplated, measurement of allergen-specific IgE in the serum is indicated. This is typically carried out using the RAST, in which discs are coated with recombinant or purified allergen (Fig. 10.6). These are incubated with test serum and, after washing, radiolabelled ^{125}I-anti-IgE antiserum is added. After a further wash, the radioactivity of the disc is read in a gamma counter, and is proportional to the amount of allergen-specific IgE. Antibodies of other classes (e.g. IgG) are not detected and do not interfere with the results. The test shows a very high correlation with skin test results.

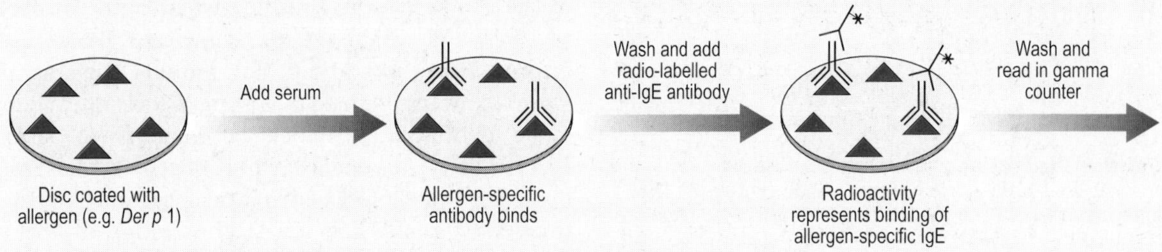

Fig. 10.6 **Radioallergosorbent test (RAST) for detection of allergen-specific IgE.**

ASTHMA

Asthma is the most common chronic disease of childhood, affecting some 5% of children and 2% of adults. The disorder is generally defined as a clinical syndrome of increased responsiveness of the bronchi to a variety of stimuli, with resultant airway narrowing which reverses spontaneously or after drug therapy and is associated with cellular inflammation. Historically it is subdivided as follows: **extrinsic** asthma is associated with positive skin tests (atopy), early onset, family history of atopy, high circulating IgE levels and a seasonal or episodic nature. The 'extrinsic' in the definition refers to the external derivation of the inciting stimulus; this form of asthma is a result of the type I hypersensitivity reactions described in this chapter. **Occupational** asthma is also essentially extrinsic in nature but is not necessarily an IgE-mediated type I hypersensitivity. Some industrial processes give rise to products which act as haptens in the induction of IgE responses (e.g. anhydrides in the plastic industry) whilst other forms of occupational asthma (e.g. toluene sensitivity in the polyurethane industry) are not IgE mediated. **Intrinsic** asthma is not associated with atopy, has an adult onset, a family history of asthma only, normal circulating IgE levels and tends to be perennial. Approximately one half of all cases of asthma have an allergic basis.

Pathogenesis

The pathogenesis of asthma undoubtedly combines the mechanisms of type I hypersensitivity and the late-phase response. The commonest allergens involved in the development of asthma are the house dust mites *Dermatophagoides pteronyssinus* and *D. farinae*, and grass pollen. The primary house dust mite allergen appears to be an intestinally derived enzyme with which the mites coat their faecal material. The cause of the bronchial hyperresponsiveness, which is a key feature of this dis-ease, is not known, although prolonged damage to the respiratory epithelium, possibly by eosinophil-derived mediators, may be important. Hyperresponsiveness manifests itself as bronchoconstriction, inflammation and mucus production with airway plugging in response to innocuous triggers that include upper respiratory tract infections, exercise, cold air, smoke and paint fumes.

Clinical and immunological features

The diagnosis of asthma rests upon the taking of a careful history, the principal complaints being cough (often nocturnal in children), wheeze and shortness of breath. Lung function tests (e.g. FEV_1) demonstrate airways obstruction, but these may be normal between attacks. Since bronchial hyperresponsiveness is an important feature, it can be assessed formally, usually as the amount of a stimulus (e.g. histamine or methacholine) to produce a fall (usually of 20%) in a lung function measurement (e.g. the FEV_1). This is termed the PC_{20} (PC, provocative concentration) (Fig. 10.7). Immunological tests (skin prick test, serum IgE levels) are usually performed to aid diagnosis and to add information gained from the history regarding triggers, so that avoidance can be optimised.

Therapy

After allergen avoidance has been optimised, there are several lines of drug therapy. Antihistamines do not have a role in the treatment of asthma. Education is an important component: some of the drugs require inhalation and optimal delivery is an acquired skill. For mild asthma, or the relief of acute shortness of breath or wheeze, the β_2-adrenoceptor agonists (e.g. salbutamol), which relax bronchial smooth muscle, are recommended. They are usually inhaled as an aerosol, powder or nebuliser, though they may also be given

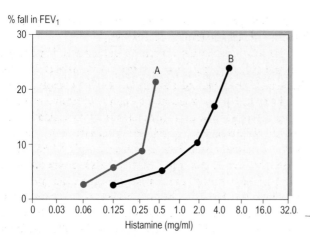

Fig. 10.7 Testing bronchial hyperresponsiveness in asthma.
The percentage fall in FEV$_1$ in a patient (A) and control (B) after
challenge with histamine. The concentration of histamine required
to lower the FEV$_1$ by 20% (PC$_{20}$) was lower in the patient (0.4 mg/
ml) than in the control (4.0 mg/ml) indicating hyperresponsiveness
in the patient.

orally in young children. If asthma is deemed severe, or
β$_2$-agonists are required regularly for symptom relief,
inhaled sodium cromoglycate may be added. An enigmatic drug, cromoglycate is still labelled as a 'mast cell
stabiliser' for want of any better concept of its mode of
action. Moderate to severe asthma requires the addition of inhaled corticosteroids, which have an important role in controlling the disease for many adults and
children. Corticosteroids have several well-identified
modifying actions in the allergic process: production of
prostaglandin and leukotriene mediators is suppressed,
inflammatory cell recruitment and migration is inhibited and vasoconstriction leads to reduced cell and fluid
leakage from the vasculature. Acute, severe asthmatic
attacks are a medical emergency and may require
hospitalisation with administration of xanthines (e.g.
theophylline) or β$_2$-adrenoceptor stimulants given intravenously and parenteral corticosteroids.

ALLERGIC RHINITIS

Although allergic rhinitis appears a somewhat trivial
disorder, it is sufficiently common and disabling to
constitute an important cause of morbidity. The annual
cost of medical services for allergic rhinitis in the USA
is estimated at in excess of $500 million. Usually begin-
ning in childhood or teenage, it affects up to 10% of
children and 20% of adolescents, and seasonal allergic
rhinitis (hay fever) has a marked effect on school per-
formance and examination achievement in this age
group. The main symptoms of rhinitis are nasal congestion, sneezing, often in paroxysms, itching and nasal
and post-nasal discharge. Allergic conjunctivitis is a
frequent association with itchiness, grittiness and excessive watering of the eyes. As with asthma, the target
organ is hyperresponsive, and smoke and paint fumes
can trigger symptoms. The rest of the upper airway
mucosa may be affected, with itchiness of the palate and
pharynx and hearing loss caused by middle ear fluid.

The pathogenesis of allergic rhinitis is similar to that
of asthma. Type I hypersensitivity to allergens, particularly grass or other pollens (seasonal), the house dust
mite and pet furs (perennial), is the initiating factor,
and a late-phase reaction can be demonstrated in many
patients on nasal challenge.

The diagnosis of allergic rhinitis or associated disorders is made on the history. Particular attention must
be paid to the geographical and temporal relationship
of the symptoms. Establishing whether the disorder is
seasonal and which season is involved (June–July for
grass pollen, July–August for moulds such as *Alter-
naria*) coupled with skin testing allows the allergens
to be identified and hence the diagnosis to be made.
Examination, particularly in children, reveals mouth
breathing, pale, blue, oedematous nasal turbinates, and
frequently a red line across the bridge of the nose
caused by the tendency to push the itchy nose upwards.
A clear fluid discharge may be visible in the middle ear.
Of less value, serum total IgE levels may be raised in
30–40% of children with allergic rhinitis, and a blood
eosinophilia may be found. The RAST, for allergen-
specific IgE, and nasal challenge are not typically required for the diagnosis. The RAST is necessary,
however, if desensitisation is being considered.

Therapy should include attempts at avoidance of
exposure, whilst the main pharmacological therapy
centres on the use of antihistamines, which are most
effective when given prophylactically, before the pollen
season starts. Newer generations of antihistamines (e.g.
terfenadine and astemizole) are specific for the H$_1$
histamine receptor and have fewer sedative side effects
than previously observed, since there is minimal transit
across the blood–brain barrier. Nasally administered
sodium cromoglycate and steroids form the second-line
treatments and when all three of these therapies are
being used, they constitute the most effective combination. Steroids are most effective in treating nasal congestion, a symptom which represents the late-phase
reaction. For conjunctivitis, prophylactic oral antihistamines and ocular drops of cromoglycate are the
best approach. Desensitisation (see below) also has an
emerging place in the management of allergic rhinitis.
Surgery to the ear, nose or throat, however, is of no
proved value in the treatment of these allergic
syndromes.

ALLERGIC ECZEMA

The term eczema is derived from Greek and means 'the
result of boiling over'. Often used interchangeably with
dermatitis, eczema defines an inflammatory skin disorder with many possible causes, the hallmark being a
histological process called spongiosis: the accumulation
of oedema fluid within and between keratinocytes in
the epidermis, giving a 'spongy' appearance. It is common, affecting between 5 and 10% of the population,
of whom 80% present at less than 1 year in age, and
90% at less than 5 years. As with other allergic dis-

orders, the incidence appears to be on the increase. Some 30% of sufferers go on to develop asthma, and 50% develop allergic rhinitis.

The main symptoms are itching or, in the infant, the appearance of dry, red patches with occasional vesicles overtaken by crusting. In infancy, the cheeks, abdomen and limb surfaces are involved, whilst in older chidren the classical distribution is on the elbow, knee and wrist flexor surfaces (Fig. 10.8). Prolonged scratching leads to the development of discoloured plaques with a leathery texture (lichenification). In approximately 75% of cases the disorder is self-limiting and clears in the first few years of life.

The diagnosis is made on history, examination and skin testing, with the total serum IgE level also usually raised. In contrast with the respiratory allergic disorders, however, the pathogenesis of allergic eczema is less clear. Skin testing itself evokes a wheal and flare response but not eczematous lesions. It is possible to replicate eczema-like plaques by patch testing with allergens such as house dust mite extracts in sensitive individuals. (Patch testing, in which the allergen is secured as a disc onto the skin surface of the back for 48 hours, is usually used for the identification of sensi-

tisers that give rise to contact dermatitis, a type IV hypersensitivity reaction; see below.)

The relationship between diet and eczema is perhaps the most intriguing and controversial aspect of the disease. Well-designed studies in which potential triggers in food (cow's milk, hen's egg protein) are avoided appear to bring about an improvement in eczema, but only in children. Skin prick tests against food derivatives are usually unhelpful. More complex and comprehensive avoidance diets run the risk of incomplete nutrition and compliance is a problem. At present, therefore, the best advice to parents of children with eczema appears to be a therapeutic trial of avoidance of hen's eggs and dairy produce, preferably followed by a period of reintroduction, with the diet to be continued if tolerated and of benefit.

URTICARIA

Urticaria (also commonly known as 'hives' or 'nettle rash') is a disorder in which well circumscribed, itchy weals erupt over different areas of the body. It is caused by localised vasodilatation and oedema occurring in the superficial dermis. Angio-oedema is a related disorder in which the oedema forms deeper within the dermis, giving larger areas of swollen tissue. Both disorders may be caused by an IgE-mediated type I hypersensitivity in which histamine is one of the dominant pathogenic mediators. However, in the majority of cases a cause for the urticaria/angio-oedema is not found. In these the disease may be chronic and idiopathic or secondary to other disease.

Urticaria associated with type I hypersensitivity is typically acute in onset and frequently occurs in children in association with foodstuffs. The first symptoms are tingling and then swelling of the lips and tongue, some of the commoner allergens being seafood, nuts, berries, eggs and chocolate. Insect stings and drug reactions may also produce the migrating wheals of urticaria. The diagnosis is frequently made by the patient or on the history, and skin testing may be helpful. Since it is often acute in onset and self-limiting, allergic urticaria is difficult to treat apart from the avoidance of provoking stimuli. Antihistamines are also of benefit in acute urticarial reactions.

ANAPHYLAXIS: DEFINITION AND GENERAL CONSIDERATIONS

The term anaphylaxis describes the clinical manifestations of an acute, generalised IgE-mediated immune reaction involving specific antigen, mast cells and basophils. The reaction requires priming by the allergen, followed by re-exposure. To provoke anaphylaxis, the allergen must be systemically absorbed, either after ingestion or parenteral injection and a range of allergens have been identified:

- foods: citrus fruits, mango, strawberry, nuts (Brazil,

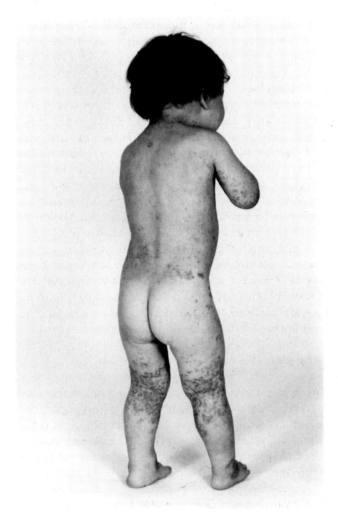

Fig. 10.8 **Typical flexor distribution of eczema in childhood.** (Courtesy of Dr E. Higgins.)

Clinical allergy

- Diagnosis by skin tests; radioallergosorbent test (RAST) and blood eosinophil count can also be performed.
- Treatment starts with avoidance of the allergen, then makes use of drugs and even desensitisation.
- Asthma is increased responsiveness of the bronchi to stimuli with resulting airway narrowing. It is treated with β_2-adrenoceptor agonists (salbutamol); cromoglycate, if moderately severe; corticosteroids to control the disease long term; and β_2-stimulants and xanthines in emergencies.
- Allergic rhinitis affects the upper airways. It can be treated with antihistamines, cromoglycate and corticosteroids.
- Eczema results from oedema between and within the keratinocytes of the epidermis (spongiosis). It most commonly presents in children under 5 years of age and may be helped by allergen avoidance.
- Urticaria (itchy wheals) and angio-oedema are both mediated by histamine, are typically acute and may be related to food.

The discovery of anaphylactic reactions

The heiroglyphics detailing the death of King Menes of Egypt following an insect sting nearly 4000 years ago are probably the first report of a fatal anaphylactic reaction. Subsequently, at the turn of this century, the term anaphylaxis was coined by Portier and Richet. These French biologists, as guests aboard the yacht of the Prince of Monaco cruising in the Mediterranean, became interested in whether it was possible to become protected against the poisonous sting of the Portugese man-of-war jellyfish. They subsequently investigated whether prior exposure of dogs to sea anemone toxin protected them from the severe reactions associated with the venom when reinjected. On the contrary, the dogs reacted even more severely the second time and died within 30 minutes, hence the term anaphylaxis which derives from the Greek and means 'anti-protection'. It became clear that not only toxic substances produced a severe reaction after reinjection: some of the most important studies on anaphylaxis were performed on individuals given more than one dose of the horse serum antitoxins used to treat tetanus and diphtheria in the 1920s. In the 1960s, it is estimated that between 100 and 500 Americans died of anaphylaxis per year when exposed to a repeated dose of penicillin. Today, penicillin and stings from insects of the Hymenoptera order (bees and wasps) are the most important causes of anaphylaxis.

cashew), shellfish (shrimp, lobster), chocolate, legumes (soya bean, peanut)
- venoms: wasps, bees, yellow-jackets, hornets
- medications: hormones (insulin, parathormone), antisera (tetanus, diphtheria), dextran.

The symptom/sign constellation ranges from widespread urticaria to cardiovascular collapse and respiratory arrest leading to death. A syndrome identical to anaphylaxis may occur in the absence of IgE-mediated responses. In this, the triggering response may occasionally be IgG mediated, as in some drug reactions. In other situations, some forms of radiological contrast media have a direct effect on complement, inducing widespread activation. The acute formation of large quantities of immune complexes intravascularly, possibly following repeated infusion of blood products, activates complement and gives an anaphylaxis-like state. These non-IgE-mediated responses are termed **anaphylactoid**.

Data on the current incidence of anaphylaxis are difficult to acquire, but the following statistics give some flavour of the size of the problem: fatal reactions to penicillin occur once every 7.5 million injections; following repeated horse antilymphocyte globulin injections used to treat organ graft rejection, anaphylaxis was observed in 2–20% of patients; between 1 in 250 and 1 in 125 individuals have severe reactions to Hymenoptera (bee and wasp) stings, and a death takes place every 6.5 million stings; such stings cause between 60 and 80 deaths per year in America, and five in the UK. There is controversy as to whether atopy predisposes to anaphylaxis, early studies indicating this to be the case, whereas latterly no association has been found.

Pathogenesis

The molecules that incite anaphylactic responses may be moderately sized proteins (>10 kDa), or they may not be sufficiently large to be antigenic in their own right but behave as haptens (see p. 146). In penicillin allergy, some of the determinants against which IgE responses can be detected by skin testing are common to penicillin derivatives, and the chance of cross-reaction with these is high. Up to 50% cross-reactivity with the cephalosporins has also been described. Animal-derived serum products, such as antilymphocyte globulin and antisera against snake venoms, are potent inducers of anaphylactic responses. The Hymenoptera order of insects contains two families: the Apidae (bees) and the Vespidae (wasps, hornets and the yellow-jackets common in North America). The major sting allergens are the forms of phospholipase A in the venom, although other sting contents may be involved. The IgE responses are not cross-reactive between wasps and bees. As a prelude to desensitisation, it is important to establish the nature of the insect from the history if possible, and RAST or skin tests should be used to identify the allergen to be used in the therapy. Skin testing in these circumstances carries a small risk of anaphylaxis and should be conducted under careful supervision.

At the heart of the pathogenesis of anaphylaxis is the activation of mast cells and basophils, with systemic release of some mediators and generation of others. The initial symptoms may appear innocuous: tingling, warmth and itchiness. The ensuing effects on the vasculature give vasodilatation and oedema. The consequence of these may be no more than a generalised flush, with urticaria and angio-oedema. More serious sequelae are hypotension, bronchospasm, laryngeal oedema and cardiac arrhythmia or infarction. Death may occur within minutes. Up to 20% of patients treated for the initial episode may have a further serious manifestation of anaphylaxis up to 8 hours later, possibly reflecting the release of mediators from recruited cells, akin to the late-phase response in other allergic conditions.

Clinical features

Early recognition and treatment are essential. Death is quick, and delay increases its likelihood. The main aim is the protection of respiratory and cardiovascular function: 1.0 ml of a 1:1000 solution of adrenaline should be given subcutaneously. The effects may be short lived and the therapy may need to be repeated at frequent intervals: as the medical maxim states, the first, second and third lines of treatment of anaphylaxis are adrenaline, adrenaline and adrenaline! Its action is to bronchodilate and vasoconstrict as well as inhibiting mast cell mediator release. Further therapies depend upon the course taken by the patient and the facilities available. Ideally, oxygen should be administered, as well as β-adrenoceptor agonists such as salbutamol or theophylline. Prolonged hypotension results from vasodilatation and fluid loss into the tissues and should be monitored in a high-dependency unit with the use of plasma expanders and inotropes as required. Monitoring should be continued for some 24 hours, and corticosteroids are usually given.

The best treatment is prevention. Avoidance of triggering foods, particularly nuts, fruits, shellfish and chocolate, may require almost obsessive self-discipline. Patient education is, therefore, important, and many are also instructed in the self-administration of adrenaline and carry pre-loaded syringes. Desensitisation has a well-established place in the management of this disorder, particularly if exposure is unavoidable or unpredictable, as in insect stings.

DESENSITISATION

Desensitisation in the context of allergy is also termed immunotherapy or hyposensitisation. It first appeared as a revolutionary treatment for allergy in 1911, but since then has run a controversial course, being favoured in America but received with less enthusiasm in the UK. The principle, as expounded in the title of the original report, is that allergy can be 'prophylactically inoculated against' in much the same way that measles or mumps can be, by giving the potentially damaging agent (in this case the allergen) in a controlled, safe encounter. It is mainly the question of safety that has influenced the use of desensitisation in the UK. In the 1980s there was an increase in interest in using this approach in a range of allergic disorders. However, a

---

Current thinking on desensitisation

In 1986, the Committee on Safety of Medicines (CSM) in the UK met to discuss the alarming figures relating death and desensitisation. Since the 1950s there had been 26 deaths, five of which had been reported during the previous 18 months. All had been associated with the use of desensitising agents, the majority being employed for the treatment of asthma. The tone of the comments of the CSM at that time put desensitisation firmly in the shade as a potential option in the physician's armament against allergy. Specific recommendations were that benefits and risks be weighed carefully; that desensitisation be carried out by experienced hands in the presence of full cardiopulmonary resuscitation facilities; and that patients be monitored for at least 2 hours. More lately there has been a resurgence in the use of desensitisation, based on some very healthy safety statistics. In the USA, in a programme treating 3236 individuals referred for Hymenoptera venom allergy, 0.25% had a severe systemic reaction on skin testing alone. Of 1410 treated with desensitisation, 12% had reactions, of which 9% were considered severe but in the whole cohort there were no deaths. In a UK series, amongst 40 adults treated for uncontrolled summer hay fever with a total of over 500 injections of a grass pollen extract, there was only one systemic reaction, rapidly reversed with subcutaneous adrenaline. It appears that desensitisation, given for the correct reasons by experienced hands, is a safe procedure.

---

number of deaths following severe generalised reactions to allergen preparations during that time led the Committee on Safety of Medicines to issue guidelines in 1986 that severely restricted the practice. In the UK, desensitisation must now be performed by highly trained staff, in specialist centres with immediate access to resuscitation equipment, and patients must remain at the centre for 2 hours after the injection.

Desensitisation is indicated for those disorders in which the hypersensitivity is clearly IgE mediated. Skin tests and RAST must be performed to demonstrate this and to confirm that there is IgE production against the allergen preparation to be used in the therapy. It is not difficult to argue for the use of desensitisation in allergy to insect stings, which in themselves are life threatening. Equally, desensitisation for drug allergy may be warranted if continued use of the drug is deemed necessary. In allergic rhinitis, the weight of potential benefits is more difficult to balance against the dangers and the lack of guaranteed efficacy. On the one hand, allergic rhinitis is a severe irritation but never killed anyone. Although up to 90% of rhinitis sufferers treated with desensitisation may benefit, up to 40% will do so with placebo injections. Desensitisation is safe and one London centre has given several thousand immunotherapeutic injections in recent years for allergies, including rhinitis, without morbidity or mortality. Desensitisation is generally not considered for asthmatics, although some studies have shown that mild asthmatics do benefit. Immunotherapeutic management of pet and multiple allergies also differs between the UK and America. Multiple allergy is not treated with multiple allergen desensitisation therapy in the UK, but may be in the USA. Equally, allergy to your cat in Britain is met with the advice to 'get rid of Tiddles'; in contrast, in America it is 'roll up your sleeve'.

Desensitisation is performed by repeated injections of an identified allergen. Most treatment regimens

Table 10.2 **Mechanism of action of desensitisation**

Mechanism	Explanation
Blocking antibodies	During repeated exposure to desensitising allergen, IgG class antibodies develop; these absorb allergens preferentially on natural exposure
Anti-IgE autoantibodies	Appear after desensitisation and could regulate production
Suppression	T cells with an allergen-specific suppressor activity are generated or expanded and down-regulate IgE allergen-specific production
Changes in effector cells	A decrease in eosinophils and mast cells in the nasal mucosa after treatment has been reported
Changes in immunoregulatory T cells	IgE production is determined by the balance of T_H1 and T_H2 CD4 lymphocyte responses: desensitisation tips the balance in favour of the T_H1 cells

begin with subcutaneous injections twice per week until the maximum dose is reached, usually after 6–10 weeks. Injections are then continued monthly for up to 1 year. It remains unclear how desensitisation works, but there are currently four main theories (Table 10.2).

Future developments in the treatment of allergic disease

Judging by the present size of the drug bill for allergy therapy, the pharmaceutical industry is unlikely to halt its large research programmes, currently aimed at providing better drugs or better modes of delivery. However, there are several alternative new approaches to allergy treatment centring on the involvement of T cells in allergy, which, though still at the experimental stage, may offer treatments for the future. One of these is surprising in this context: the use of cyclosporin, a drug usually associated with treating organ graft rejection. The rationale for the use of cyclosporin is based on the recent demonstration that activated T cells, expressing the IL-2 receptor on their surface, are a dominant feature in the blood and bronchial biopsies of patients with acute severe asthma and are likely to be responsible for recruiting and activating inflammatory cells. Activated T cells are inactivated by cyclosporin specifically through its ability to inhibit the IL-2 receptor/IL-2 autocrine loop. In a recent randomised, double-blind, placebo-controlled trial, asthmatic patients receiving cyclosporin had improved peak air flow and a reduced dependence on steroids. A second strategy is to block the functioning of CD23, the low-affinity IgE receptor on B lymphocytes that is involved in up-regulating IgE production. Antibody to CD23 injected into a rat model of allergy stops the production of allergen-specific IgE and could be applicable in humans. Finally, peptide immunotherapy (see p. 311) is an approach that is gaining credence as a future treatment of disorders in which tissue damage is largely orchestrated by clones of T lymphocytes recognising particular peptide antigens presented by selected class II HLA molecules. In allergy, recent evidence supports the existence of such clones. In one patient with house dust mite-induced perennial allergic rhinitis, a T cell clone was isolated that reacts with extract of *Dermatophagoides farinae*. The sequence of the T cell receptor V_β chain of this clone was obtained: 6 years later the patient still had T cells bearing the same receptor sequence in the peripheral blood. Targeting of these long-lived, allergen-reactive clones could be an important first step in peptide immunotherapy.

Generalised anaphylaxis and desensitisation

- Occurs after re-exposure to a systemically absorbed allergen, e.g. food, venom, medication.
- It is caused by activation of mast cells and basophils.
- Symptoms range from urticaria to cardiovascular collapse and respiratory arrest; further episodes can occur up to 8 hours later; death may occur within minutes.
- Treatment involves protecting respiratory and cardiovascular function and administering subcutaneous adrenaline (often repeated at intervals).
- Prevention can involve avoiding the trigger, carrying adrenaline and undergoing desensitisation.

OTHER TYPES OF HYPERSENSITIVITY

TYPE II HYPERSENSITIVITY: ANTIBODY TARGETS CELL SURFACE ANTIGENS

Hypersensitivity reactions types II and III are initiated by the interaction between antibody and antigen but in these cases IgE is not involved. The distinction between the types is based on where the complex of antibody and antigen form: in type II, the target is fixed in the tissues or on the cell surface; in type III the target is soluble and circulating immune complexes are formed.

The consequences of antibody binding to a cell surface antigen are predictable: (1) complement is activated leading to cell lysis, mast cell activation and neutrophil recruitment; (2) the antigen–antibody complex recruits cells directly through Fc interactions (Fig. 10.9). The arrival of cells with cytotoxic capability (neutrophils, eosinophils, monocytes, killer cells) may lead to a mechanism of damage described as antibody-dependent cell-mediated cytotoxicity (ADCC). There is also the possibility that if the cell surface target is a receptor, binding of antibody will have an effect on cell function: this could be directly inhibitory, could block binding of the natural ligand or be excitatory. The best known examples of the effects of antibodies on physiological receptor function are in autoimmune thyroid disease (see Ch. 13).

The diseases that arise as a result of tissue damage in a type II hypersensitivity reaction are varied and the clinical picture depends upon the target tissue:

- organ-specific autoimmune diseases
  - myasthenia gravis
  - antiglomerular basement membrane glomerulonephritis
  - pemphigus vulgaris
- autoimmune cytopenias (i.e. blood cell destruction)
  - haemolytic anaemia
  - thrombocytopenia
  - neutropenia
- transfusion reactions
- haemolytic disease of the newborn (rhesus isoimmunisation)
- hyperacute allograft rejection.

The diseases will be described in detail in their respective chapters. In some, the antibodies target self cell surface proteins, resulting in an autoimmune disease. In others, the targets are on exogenous cells, perhaps in an incompatible blood transfusion or organ graft. In some type II hypersensitivity diseases, the pathogenetic mechanisms are known: for example, several forms of haemolytic anaemia follow infectious disease or drug reactions (see p. 287). In these the red blood cell surface antigen may be targeted as a result of cross-reaction with the provoking stimulus. Alternatively, drugs can modify cell surface proteins and render them immunogenic. In haemolytic disease of the newborn (rhesus isoimmunisation) (see p. 292), transfusion reactions and hyperacute graft rejection (see p. 149), antibodies against cell surface targets arise during a previous encounter, whether it be a previous pregnancy, in the case of rhesus isoimmunisation, or a previous transfusion or transplant. In other conditions, particularly the organ-specific autoimmune diseases, it remains unknown why the antibodies arise.

TYPE III HYPERSENSITIVITY: ANTIGEN AND ANTIBODY INTERACT IN THE CIRCULATION

In type III hypersensitivity, antigen–antibody complexes form. To initiate a type III hypersensitivity reaction, the complexes become deposited in a tissue and there the process of complement and cellular recruitment and activation takes place, with resulting tissue damage. The typical histological appearance of an immune complex lesion frequently includes deposition of fibrin (so-called 'fibrinoid necrosis') suggesting that activation of the clotting cascade also has a role in tissue damage.

There are two forms of type III hypersensitivity reaction: complexes may form in the circulation and become deposited in the tissues, or they may actually form within tissues. The latter mechanism is also termed the 'Arthus' reaction, after Maurice Arthus who injected foreign proteins under the skin of animals that he had already immunised with the same protein. The antigen–antibody complexes forming within the tissue incited an erythematous lesion after 3–6 hours.

Immune complex formation in itself is not an exceptional or dangerous occurrence, since immune complexes are carried through the circulation during many diseases ranging from the common cold to cancer. This process is a physiological mechanism for removing antigen. Immune complexes in the circulation recruit complement and are carried to the spleen or liver on complement receptors embedded in the red blood cell membrane (see Ch. 21). Within the tissues, small numbers of complexes being deposited are easily removed. For a type III hypersensitivity reaction to occur, then, something must disturb this homeostatic mechanism. Several factors are known to be capable of predisposing to the excessive and damaging formation of immune complexes, and these relate to the antigen, the host response and the tissue.

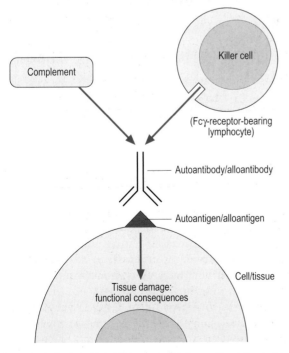

Fig. 10.9 Mechanism of type II hypersensitivity reactions. See text for details.

Factors relating to the antigen include **charge** and **persistence**. A charged molecule, such as DNA, is more likely to be attracted to, and become attached to, charged areas within the body, such as the glomerular basement membrane (DNA is an important target antigen of autoantibodies in systemic lupus erythematosus (SLE)). Persistent production of antigen will lead to a continuous supply of complexes, overloading the removal process and amplifying the opportunities for deposition and damage. Examples of antigen persistence include the bacterial proteins continuously cast off the heart valves during infective endocarditis, and similar proteins emanating from infected ventriculoperitoneal shunts used to relieve high intracranial pressure.

The host response is important in determining the potential pathogenicity of immune complexes. The **isotype** of antibody in a complex influences complement fixation and, thus, its solubility. The integrity of the complement cascade is also an important determinant of whether complexes are solubilised and removed. Function of the classical pathway, which requires C2 and C4, is critical in solubilising antigen–antibody complexes. Genetically determined deficiency of complement component C4 is found in approximately half of patients with SLE, one of the best examples of a disease in which immune complexes contribute to the pathogenesis. C2 deficiency is much rarer, but almost all patients with this defect have an SLE-like syndrome. Patients with SLE also have impaired immune complex transport, since a reduction in the density of complement receptors on the surface of their erythrocytes has been reported.

The tissues typically exposed to injury by immune complexes are the renal glomerulus and the joint synovium. These are tissues in which plasma from the blood is ultrafiltrated to form urine and synovial fluid, respectively. The hydrostatic pressure involved in such a process and the filtrative function of the glomerular basement membrane are likely to contribute to the retention and, therefore, the pathogenicity of immune complexes.

Finally, there are the characteristics of the complexes themselves, which determine the extent of tissue damage (Table 10.3). Much of the research in this area

Table 10.3 **Factors contributing to immune complex disease**

Factors	Mechanisms
Relative proportions of antigen and antibody	Complexes formed in antigen or antibody excess are less likely to deposit
Impaired classical complement pathway function	Classical pathway has key role in solubilising and transporting complexes
Isotype of antibody	Isotype dictates ability to fix complement
Rate of complex formation	If rate of formation exceeds clearance, complex deposition is enhanced

has been carried out using animal models, in which a source of foreign antigen is injected as a bolus (see box 'Serum sickness as a model of immune complex disease').

The variety of factors capable of influencing immune complex deposition is paralleled by the variety of diseases which are known to be immune complex mediated. There are three broad categories of immune complex disease (Table 10.4; Fig. 10.11). In some, the immune complexes formed in the circulation deposit in the tissues, leading directly to nephritis, synovitis or iritis. In a second group, complex deposition is predominantly into the walls of medium or small-sized arterioles, and the vasculitis that ensues is the cause of organ damage in the kidney, skin or other organs. In others, particularly the type III hypersensitivity lung diseases, antigens and antibody combine within the tissue, resembling an Arthus reaction.

The lung disorders are an interesting group of occupation and 'pastime-related' diseases. Exposure over many months or years to excessive amounts of inhaled antigen leads to the generation of large concentrations of antibodies within the lung interstitium. At a subsequent exposure, immune complex formation takes place on a large scale in the alveoli. Typically, patients with this disease, termed **extrinsic allergic alveolitis**, present 3–6 hours after loading mouldy hay, cleaning the pigeon loft or packing the sugar cane, with symptoms of fever, chills, malaise and dyspnoea. They may admit to milder episodes leading up to the presenting illness. Symptoms usually remit within 24 hours, but chronic exposure can lead to progressive shortness of breath, with cyanosis, lung fibrosis and the development of cor pulmonale. The diagnosis is made on the history and the demonstration of circulating IgG antibodies (called **precipitins**) to the provoking antigen.

TYPE IV HYPERSENSITIVITY: TISSUE DAMAGE BY T$_H$1 CELLS

The type IV (delayed) hypersensitivity category is perhaps the one that has least stood the test of time during the years after the original classification of tissue-damaging reactions by Gell and Coombs. At the time they wrote, little was known of T cell physiology, the processes of antigen presentation, cytokines or the cognate interactions between T and B lymphocytes. The description of type IV hypersensitivity was based upon the observation that certain inflammatory conditions associated with tissue damage are characterised by cellular infiltrates, composed in the main of a combination of lymphocytes and macrophages. Such inflammatory infiltrates arise at least 24 hours after challenge with the provoking stimulus, and macrophages in the lesion frequently fuse to form giant cells and epithelioid cells.

Some of the best examples of type IV hypersensitivity include reactions to mycobacteria and other similar

---

Serum sickness as a model of immune complex disease

The possibility that antigen–antibody complexes could result in disease was proposed by von Pirquet in 1911. At that time, a common therapy was the injection of hyperimmune antiserum against pathogenic toxins such as those produced by diphtheria and tetanus. These antisera were produced by raising the antibodies in horses, but a high proportion of patients developed reactions after the injections. The reaction typically comprised a transient arthritis, skin rash and fever arising a week after the first injection and then more rapidly after subsequent doses. Von Pirquet showed that the reactions could be induced by normal horse serum not containing the antitoxin, and he proposed that antibodies formed against the foreign proteins in horse serum were responsible for the reaction. Studies some 40 to 50 years later reproduced similar effects after a bolus injection of foreign protein into rabbits (Fig. 10.10). This model is termed **acute** serum sickness and probably represents the processes seen in post-streptococcal nephritis, with antibody levels rising rapidly in response to a large bacterial load. Another model, **chronic** serum sickness is generated by repeated intermittent injection of foreign antigen and could represent the processes seen in immune complex diseases such as shunt nephritis and SLE.

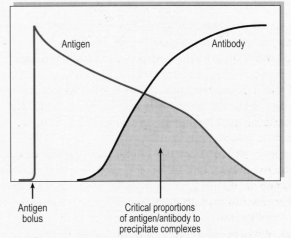

Fig. 10.10 **Immune complexes arise in immune complex disease.** See text for details.

Table 10.4 **Immune complex-mediated disorders**

Immune complex deposits	Antigen	Disorder	Pathology
Deposited or formed in tissue	Group A streptococci	Post-streptococcal nephritis	Nephritis
	DNA	Systemic lupus erythematosus (SLE)	Nephritis, serositis
	Bacterial antigens	Subacute bacterial endocarditis (SBE); shunt nephritis	Nephritis
Vessel deposition	HBsAg	Polyarteritis nodosa	Vasculitis
	DNA	SLE	Vasculitis
	Bacterial antigens	SBE	Vasculitis
Form in tissues	Mouldy hay	Farmer's lung	Extrinsic allergic alveolitis (EAA)
	Mouldy sugar cane	Bagassosis	EAA
	Avian droppings	Bird breeder's lung; pigeon fancier's lung	EAA

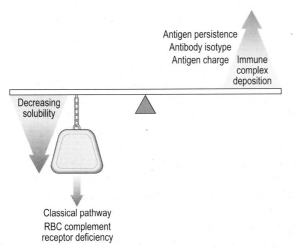

Fig. 10.11 **Factors contributing to immune complex-mediated damage.**

organisms, which the immune system has difficulty eliminating. Reactions range from the local redness and swelling seen at the site of intradermal tests for tuberculosis immunity (e.g. Heaf test, Mantoux test), in which an extract from the organism is injected, to the caseating necrosis that occasionally results from a host's attempts to deal with *Mycobacterium tuberculosis* infection. Granulomata, which 'wall off' the infective focus, may also arise in response to other infections, such as the parasitic worm infestation of schistosomiasis. Within the granulomata, there is extensive tissue damage, with fibrosis and calcification. This type of reaction can have serious clinical consequences if the site of damage is the lung, liver or bone. In these circumstances, the immune system is caught between the repercussions of not dealing with the infection, and the tissue damage that is caused by activated and differentiated macrophages. Macrophages are activated by CD4$^+$ T$_H$1 lymphocytes and release powerful hydrolytic enzymes and toxic oxygen metabolites (see Ch. 6). Other factors released within the infiltrate encourage fibrosis and angiogenesis.

Another example of type IV hypersensitivity is that resulting in some individuals from exposure to contact with nickel in jewellery, dichromate in the leather industry or *p*-phenyldiamine in sunscreens and hair dyes. The reaction is confined to the skin and is frequently termed **contact dermatitis**. Typically there is an eczematous reaction with erythema, oedema, vesicles and scaling. Since there are many potential irritants and the lesions usually require 48 hours to appear, the diagnosis of such reactions is often a painstaking piece of detective work. This may be helped by **patch testing** in which potential contact sensitisers are placed in contact with the skin on the back for 48 hours.

Application of sensitising agents to the skin in animal models has allowed some of the pathogenetic aspects of contact dermatitis to be studied. As early as 1942, Landsteiner and Chase demonstrated that cells, but not serum, could transfer contact sensitivity from an affected to an unsensitised animal. Prior to this, Landsteiner had coined the term **hapten** to describe substances incapable, because of their small size, of provoking the formation of antibodies without conjugation to carrier proteins, and this concept is at the heart of the process involved in contact dermatitis. It is believed that the metals or compounds in the sensitising agent become conjugated to tissue proteins. An intact local lymphatic system and lymph node are required for the reaction to be initiated, and the hapten–carrier compound is probably transported to the node by Langerhans cells in the skin.

In vitro, type IV hypersensitivity reactions are recreated in assays termed lymphocyte transformation or proliferation assays (see Ch. 7). Culture of lymphocytes from a reactive individual with the provoking agent (mycobacterial extract, schistosomal proteins, nickel) results in measurable T cell responses. Some of these, such as the production of IFN-γ are of direct relevance to the pathogenetic processes (Fig. 10.12).

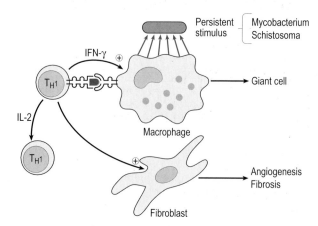

Fig. 10.12 **Diagram illustrating the cellular/molecular basis of a type IV hypersensitivity response.**

Other types of hypersensitivity (II–IV)

- Antibody, recruiting complement and cytotoxic cells with Fc receptors can cause tissue damage. This is frequently an autoantibody. The antigenic targets may be tissue-fixed (type II) or in the circulation (type III).
- In type II, the target cell surface antigens may be altered self or exogenous cells (e.g. hyperacute graft rejection).
- In type III the immune complex may be deposited in tissues or vessels (SLE) or may form in tissues (farmer's lung).
- Hypersensitivity resulting from T lymphocyte reactions is usually delayed in onset. The central cells in this type IV hypersensitivity are the CD4$^+$ T lymphocyte and the macrophage.
- Granulomata are characteristic and contact dermatitis is a typical clinical example.

Transplantation

The obvious reason for transplantation is to re-establish a function lost following end-stage disease (or physical loss) of a given organ or tissue. That was not the reason for one of the first grafts on record. To free himself from captivity in Crete, Daedalus aimed to acquire a new function — that of flying — through the xenogeneic transplant of bird feathers. His attempt succeeded and he landed safely in mainland Greece. His son, Icarus, failed in the same attempt. His transplant failed, reportedly from the melting of a thermolabile adhesive — perhaps the first reported case of hyperacute rejection — even though we are now aware of immunological reasons (see box: 'Xenogenic transplantation') for the failure of a **xenograft**, a transplant between members of different species. The outcome of an **autograft** is different, as depicted in Byzantine iconography. In one such example, a doubting witness to the Virgin Mary's ascension into heaven finds his arm severed by an impatient Angel. An intervention of the Virgin Mary re-establishes the anatomy and physiology of the severed limb. This successful outcome may not be the result only of the skills of the operator but also of the fact that in this type of intervention, an

---

Xenogenic transplantation

The shortage of organs for transplantation has [re]search on the possibility of animal donors. A [choi]ce is represented by pigs, since their organs [are h]uman equivalents for size. When trans[planted into h]umans, however, pig organs undergo [rejec]tion. This is because of the presence of [natural] antibodies in the human circulation, [which bind] swine endothelial cells, activate [complement] ively and provoke graft destruction [during] surgery. Various approaches have [been tried] to overcome these limitations in[cluding removal] tion of the 'natural' antibodies and [com]plement activation.

[The antibodies re]cognised by the human anti-swine [serum have bee]n identified as a single carbohydrate [structure havin]g a terminal trisaccharide: galactosyl α-1,3-galactosyl β-1,4-N-acetylglucosaminyl. The proposition to construct an immunosorbent device containing beads coated with this carbohydrate antigen and aimed at removing damaging antibodies from the patient's serum is being actively pursued. Another suggestion is to generate 'knock-out' pigs in which the gene encoding the enzyme responsible for the

generation of the damaging epitope, α-1,3-galactosyl transferase, is crippled, with the consequent 'silencing' of the target antigen. An alternative approach focuses on the control of complement activation, the main mediator of damage. This has already produced results. In xenogeneic transplants, the endothelial cell damage is ultimately caused by unrestrained complement activation. The activation is unrestrained because pig cell membrane-bound complement inhibitors cannot control activation of human complement. Transgenic pigs, expressing human complement inhibitors have now been generated. When their hearts are transplanted into baboons the hyperacute rejection is abolished. Instead of minutes, the transplanted hearts survived up to 30 hours.

The next step will probably be the establishment of genetically engineered pigs, in which expression of human complement inhibitors is induced and that of the antigen target of natural antibodies silenced. Once these hurdles have been overcome, there will still be problems of cellular and humoral reactions to xenoantigens, but these are for the future.

autograft, a tissue or organ is transplanted within the same individual; in clinical practice the tissue is usually transplanted to a new site. In an autograft, as Hindu physicians knew some 2500 years ago, the graft invariably 'takes'. During experimental attempts in the early 1950s to transfer kidneys between humans, surgeons were faced with the natural outcome of an **allograft** — a graft between genetically non-identical members of the same species — namely invariable **rejection**. These experimenters noted that rejection can be partly controlled by drastically restraining the immune system with **immunosuppression**. During these initial attempts at kidney transplantation, it was also noted that a **syngraft**, a graft between genetically identical subjects, such as monozygotic twins, would not undergo rejection. The study of why genetically different individuals are histoincompatible, i.e. reject each other's tissues, led to the identification of glycoproteins encoded by the MHC as the key to incompatibility. As discussed elsewhere (see p. 58), the enormous variability of the MHC molecules within a species must confer some evolutionary advantage. If that species were confronted, say, by a pandemic with a lethal virus, it would be advantageous for some individuals to have a set of MHC molecules — missing in the remaining dying population — able to present a peptide of the processed virus to the immune system in such a way that the virus was eliminated and the individuals survived. A downside to this evolutionary advantage is the fact that a grafted tissue, by virtue of the unrelatedness of its MHC molecules to those of the recipient, elicits in the latter a most vigourous anti-donor-MHC immune response. The nomenclature used to describe different types of transplant is summarised in the box: 'Nomenclature'.

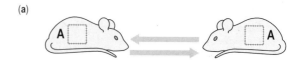
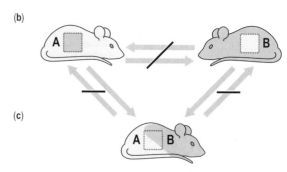

Fig. 11.1 Rules of transplantation.
(**a**) A syngeneic transplantation, within individuals of an inbred strain always succeeds. (**b**) An allogeneic transplantation, between individuals of different inbred strains always fails. (**c**) A transplantation from an inbred parent to a hybrid (F₁) offspring succeeds, but grafts from the offspring to either parent will fail. Moreover, whilst the immunocompetent cells of AB react with neither of the alloantigens encoded by A or B, the cells of A or B can react against alloantigens present in AB. In the last example, the graft is not rejected itself but provides immunocompetent cells that attack the host, through the recognition of alloantigenic differences, in what is known as graft-versus-host (GVH) reaction. GVH occurs when immunocompetent cells are tranferred into an animal that cannot reject them either for genetic reasons, as in the case depicted, or following immunosuppression.

- transplantations within inbred strains will succeed
- transplantation between inbred strains will fail
- transplantations from an inbred parent to a hybrid (F1) offspring will succeed, but grafts from the offspring to either parent will fail.

Using inbred animals it has been possible to define the dynamic process of rejection (Fig. 11.2). Transplanting a segment of skin from mouse A into the genetically unrelated mouse B (allotransplantation), the skin is rejected in 7–14 days (first-set or primary rejection). If mouse B is transplanted again with skin of mouse A, the rejection occurs much more speedily

---

Nomenclature

- Autograft or autologous transplant: the organ/tissue is transplanted within the same individual. It does not undergo rejection.
- Syngraft or syngeneic transplant: the organ/tissue is transplanted between genetically identical subjects, such as monozygotic twins or inbred laboratory animals. It does not undergo rejection.
- Allograft or allogeneic transplant: the organ/tissue is transplanted between genetically non-identical members of the same species. It is rejected unless immunosuppression is instituted.
- Xenograft or xenogeneic transplant: the organ/tissue is transplanted between members of different species. It is rejected hyperacutely.

Introductory points

- Transplantation is used to replace organs that have undergone an irreversible pathological process which threatens the patient's life or considerably hampers the quality of life.
- In humans, the organ usually derives from a genetically unrelated individual (allograft), rarely from a monozygous twin (syngraft); in the future it may derive from a member of a different species (xenograft).
- An allograft would normally be rejected. This is prevented by immunosuppression. A syngraft is never rejected, while a xenograft is rejected hyperacutely.

On the basis of studies in genetically identical inbred animals some rules of transplantation have been established (Fig. 11.1):

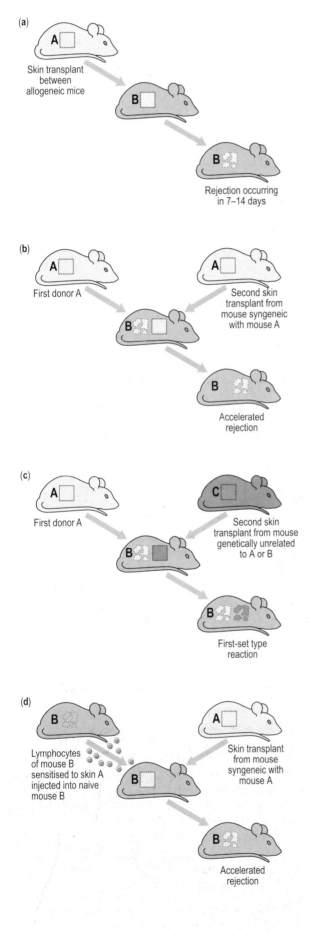

(a)

Skin transplant
between
allogeneic mice

Rejection occurring
in 7–14 days

(b)

First donor A

Second skin
transplant from
mouse syngeneic
with mouse A

Accelerated
rejection

(c)

First donor A

Second skin
transplant from mouse
genetically unrelated
to A or B

First-set type
reaction

(d)

Lymphocytes
of mouse B
sensitised to skin A
injected into naive
mouse B

Skin transplant
from mouse
syngeneic with
mouse A

Accelerated
rejection

Fig. 11.2 **Types of rejection.**
(**a**) Transplantation of a skin graft from mouse A to the genetically unrelated mouse B (allograft) results in rejection of the skin graft. This starts manifesting itself 1 week post-transplant and leads to the elimination of the graft though a process of primary — or first-set — rejection. (**b**) If a mouse B is grafted a second time with skin from mouse A or from a mouse genetically identical to A, the ensuing rejection is accelerated. (**c**) If mouse B is grafted a second time but with skin from a mouse C, unrelated to B or A, the ensuing rejection has the features of a primary rejection. (**d**) The lymphocytes of a mouse that has undergone rejection are able to transfer the memory of sensitisation to a naive mouse, such that on engraftment of skin a second-set rejection occurs.

(second-set or secondary rejection). A second-set rejection occurs even if the skin derives not from the very same mouse A but from a mouse of the same inbred strain, a syngeneic mouse. If the transplanted tissue, however, derives from a third-party mouse C, genetically unrelated to both mouse A and B, the skin is eliminated following the pattern of a first-set type of rejection. In common with conventional immune responses, therefore, antigraft immunity has the characteristics of memory and specificity.

MECHANISMS OF REJECTION

In an attempt to understand the mechanisms of rejection, tissues of the rejecting organs obtained by biopsy have been analysed. They invariably contain an inflammatory infiltrate predominantly composed of mononuclear white blood cells, i.e. lymphocytes and macrophages. The analysis of such infiltrates with monoclonal antibodies has demonstrated their composition to be heterogeneous, with CD4 cells, CD8 cells, macrophages, B lymphocytes and natural killer cells all being represented. Therefore, the analysis of the infiltrate characterising cellular rejection (see below) that occurs 7–14 days post-operatively does not suggest the involvement of a single type of immunocompetent cell, or indeed a single mechanism, in the development of rejection.

There is evidence to suggest that the mechanisms prevailing during physiological immune responses also apply to graft rejection (Fig. 11.3). As in classical immune responses, it is the balance between the different components of the immune system that decrees the magnitude and manifestations of the rejection process. Once a virgin (or naive) helper CD4 cell designated T_H0 has recognised an alloantigen, presented by a professional antigen-presenting cell such as a dendritic cell, which is singularly competent in providing the co-stimulation signals needed to arouse virgin cells, it can become either a T_H1 or a T_H2 cell according to the microenvironment it encounters and the nature of the alloantigenic stimulus. If the surrounding medium is rich in IL-12, a macrophage-derived cytokine, the

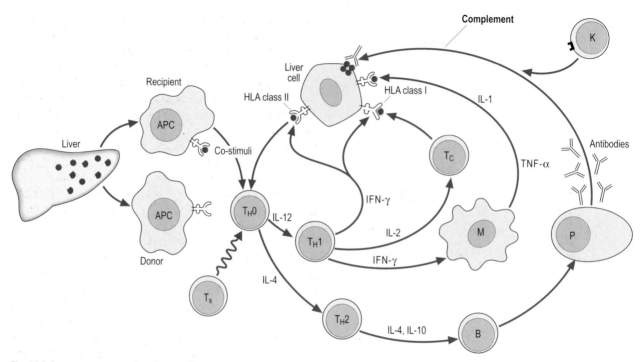

Fig. 11.3 Immune responses to a liver graft.
Intact alloantigens present on donor APCs or allopeptides present in the groove of the recipient's HLA molecules are presented to an uncommitted T helper (T_H0) lymphocyte. T_H0 cells become activated and, according to the nature of the alloantigen and the presence in the microenvironment of IL-12 or IL-4, differentiate into T_H1 or T_H2 cells to initiate a series of immune reactions. These are determined by the cytokines produced: T_H2 cells secrete mainly IL-4 and IL-10 and direct alloantibody production by B lymphocytes; T_H1 cells secrete IL-2 and IFN-γ, which stimulate cytotoxic T lymphocytes (T_C), enhance expression of class I and induce expression of class II HLA molecules on hepatocytes and activate macrophages. Activated macrophages release IL-1 and TNF-α. If T suppressor (T_S) lymphocytes do not oppose, a variety of effector mechanisms are triggered: liver cell destruction could derive from the action of T_C lymphocytes; cytokines released by T_H1 cells and recruited macrophages; complement activation; and/or engagement of FcR-bearing killer (K) lymphocytes by the alloantibody bound to the hepatocyte surface.

virgin T_H0 CD4 cell will commit itself to the T_H1 phenotype and function and orchestrate the activation of CD8 cytotoxic T cells and of macrophages through the release of IL-2 and IFN-γ. If, however, the prevailing cytokine is IL-4, the virgin cell will differentiate into the T_H2 phenotype, and through the secretion of IL-4 and IL-10 will direct the activation of B lymphocytes and antibody production. The study of proteins and RNA transcripts within the graft during cellular rejection has consistently shown the presence of IL-2 and IFN-γ and of granzyme B, a specific marker of cytotoxic T cells, but not of IL-4, suggesting the execution of a T_H1-directed programme during rejection episodes. IFN-γ would recruit and activate macrophages and enhance MHC expression on the graft, making it particularly susceptible to the cytotoxic action of CD8 cells; IL-2 would, in turn, favour the activation of cytotoxic T cells. There is some evidence indicating the involvement of cells of the T_H2 phenotype in the induction of graft tolerance.

ALLOANTIGEN RECOGNITION

Within the context of clinical and experimental transplantation, performed between unrelated individuals of the same species, the antigens recognised during rejection are referred to as **alloantigens** and, as mentioned

earlier, the key alloantigens are those encoded by the MHC. In humans these are known as HLA molecules. The physiological function of such molecules is to present peptide antigen to a complementary T cell receptor. The key question arises as to how MHC-derived alloantigens are recognised. Two possibilities exist (Fig. 11.4). First, the recipient's immune system could recognise an intact MHC molecule (**direct allorecognition**). Second, a peptide (allopeptide) derived from the foreign MHC molecule could be presented within the groove of the recipient's MHC molecule (**indirect allorecognition**). It has been established that cells capable of recognising intact donor-MHC molecules outnumber those recognising processed allopeptides by 1000–10 000. The reason for this difference has been attributed to the fact that intact MHC molecules derived from the donor, the targets of direct allorecognition, carry in their grooves peptides originating from antigenic encounters that occurred in the donor. Therefore, the alloantigens recognised by the recipient's immune system consist not only of donor MHC molecules but also of MHC molecules loaded with peptides generated within the donor before transplantation. In addition to providing supplementary alloantigenic stimuli, the 'carry-over' peptides stabilise the conformation of the donor's MHC molecules. A stable MHC conformation has an important role in

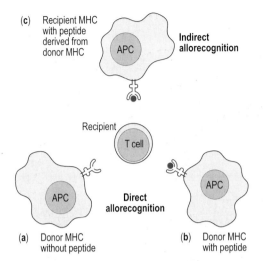

(c) Recipient MHC with peptide derived from donor MHC — Indirect allorecognition

Recipient T cell

Direct allorecognition

(a) Donor MHC without peptide

(b) Donor MHC with peptide

Fig. 11.4 **Types of allorecognition.**
The recipient's T cells have the potential of recognising HLA molecules as they are (**a**) or loaded with 'carry-over' peptides (**b**), the latter generated through the processing of antigens that occurred in the donor until the day of donation. The carry-over peptide magnifies enormously the range of alloantigens to be recognised by the recipient's immune system. (a) and (b) depict the two forms of direct allorecognition. (**c**) An alloantigen, typically an HLA molecule, can be taken up and processed by the recipient's APC and then be presented to autologous T cells. This exemplifies indirect allorecognition.

allorecognition, since empty donor's MHC molecules have been shown to provide a poor allogeneic stimulus.

CLASSIFICATION OF REJECTION REACTIONS

In clinical practice, the vast majority of transplanted organs are allogeneic and, in spite of immunosuppression therapy, tend to undergo episodes of rejection of different severity. Rejection can be classified according to the timescale of its appearance and to the immune mechanisms involved (Table 11.1).

Hyperacute rejection

Hyperacute rejection is mediated by pre-formed antibodies in the recipient that are directed against antigens of the donor organ; it occurs within minutes to a few hours after implantation, depending on the concentration and type of the 'anti-donor' antibody present in the recipient. Transplants across the ABO blood group barrier provide examples of hyperacute rejection, which can be particularly dramatic when an organ from a group A or B donor is transplanted into an O recipient,

Table 11.1 **Classification of rejection**

Type	Time after transplantation	Probable mechanism
Hyperacute	Minutes	Preformed antibodies
Accelerated acute	1–5 days	T lymphocytes
Acute	From 2nd week	T lymphocytes
Chronic	Months to years	Antibodies, complement, adhesion molecules

whose circulation contains anti-A and anti-B antibodies (isohaemagglutinins). Remember that ABO blood group antigens are abundantly expressed on endothelial cells. Hyperacute rejection can also be mediated by antibodies directed against donor HLA class I molecules, the origin of which can be traced to previous leukocyte-containing blood transfusions, previous transplants or pregnancies. The recipient's preformed antibodies bind to the endothelium in vessels and activate complement and the clotting cascade, leading to the formation of thrombi and necrosis of the implanted organ. In addition to antibodies and complement, a heavy polymorphonuclear leukocyte infiltration characterises hyperacute rejection.

Acute rejection

Acute rejection is mediated by T lymphocytes and becomes apparent some 7 days post-operatively. The recipient's T cells recognise alloantigens mainly through the mechanism of direct allorecognition (see above). Lymphocyte- and monocyte-rich cell infiltrations characterise this type of reaction. An accelerated form of acute rejection that occurs within 1–5 days post-transplant is probably mediated by T lymphocytes that have been previously sensitised to alloantigens (e.g. through transfusions, pregnancies).

Chronic rejection

Chronic rejection appears months or years after successful transplantation. It is the major cause of long-term graft loss, but its pathophysiology is poorly understood. It is thought that an early damage to the vascular endothelium, whether or not immune in nature, is a predisposing factor to this late complication. The endothelium may be further damaged by antibodies to alloantigens, deposition of immune complexes, activation of complement, exposure of collagen and activation of the clotting cascade. This would favour endothelial cell proliferation and narrowing of the vascular lumen. Cell infiltration is not a major feature of chronic rejection, although macrophages are deemed to play an important role through cytokine release (IL-1, IL-6, TNF-α). Adhesion molecules are up-regulated on endothelial cells.

GRAFT-VERSUS-HOST REACTIONS

A singular immunological condition arises when grafts containing immunocompetent cells are engrafted into immunologically incompetent recipients. Immunocompetent cells from the graft recognise alloantigens of the recipient and the recipient develops a disorder known as the graft-versus-host (GVH) reaction. This reaction is common after transplantation of bone marrow, even when the matching between donor and recipient has been stringent. When GVH becomes symptomatic the term graft-versus-host disease (GVHD) is more appropriate. GVHD has been described not only following bone marrow transplantation but also, occasionally, after liver transplantation and even after blood transfusions. GVHD can be divided into two distinct entities: acute disease, occurring in the first 1 or 2 months after transplantation, and chronic disease, developing at least 2 or 3 months after transplantation. In humans, GVHD typically affects the skin, liver, intestinal tract and immune system and appears within days or weeks after bone marrow transplantation. In mild GVH reactions, patients manifest erythema of the palms, soles and ears. Hepatic signs of mild reactions are limited to asymptomatic hyperbilirubinaemia, and gastrointestinal involvement is indicated by mild diarrhoea. In the case of severe GVHD, the skin lesions can include a necrolytic disorder, characterised by blister formation and desquamation. Severe liver abnormalities include jaundice, elevation of alkaline phosphatase, which denotes cholestasis, and of transaminases, a sign of liver cell damage. Severe gastrointestinal GVHD includes abdominal pain and diarrhoea, with life-threatening electrolyte abnormalities. These manifestations are the result of injury to the epithelial cells of the target organs. Mild GVH may resolve spontaneously or with mild immunosuppressive treatments. Severe GVH is usually unresponsive to treatments and has a fatal outcome. The chronic form of the disease shares certain clinical characteristics with systemic sclerosis (see p. 179).

The most effective treatment to prevent acute GVHD is a combination of methotrexate and cyclosporin. Treatment of established acute GVHD is with methylprednisolone, cyclosporin and/or antithymocyte globulin.

TISSUE TYPING

Matching for molecules of the HLA is the ideal criterion for selection of donors for allografts. This is regularly performed in kidney transplantation and focuses on the products of the alleles at the class I *HLA-A* and *HLA-B* loci, which are currently determined serologically, and on those encoded by class II *HLA-DR*, which are now identified mainly by molecular techniques (see p. 57). The benefit of HLA matching has been clearly demonstrated in large series of kidney transplants and is also becoming apparent in heart transplants. HLA matching, even if highly desirable, is currently precluded by time constraints in allotransplantation of organs such as the heart. While 48 hours of cold ischaemia (i.e. the period in which the explanted organ is preserved in the cold) can elapse between explant and reimplantation of kidneys without major prejudice to their viability or function, a period of 4 hours of cold ischaemia is the longest considered safe in heart transplantation. Therefore, a full work-up is logistically feasible for the transplantation of kidneys but not yet for heart and other organs. In the context of renal transplantation, the clinical benefits of matching have been demonstrated unambiguously in a large prospective study based on cadaveric donors. The 1-year

graft survival was 88% for HLA-matched kidneys and 79% for mismatched kidneys. This advantage was heightened beyond the first year after transplantation (Fig. 11.5). Increasing degrees of HLA-A, HLA-B and HLA-DR antigen matching improves graft survival in a gradual fashion (Fig. 11.6); this benefit is amplified further if the DR specificities are identified by DNA typing, which allows finer resolution. The analysis of some 8000 patients who underwent cardiac transplantation also demonstrates an impressive correlation between matching for HLA-A, HLA-B and HLA-DR and graft survival.

On the basis of the above results, national and regional policies are being implemented or devised. For

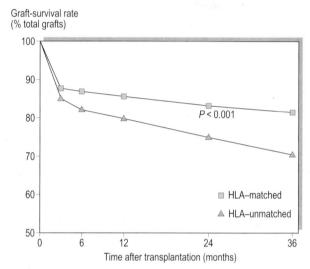

Fig. 11.5 Tissue typing and graft survival.
Effect of matching for HLA A, B and DR on graft survival. Graft-survival rates in HLA-matched compared with those in HLA-unmatched cadaveric renal transplants. (Modified from Takemoto (1992) New England Journal of Medicine, 327: 834–839.)

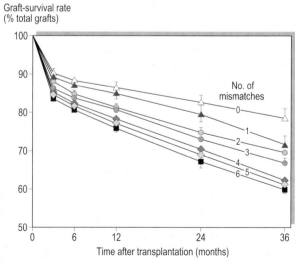

Fig. 11.6 Influence of the number of matches on graft-survival rates in cadaveric renal transplants.
The survival rate falls with the number of mismatches of HLA A, B and DR antigens. (Modified from Terasaki (1991) Clinical transplants. Los Angeles CA, UCLA Tissue Typing Laboratory, pp. 409–430.)

example, in the USA a national policy states that organ sharing amongst transplantation centres is mandatory for kidneys with a six-antigen match. The proposal to extend this policy to heart transplantation encounters the problem of the short cold-ischaemia time. This places serious limitations on the distance over which transport is feasible. Prospects for the future are favourable, however, in view of the development of DNA typing techniques soon to be implemented on a routine basis to speed HLA typing results. Potential recipients in a given region will be typed in advance to create a sufficiently large pool of candidates to receive the best HLA match.

PRE-SENSITISATION

The presence of antibodies that react with antigens of the graft may have disastrous results. Hyperacute reactions, which are mediated by complement-fixing antibodies, are virtually irreversible. The existence of pre-sensitisation is tested for by incubating the serum of the recipient and the T lymphocytes of the donor (or a panel of normal lymphocytes) in the presence of rabbit complement. The lysis of the lymphocytes indicates the presence of preformed anti-donor HLA class I antibodies, a 'positive cross-match'. Pre-sensitisation is considered an absolute contraindication in renal transplantation, where a positive cross-match is usually predictive of hyperacute rejection. Currently, pre-sensitisation is not routinely evaluated in cardiac and liver transplantation. Low-titre pre-sensitisation to antigens expressed on B lymphocytes, but not T lymphocytes, is not a contraindication to renal trans-

plant. In some rare cases of hyperacute renal rejection, antibodies with reactivity to renal endothelium and monocytes have been detected in the circulation and eluted from the rejected kidney. The role of cyto-fluorimetry (see p. 83) in the assessment of pre-sensitisation is currently under investigation. As in the cross-match assay described above, this technique allows detection of low-level complement-fixing antibodies and also of antibodies that do not fix complement.

IMMUNOSUPPRESSIVE THERAPY

DRUGS

The action of the immunosuppressive drugs discussed here is not specifically 'antirejection'. These drugs are widely used in a range of conditions in which a 'dampening down' of the immune system is required. However, several of them, most notably cyclosporin A, have transformed clinical transplantation and for this reason it is appropriate that the pharmacological approach to controlling rejection be discussed here (Table 11.2). In Chapter 22, these drugs and their modes of action are discussed in greater detail.

Azathioprine. The antimetabolite azathioprine acts as a purine antagonist and functions as an effective anti-proliferative agent. It was for two decades the keystone to immunosuppressive therapy in humans.

Corticosteroids. Corticosteroids have multiple effects on the immune system, including a decrease in the numbers of circulating B lymphocytes and inhibition of monocyte trafficking, T cell proliferation and cytokine gene expression (i.e. transcription of IL-1, IL-2 , IL-6, INF-γ and TNF-α). Side effects of these drugs on skin, bones and other tissues continue to present problems in clinical transplantation. Glucocorticoids are important adjuncts to immunosuppressive therapy in transplantation. **Prednisone** is given immediately before or at the time of transplantation, and its dosage is gradually reduced. **Methylprednisolone** is administered immediately upon diagnosis of beginning rejection and continued once daily for 3 days. Although azathioprine and prednisone can be used successfully to control graft rejection, both of these agents act non-specifically on the immune system.

Mechanisms of rejection

- There are different types of rejection. Hyperacute rejection results from pre-formed antibodies to HLA class I antigens or antigens of the ABO blood group. Acute and accelerated acute rejections are caused by cellular allorecognition of the graft. The mechanisms of chronic rejection are unknown.
- The transfer of immunocompetent allogeneic cells into an immune depressed individual leads to these rejecting the recipient (graft-versus-host reaction). This is known as graft-versus-host disease when accompanied by clinical manifestations.
- Good HLA matching prolongs graft survival. Pre-operative matching is routinely done for renal transplants, but not for liver, heart and lung transplants because of the short periods for which the latter organs maintain their function when explanted. This limitation will soon be remedied by use of rapid molecular HLA typing techniques.
- Pre-sensitisation, i.e. the presence of pre-formed antibodies to HLA class I or ABO antigens in the recipient's blood, is tested for in renal but not other types of transplantation. This policy is currently under review.

Table 11.2 **Mechanisms of action of immunosuppressive drugs**

Agent	Mode of action
Azathioprine	Inhibits purine synthesis
Corticosteroids	Block cytokine gene expression
Cyclosporin A; tacrolimus	Block Ca^{2+}-dependent T cell activation pathway
Sirolimus	Blocks IL-2 triggered proliferation and CD28/CTLA-4 mediated co-stimulatory signals

Cyclosporin A. Cyclosporin A is a small fungal cyclic peptide that has had a major impact on clinical transplantation since the early 1980s, significantly increasing graft survival rates and reducing the incidence of severe GVHD following bone marrow transplantation. The major effects of cyclosporin A on T cells is through the inhibition of IL-2 secretion. Another possible mode of action of cyclosporin A is the stimulation of production of cell growth-inhibitory cytokines, such as TGF-β. Because TGF-β inhibits both T cell proliferation and the generation of cytotoxic lymphocytes, a heightened production of TGF-β may contribute to the immunosuppressive activity of cyclosporin A. A common, dose-dependent and reversible side effect of cyclosporin A is nephrotoxicity.

Tacrolimus. Tacrolimus, previously known as FK506, is a macrolide antibiotic isolated from a Japanese soil fungus, *Streptomyces tsukubaensis*, with similar immunosuppressive effects and mechanisms to those of cyclosporin. Contrary to early claims, it has been shown that tacrolimus has similar nephrotoxicity to that of cyclosporin.

Sirolimus. Sirolimus, previously known as rapamycin, is a macrolide that has a similar mode of action to tacrolimus.

Antibodies

Antibodies can be used to target specific cells. The function of the targeted cells is abolished or lessened either through antibody-directed cell lysis or modulation of surface molecules. Polyclonal and monoclonal antibodies can be made that react with cell surface molecules expressed by all lymphocytes, by T cells but not B cells, by some T cells, for example CD4$^+$ or CD8$^+$ subsets, or by activated but not resting T cells, for example those expressing IL-2 receptor (CD25).

Monoclonal antibodies have the advantage of monospecificity and can be purified to homogeneity. Not all monoclonal antibodies specific for the same molecule may have the same effects in vivo since (1) they may react with different epitopes and deliver a different signal to the cell, and (2) antibodies with specificity for an identical epitope, but with different Fc regions, may have different properties.

Polyclonal antilymphocyte and antithymocyte globulin. Since the early 1980s, antilymphocyte globulin (ALG) and antithymocyte globulin (ATG) have been used by many transplant centres for the treatment of rejection episodes. These polyclonal antisera are composed of multiple antibodies specific for a variety of lymphocyte cell surface molecules. Both ALG and ATG are prepared by injecting lymphocytes or thymocytes into horses, rabbits or goats to produce antilymphocyte serum, from which the globulin fraction is then separated. The thymus is greatly enriched in T cells. One problem is variation between different preparations of

antisera. The main adverse effect is fever, which results from the release of pyrogens owing to the rapid breakdown of lymphoid cells.

Monoclonal anti-CD3. The mouse monoclonal antibody OKT3, which recognises the human CD3 molecule, has been used to treat recipients of allografts in clinical transplantation. Intravenous administration of OKT3 clears T cells from the circulation very efficiently, presumably by opsonisation. An increase in the number of circulating lymphocytes that are unreactive with OKT3 but are reactive with antibodies directed at other T cell markers is also observed, suggesting that one mode of action of OKT3 is modulation of the CD3 molecule from the surface of T cells. The major disadvantages of anti-CD3 monoclonal antibody treatment are its side effects and the development of anti-mouse Ig antibodies in approximately 75% of patients. As a result, OKT3 therapy can only effectively be used to treat a rejection episode after transplantation.

Monoclonal anti-CD4 and anti-CD8. Monoclonal antibodies specific for the two major subsets of T cells are also available. The immunosuppressive properties of monoclonal antibodies specific for the human CD4 molecule, OKT4, have been tested in a primate model; however, the results obtained were not very encouraging. Nonetheless, clinical trials of anti-CD4 monoclonal antibody therapy are currently in progress.

Monoclonal antibodies specific for activation antigens. When T cells respond to antigen and become activated, they express the IL-2 receptor. Targeting this receptor may allow more selective immunosuppressive therapy.

Side effects of antibody therapy. Significant untoward events are associated with clinical use of OKT3 and antilymphocyte ALG/ATG. Soon after administration, some patients experience a syndrome of fever and myalgia that is believed to be caused by systemic release of cytokines. The second major adverse event is development of lymphomas. These account for about 65% of all tumours that develop in transplantation recipients, and they occur in 1–2% of all recipients of transplanted organs. Like other immunosuppressive drugs, immunosuppressive antibodies also increase the risk of infectious complications in recipients.

IMMUNOSUPPRESSIVE REGIMENS

Typical immunosuppressive regimens involve the use of multiple immunosuppressive drugs acting at different levels of T cell activation. A standard triple-drug choice includes cyclosporin, azathioprine and corticosteroids. Tacrolimus has been used instead of cyclosporin with some success in recent studies.

Antilymphocyte antibodies are used in some centres before transplantation to prevent the activation of anti-graft immune responses or during episodes of rejection.

The treatment is effective but is accompanied by an increased incidence of lymphoproliferative disorders and possibly of infections. The administration of the murine anti-CD3 antibody OKT3 is associated with an early cytokine-mediated set of manifestations that include fever, chills and, in some cases, hypotension, pulmonary oedema, encephalopathy and nephropathy; these together constitute a capillary leak syndrome. Furthermore, because of its murine nature, OKT3 is the target of the recipient anti-murine Ig immune response that can reduce the antibody efficacy during the first cycle of treatment and prevent its use in future episodes of rejection. Attempts are being made to 'humanise' murine monoclonal antibodies, such that the murine antigen-recognising elements of the immunoglobulin are inserted onto a human immunoglobulin background.

COMMON COMPLICATIONS OF ALLOTRANSPLANTATION

As a consequence of the vigourous immunosuppression required to avoid allograft rejection, a number of complications, including infections and malignancies, commonly arise after transplantation. Bacterial, fungal or viral infections are frequent and may be life threatening early after surgery. After the first post-operative month, those opportunistic infections that typically emerge when the cellular immune system is impaired start appearing. Agents frequently responsible include

---

Blood tranfusions

Since the advent of powerful immunosuppressants, the use of blood transfusion in the prevention of graft rejection has become of historical relevance. That blood transfusion has a beneficial effect on graft survival may sound surprising. It certainly astonished the researchers who first noted this phenomenon. In the 1960s, the belief that transfusion-induced *sensitisation* against a random lymphocyte panel would lead to a high graft-failure rate convinced a number of transplantation units to restrict blood transfusions to as few dialysis patients as possible. The analysis of the data collected from several centres gave a result that was opposite to that expected: the graft survived longer in the patients transfused than in those non-transfused. Immunological mechanisms, such as clonal anergy, have been invoked. Clonal anergy occurs when cells with the potential to react against an antigen are inactivated but not deleted from the recipient. It has also been suggested that the unresponsiveness induced by transfusions is prolonged by **chimerism**, the phenomenon whereby donor cells survive within the recipient. Neither mechanism, however, has been conclusively demonstrated to be responsible for blood transfusion-induced immunosuppression.

---

cytomegalovirus (see below), herpes viruses, fungal organisms (*Aspergillus* and *Nocardia* spp., cryptococcal infection), mycobacteria and parasites (*Pneumocystis, Toxoplasma* spp.).

Cytomegalovirus infection

This is the most frequent and pathologically important post-transplant infection. Cytomegalovirus (CMV) belongs to the β herpes virus group, has a worldwide distribution and its spread normally requires repeated or prolonged intimate exposure. Transfusions containing viable leukocytes also transmit CMV. CMV infection probably lasts for life and usually remains latent. In patients with impaired T cell immunity (e.g. the recipients of organ transplants), CMV frequently reactivates. Primary CMV infections also occur in recipients of organ transplants and derive from the graft itself. Reactivation of latent virus or, occasionally, reinfection with a new strain accounts for the infection in CMV-seropositive transplant recipients.

Chronic antigen stimulation provided by the allograft in association with immunosuppression appears to be an ideal setting for CMV activation and CMV-induced disease. In renal, cardiac, lung, liver and bone marrow transplant recipients, CMV is responsible for several manifestations including fever, leukopenia, hepatitis, pneumonitis, oesophagitis, gastritis and colitis, typically starting 1 month after surgery. CMV retinitis can appear later. The transplanted organ is peculiarly susceptible to CMV, with hepatitis arising after liver transplantation and CMV pneumonitis after lung transplantation. A number of measures are implemented to reduce the impact of CMV infection in transplantation, including using blood and organs from seronegative donors for seronegative recipients and matching of organ or bone marrow transplants by CMV serology.

Ganciclovir, a guanosine derivative, is used in the treatment of CMV infection, since it is a selective inhibitor of CMV DNA polymerase.

Malignancies

With the improved survival of patients receiving an allograft, an increase in the incidence of malignancies has also been observed. The use of multiple immunosuppressive drugs has been implicated as a strong contributing factor for this increased susceptibility to malignancy. The most common cancers seen after organ transplantation are lymphoma, skin cancer and Kaposi's sarcoma. The increased incidence of malignancy is a major factor in the increased morbidity and late failure rates in transplant recipients. That immunosuppression has a key role in predisposing to malignant tumours is demonstrated by the relatively common occurrence of malignancies such as Kaposi's sarcoma and lymphomas in patients with AIDS. Immunosuppressive therapy is likely to favour growth of neoplastic cells by reducing mechanisms of immune surveillance. The overall incidence of skin cancer in kidney transplant patients is about 100 times higher than in control populations, with cutaneous carcinomas accounting for about 50% of cancers and the incidence increasing with time after renal transplantation. Squamous cell carcinoma is more frequent than basal cell carcinoma, at variance with the general rule. Kaposi's sarcoma has been reported in liver transplant recipients with a high prevalence, especially in male patients of Mediterranean origin. The human papilloma virus has been implicated in the aetiology of post-transplant skin cancers.

The development of **lymphoproliferative diseases** is also dependent on immunosuppression, induced by drugs such as cyclosporin, tacrolimus and OKT3. In the setting of allotransplantation, these disorders are particularly aggressive, with a high incidence of central nervous system and extranodal involvement; they are mainly classified as B cell-derived, large-cell non-Hodgkin's lymphomas and can be polyclonal or monoclonal. Their outcome is poor, unless immunosuppressive therapy can be stopped. The origin of these lymphoproliferative diseases has been ascribed to the effect of the oncogenic Epstein–Barr virus over B cells constantly stimulated by the allograft. Immunosuppression would play a catalysing role.

Immunosuppressive therapy

- The use of immunosuppression controls rejection episodes. The introduction of cyclosporin A in the 1980s has dramatically improved the outcome of allotransplantation.
- Immunosuppressive regimens typically include the use of multiple drugs (e.g. corticosteroids, azathioprine and cyclosporin) acting at different levels of the T lymphocyte activation pathway.
- Episodes of rejection resistant to conventional immunosuppressive regimens are controlled by the use of high-dose steroids, tacrolimus or antilymphocyte antibodies.
- Side effects of immunosuppression include infections with opportunistic microorganisms and malignancies.

CLINICAL TRANSPLANTATION

KIDNEY TRANSPLANTATION

The indications for kidney transplantation include end-stage renal disease caused by insulin-dependent diabetes mellitus, chronic glomerulonephritis, polycystic kidney disease, nephrosclerosis, systemic lupus erythematosus, interstitial nephritis, IgA nephropathy and Alport's syndrome. The use of cyclosporin has improved cadaveric graft survival rates to over 80% at 1 year and to 70% at 5 years. Graft loss from rejection is much slower after the first year. Donors can be cadavers or volunteer blood-related living donors: in Europe up to 85% of kidneys come from cadavers.

Preservation for at least 48 hours is achieved by flushing the kidney with appropriate solutions and by storage in ice. The surgical procedure differs according to the age of the recipient. In adults, the renal graft is placed extraperitoneally in the iliac fossa; in small children, it is placed retroperitoneally.

HLA matching is routinely practised for selection of donors for renal allografts, and potential recipients are normally screened for preformed antibodies to HLA class I antigens. The histological appearance of acute renal rejection, typically occurring 7–14 days post-transplant, is shown in Figures 11.7 and 11.8.

The failure of transplanted kidneys after several years of adequate function is attributed to 'chronic rejection'. This is characterised by the development of nephrosclerosis, with proliferation of the vascular intima of renal vessels, and intimal fibrosis, resulting in decrease in the lumen of the vessels (Fig. 11.9). Current modes of treatment have little effect on the progression of chronic rejection, which remains the most common cause of failure of long-term allografts.

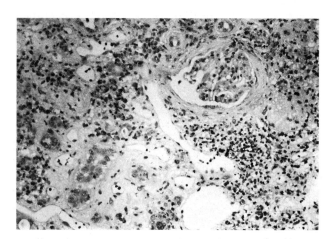

Fig. 11.7 **Mononuclear cells, including lymphocytes, macrophages and plasma cells, infiltrate the renal interstitium and tubular epithelial cells (lymphocytic tubulitis) in acute cellular rejection.** (Courtesy of Dr P. J. O'Donnell)

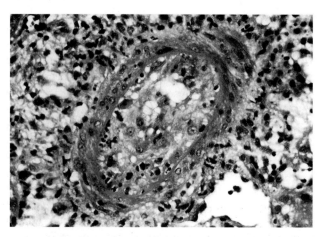

Fig. 11.8 **A small artery shows oedema and mononuclear cell infiltration of the intima with disruption of the endothelial lining in acute vascular rejection of the kidney.** (Courtesy of Dr P. J. O'Donnell)

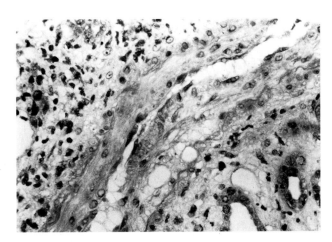

Fig. 11.9 **A medium calibre artery shows considerable luminal narrowing due to intimal fibrosis, mucoid change and smooth muscle proliferation in chronic renal rejection.** (Courtesy of Dr P. J. O'Donnell)

Amongst other complications, dyslipidaemia is frequently observed, with cardiovascular disease being the most common cause of long-term mortality in these patients. The original disease recurs in 10 to 20% of grafts, recurrent glomerulonephritis in the transplanted kidney being common. The nephritides that recur most commonly are membranous glomerulonephritis, mesangiocapillary glomerulonephritis and IgA nephropathy.

LIVER TRANSPLANTATION

The indication for liver transplantation is irreversible liver disease. The aetiology of this can differ in children and adults. Indications common to both age groups include end-stage cirrhosis and fulminant liver failure of whatever origin. Biliary atresia, inherited or genetic metabolic disorders associated with liver failure are characteristic of childhood, while primary biliary cirrhosis and alcoholic cirrhosis are typical of adults. Contraindications to transplantation include systemic diseases, extrahepatic infections and pre-existing advanced cardiovascular or pulmonary disease. Since the introduction of cyclosporin, 1-year survival rates approach 80–85% while the 5-year survival rates are approximately 60%. Donors are selected on the basis of negativity for bacterial or fungal infections and exclusion of hepatitis B and C viruses and human immunodeficiency virus (HIV). Compatibility for ABO blood groups is assessed even though ABO-incompatible donors are used in emergencies. Tissue typing for HLA matching is not routinely performed, and pre-sensitisation is not an exclusion criterion in liver transplantation. There are studies to demonstrate, however, that histocompatibility testing and assessment of pre-sensitisation would also improve the outcome in liver transplantation.

Liver preservation can last up to 24 hours with the use of graft preservers such as 'University of Wisconsin solution', which is rich in lactobionate and raffinose.

Acute rejection of the transplanted liver occurs in the majority of patients, beginning 1 to 2 weeks after

News in liver transplantation

A number of new approaches are currently being implemented in liver transplantation.

Reduced liver transplantion. This refers to the use of liver segments to transplant small recipients. This procedure allows infants with end-stage liver disease to receive a graft, which would be otherwise impractical because of space constraints. Babies as young as 2 weeks of age have been transplanted by this technique.

Auxiliary orthotopic transplantation. This refers to the transplantation of a segment of donor liver in a recipient who has undergone hemi-hepatectomy to make room for the graft. Orthotopic means that the graft is placed in its correct anatomical location. This procedure is used to offset enzymatic liver defects that are not accompanied by structural hepatic damage (e.g. Crigler–Najjar syndrome, propionic acidaemia, urea cycle defects) but are responsible for lethal systemic effects. In this setting, if the donor's liver fails, the recipient's own organ can function as a backup until a new liver is found. Auxiliary transplantation is also used as a temporary measure in fulminant liver failure, where the recipient's liver has the potential of regeneration and full functional recovery. This avoids life-long immunosuppression.

'Split' livers. This refers to the use of one liver for two recipients. This procedure helps in tackling organ shortage and in shortening the time on the waiting list. The operation is technically demanding and requires the simultaneous work of two transplant teams.

Living related donors. The donor of the liver segment is typically a first-degree living relative. The operation can be carefully planned and it is usually performed when the recipient is still in relatively good condition. When the organ donation comes from a blood relative — and not from a spouse — rejection is less frequent and less severe. This procedure avoids damage to the liver resulting from preservation but does present some risks for the donor.

surgery and is accompanied by increases in serum bilirubin and aminotransferase levels. These tests, however, lack specificity. Liver biopsy is often performed to establish the correct diagnosis. The histological appearance shows mononuclear cell portal infiltration, bile duct injury and endothelial inflammation ('endothelialitis') (Figs 11.10 and 11.11).

Chronic rejection is characterised by progressive cholestasis, focal parenchymal necrosis, mononuclear infiltration, vascular lesions and fibrosis (Fig. 11.12).

Recurrence of the initial condition is almost invariable for hepatitides B and C, if sufficiently sensitive virus markers are used to document the presence of the

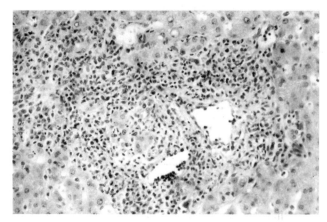

Fig. 11.10 Mononuclear cells including lymphocytes, lymphoblasts and macrophages infiltrate a portal tract during acute liver rejection.
Lymphocytes damage the endothelial lining of portal vein radicles. Bile duct epithelial cells are swollen and damaged. (Courtesy of Dr B. Portmann)

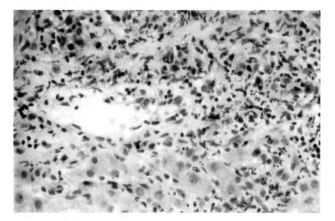

Fig. 11.11 Magnified view of endothelitis affecting a portal vein radicle. (Courtesy of Dr B. Portmann)

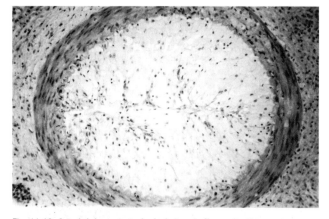

Fig. 11.12 Arterial damage typical of chronic liver rejection.
The arteriole is occluded by 'foamy' cells, inflammatory cells and fibrin. (Courtesy of Dr B. Portmann)

infections. Diseases with a putatative immune pathogenesis, such as primary biliary cirrhosis, sclerosing cholangitis and autoimmune hepatitis, have also been reported to recur occasionally.

PANCREAS TRANSPLANTATION

Pancreas transplantation has not yet become a standard mode of treatment. It is a life-enhancing not a life-saving procedure, as the transplantation of other organs is. The main indication is insulin-dependent diabetes, where the graft would improve not only the metabolic imbalance but also help in preventing late diabetic complications. It has been typically performed in nephropathic diabetic patients in association with a kidney allograft. Transplantation of the pancreas as a whole or as a segment has succeeded in curing diabetes in a number of cases. The transplantation of isolated islets of Langerhans has been repeatedly attempted with relatively unrewarding results. The transplantation of a segment of pancreas from a healthy diabetic twin into his monozygous co-twin, suffering from long-standing insulin-dependent diabetes, has resulted in the cure of the metabolic disorder. As expected, tissue rejection did not occur. Insulin-dependent diabetes did recur, however, accompanied by a lymphocytic and monocytic infiltration of the islets of Langerhans. This episode illustrates the long-lasting memory of β cell-specific autoimmune responses, which caused diabetes originally and re-enacted the disease in the syngeneic graft. It also outlines the potential obstacles to pancreas transplantation in insulin-dependent diabetes, since β cells of allogeneic origin may become the targets of both autoimmunity and allorecognition (see Ch. 13).

HEART TRANSPLANTATION

The indication for heart transplantation is a cardiac disease unresponsive to conventional medical or surgical treatment and likely to cause the patient's death within 6–12 months. Cardiomyopathy and congenital uncorrectable defects are the main indications in children, while coronary heart disease and dilated cardiomyopathy are the main indications in adults. Since the introduction of cyclosporin, 1-year survival ranges between 80 and 90%, while 5-year survival is between 60 and 70%. The cardiac transplant recipient can achieve approximately 70% of the maximal cardiac output.

Tissue typing for HLA matching is not routinely performed because of difficulty in obtaining good matches and the notion that there is a lack of correlation between match and outcome. This notion has been recently challenged. HLA typing is, therefore, likely to be added to the criteria for optimising heart transplantation, which currently focus on organ size, ABO matching and avoidance of transferring organs from a CMV-positive donor to a CMV-negative recipient. Assessment of pre-sensitisation is also conventionally disregarded. Recent studies have demonstrated that patients with preformed antibodies directed at one or more of the HLA antigens have a poorer overall rate of graft survival than non-sensitised recipients. This differential graft survival will provide the stimulus for assessing systematically pre-sensitisation in potential recipients.

Histology plays a key role in the diagnosis of acute rejection and repeated endomyocardial biopsies are normally performed for monitoring ongoing rejection. The prolongation of isovolumic relaxation time, measured by echocardiography, is also compatible with rejection. Biopsies, taken every 1 to 2 weeks early after transplantation, and with gradually widening intervals thereafter, demonstrate changes suggestive of rejection (Fig. 11.13). An accelerated coronary vascular disease appears later and is referred to as chronic rejection, even though the involvement of the immune system in its causation still remains to be demonstrated. This diffuse vascular process affects both distal and proximal coronary vessels so that conventional modes of intervention such as angioplasty or coronary artery bypass grafting are ineffective (Fig. 11.14).

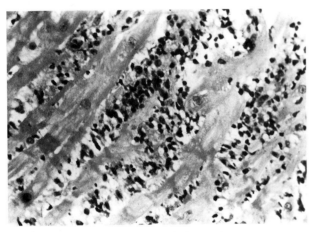

Fig. 11.13 **Focus of acute cellular rejection in a heart transplant recipient.**
A mononuclear cell infiltrate composed of lymphocytes and macrophages characterises an episode of acute cellular rejection (High magnification — Courtesy of Dr N. Cary)

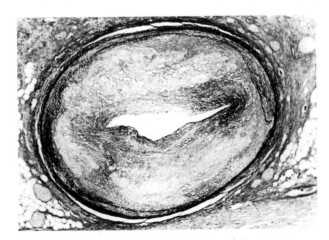

Fig. 11.14 **The principal manifestation of chronic rejection in heart transplantation is coronary graft vascular occlusive disease.**
This is characterised by intimal thickening which tends to be more diffuse and concentric than conventional atherosclerosis. The thickening seen here is concentric and muscular elastic in nature. (Courtesy of Dr N. Cary)

LUNG TRANSPLANTATION

End-stage pulmonary disease represents the indication for lung transplantation. The most common diagnoses that have required lung allograft include chronic obstructive pulmonary disease, emphysema caused by α_1-antitrypsin deficiency, idiopathic pulmonary fibrosis, cystic fibrosis and primary pulmonary hypertension. Lung transplantation improves lung function in patients with restrictive or obstructive disease and alleviates pulmonary hypertension in patients with pulmonary vascular disease.

ABO group compatibility and lung size are the only factors that are routinely matched between the donor and recipient.

Complications occurring soon after lung transplantation may have a primary technical cause, but after the very early stages, rejection and infection are the predominating complications. A majority of recipients have early episodes of acute rejection that are characterised by non-specific manifestations, including cough, dyspnoea, fever, radiographic infiltrates and worsening of pulmonary function and oxygenation. Rejection episodes are documented by transbronchial lung biopsy. A quarter of patients develop chronic rejection, characterised by airflow limitation and histologically by obliterative bronchiolitis and vascular sclerosis (Fig. 11.15). A possible immunological cause is suggested by the clinical improvement following an increase in immunosuppression.

The lung as an allograft is especially susceptible to infections. It originates from a brain-dead donor connected to a ventilator and exposed to nosocomial microorganisms. Its natural defence mechanisms are impaired including a decrease in mucociliary clearance and depression of the cough reflex, since the transplanted lung is denervated.

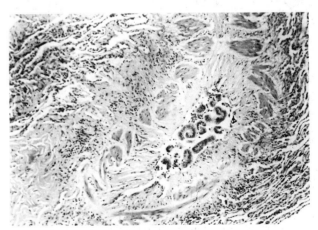

Fig. 11.15 **The principal manifestation of chronic rejection following lung transplantation is the development of obliterative bronchiolitis.**
This is characterised by occlusion of bronchioles by fibrous connective tissue. In its developing phases this may show inflammatory infiltration. In this case there is subtotal obliteration of the bronchiolar lumen due to a thick layer of pale-staining submucosal fibrosis, seen here between the partially detached bronchiolar epithelium (artefact) and the darker-staining smooth muscle bundles. (Courtesy of Dr N. Cary)

BONE MARROW TRANSPLANTATION

Bone marrow transplantation involves the transfer of pluripotent haematopoietic stem cells capable of regenerating all cellular elements of the blood and immune system. It has become the conventional form of treatment for congenital immunodeficiency diseases, selected malignancies and aplastic anaemia for patients who have an HLA-identical sibling or an identical twin. For patients who lack an HLA-matched sibling, a closely HLA-matched unrelated individual or an imperfectly HLA-matched relative may act as donors.

The reason why HLA matching needs to be especially stringent in bone marrow transplantation is because the recipient is either immunodeficient or needs to be 'conditioned', i.e. undergo profound chemoradiotherapy to eliminate residual disease and create space for the new marrow. This results in ablation of the recipient's immune system. The immunoincompetent recipient is, therefore, at high risk of developing life-threatening GVHD.

Donor selection is done in sequential steps starting from the search for the best match, namely a genotypically identical sibling. Information regarding genotypic identity for HLA class I and II determinants can be readily obtained within families by determining the HLA class I and class II antigens of the four parental haplotypes and analysing their segregation in the family. If genotypically identical siblings are unavailable, the second best choice is to obtain bone marrow from HLA-haploidentical relatives. Parents and offspring are always HLA haploidentical. The degree of disparity between HLA-haploidentical donor–recipient pairs depends on the similarity of the non-shared haplotypes. The risk of GVHD increases progressively with the number of HLA disparities in the recipient compared with the donor. Bone marrow can be obtained from unrelated donors, if neither genotypically identical siblings nor haploidentical relatives are available. In this case, the donors are HLA phenotypically identical unrelated volunteers. But, whilst HLA genotypically identical siblings have complete genetic identity at all loci between *HLA-A* and *HLA-DP*, HLA phenotypically matched pairs can have disparities resulting from MHC polymorphisms that will not be detectable by conventional typing methods. As a consequence, patients transplanted with marrow from an HLA phenotypically identical unrelated donor have a much higher risk of acute GVHD than patients transplanted from an HLA genotypically identical sibling. In view of the large number of HLA loci and their extreme polymorphism, marrow donor registries have been established to augment the probability of finding a closely matched donor for any patient who lacks genotypically or haploidentical relatives as potential donors.

The indications for bone marrow transplant are numerous and are increasing. Allogenic bone marrow transplantation has been successful in treating children with immunodeficiency disorders such as severe combined immunodeficiency, Wiskott–Aldrich and Chédiak–Higashi syndromes. In **aplastic anaemia**, marrow transplantation is the preferred method of treatment if an HLA-identical sibling is available, and in this setting 85% long-term survival is achieved. In children with homozygous **β-thalassaemia**, allogenic bone marrow transplantation has led to disease-free 1-year survival of 75%. Non-transplanted patients undergo iron overload and usually die in their twenties.

In **haematological malignancies**, long-term survival and cure rates of up to 70% have been reported. In **acute lymphoblastic leukaemia**, bone marrow transplantation is indicated in those 50% of children who are not cured by a primary chemotherapy regimen. Interestingly, patients with leukaemia treated with bone marrow transplantation experience the beneficial graft-versus-leukaemia (GVL) effect (see box: 'Graft-versus-leukaemia'), that occurs in association with GVHD.

In **chronic myelogenous leukaemia** (CML), allogenic transplantation with marrow from an HLA-matched sibling donor is the treatment of choice for patients who are in the stable phase. If the patient with CML has no HLA-identical family donor, transplantation should be undertaken only when the clinical condition deteriorates, in order to justify a riskier procedure. Long-term disease-free survival has been achieved in patients with both **Hodgkin's disease** and **non-Hodgkin's lymphoma**. In both conditions, the results are better when the treatment is performed soon after a relapse, at a time when the disease is minimal. Under these circumstances, a disease-free survival of up to 70% can be achieved. A lower mortality rate is associated with the use of an autologous graft, and this is the preferred mode of treatment in most centres. Bone marrow transplantation is being tested in non-haematological malignancies, where extremely aggressive, bone marrow impairing chemotherapeutic regimens may be desired to treat the original malignancy. Anecdotal successes have been reported in neuroblastoma, breast cancer, testicular tumours and gynaecological cancers.

Standard criteria for bone marrow harvesting indicate that 100–300 million cells (10 to 15 ml of bone marrow) per kg of recipient weight is the optimal number of cells to be obtained from the donor. The

---

Graft-versus-leukaemia

Patients with leukaemia treated with bone marrow transplant are said to have a lower rate of leukaemic relapses if their transplant is accompanied by GVHD. Those patients who receive bone marrow depleted of T lymphocytes — and do not experience GVHD — appear to suffer from an increased rate of relapses. The beneficial antitumour effect associated with GVHD is known as the graft-versus-leukaemia effect (GVL). The mechanisms at the basis of GVL are unknown.

harvested preparation is then passed though a stainless steel mesh to achieve a monodispersed cell suspension. Depletion of malignant cells, or positive selection of bone marrow stem cells, may be used in patients with malignancies with metastases located in the bone marrow if autologous marrow is to be infused. If donor and recipient are ABO incompatible, erythrocytes are eliminated to prevent haemolytic reactions. At this stage, the pluripotent haematopoietic stem cell-containing suspension is either infused intravenously or cryopreserved for later infusion.

Before bone marrow is infused, the recipient must undergo chemotherapy and/or radiotherapy — **conditioning** — to suppress the immune system, to create space in the bone marrow and to eliminate malignant cells in cases where malignancy was the reason for the transplantation. Most preparative regimens consist of radiotherapy combined with alkylating agents: etoposide and cytarabine.

The major complications of marrow transplantation are graft rejection, GVHD, opportunistic infection and recurrence of malignancy. Graft rejection is the graft destruction by immune competent cells in the host. This is a serious complication because second grafts rarely succeed and death of the recipient is the expected outcome. In the setting of recipients receiving marrow from an HLA-identical sibling, this complication is fortunately rare. Predisposing factors include

previous blood transfusions and insufficiently aggressive conditioning regimens. A complication peculiar to bone marrow transplantation is veno-occlusive disease of the liver, which consists of three main symptoms: jaundice, tender hepatomegaly and ascites. It is present in up to 50% of the patients. Progressive liver failure can develop and a fatal outcome is not unusual. Thrombolytic therapy has been used recently with some success.

TRANSPLANTATION: AN OUTLOOK

Organ transplantation faces a number of problems, ranging from organisational to philosophical. Organs are in short supply, and graft failure of non-paired organs is synonymous with death if a new organ is not found promptly. The rate of malignancies is increased by the aggressive immunosuppressive regimens needed for long-term graft survival. The concept of heart-beating cadaveric donors sounds like an oxymoron and poses ethical problems. Only grafts from living donors are culturally acceptable in some societies. Moreover, several cases are known to have occurred in which poverty and not a close family link was the reason to part with one kidney. Can any of these issues be addressed in the near future?

The organ shortage will soon be tackled by the use of organs obtained from genetically 'humanised' animal donors. Additionally, the manufacture of artificial devices to pump blood around the body or to control sugar levels may provide an answer to shortage of hearts and pancreata. The possibility of more specific modes of treatment to silence allorecognition is being vigorously explored, although current evidence suggests that effective immune intervention needs to be tailored to an individual patient, raising economical question marks over the large-scale feasibility of such an approach. The prospect of subduing universal mediators of inflammatory damage, such as complement and cytokines, with specific antagonists appears to be more promising in the short term. Ethical issues will remain. The question asked will probably be: 'Do we have the right to use animals as a source of spare parts for our own survival?'.

Clinical transplantation
- Graft-versus-host disease is typically seen in bone marrow transplantation, where the grafted tissue comprises immunocompetent allogeneic cells. GVHD can be observed in other settings when the organ transplanted contains a sufficient number of immunocompetent cells.
- Indications for clinical transplantation expand steadily. This expansion is challenged by organ shortage.
- Organ shortage is currently tackled by effective use of available resources (e.g. organ-sharing programmes, use of split livers, donations from relatives). 'Humanised' xenogenic grafts should soon alleviate this problem.

Rheumatic diseases

This chapter describes a number of diseases with a proved or supposed immune pathogenesis; they are variably referred to as **rheumatic, connective tissue** or **collagen diseases**. Rheumatic denotes the migratory nature of the pain (ρέω, reads reo, Greek for flowing), whilst the terms 'connective tissue' and 'collagen' indicate the components typically affected. In these disorders, collagen may have dual relevance: as a target for autoimmune reactions and as a component of connective tissue produced in excess. Clinical manifestations centre around the joints and muscles, but other systems are involved to differing degrees in the different conditions. In systemic lupus erythematosus, for example, systemic manifestations frequently predominate over those localised to the joints, whereas a disease such as ankylosing spondylitis is mainly focused on a particular region, in this case the sacroilium.

SYSTEMIC LUPUS ERYTHEMATOSUS

Systemic lupus erythematosus (SLE, also often shortened to **lupus**) is a multisystem disease that follows a fluctuating course, with exacerbations and spontaneous remissions. It is identified by its clinical features and by a variety of circulating autoantibodies. In particular, autoantibodies directed against components of the cell nucleus play a pivotal diagnostic — and pathogenic — role. SLE affects 40 in 100 000 North European or American Caucasians. The incidence appears to be higher in black populations and higher still in Orientals. Nine of ten SLE patients are women, 80% of them being of childbearing age. Possession of certain HLA class II alleles — *DR3* in Caucasians, *DR2* in Orientals — confers susceptibility to the disease. The role of genes in the causation of the disease is indicated by the higher concordance for SLE in monozygotic when compared with dizygotic twins.

Pathology

Renal failure is a major cause of morbidity and mortality in SLE, and its pathogenesis is discussed in full in Chapter 16. A renal biopsy is taken when the information it can provide is useful for treatment. The localisation and type of immune complex, as well as the activity and chronicity of the histological lesions are all important for guiding treatment and assessing prognosis. Detection of immune complexes, also called immune deposits, is carried out on frozen tissue sections using a direct immunofluorescence technique. In between one half and all cases of active SLE, such immune deposits can also be seen at the dermoepidermal junction in the skin.

Pathogenesis

Akin to other autoimmune diseases, the pathogenic scenario for SLE sees environmental factors interacting with suceptibility genes to produce an overactive, autoaggressive immune response: the main effectors of tissue damage are autoantibodies and immune complexes. To examine the genetic link first; HLA class II gene products have been implicated in predisposition to SLE, presumably at the level of T helper lymphocyte recognition of a 'lupus peptide', but the relative risks associated with possession of HLA-DR2 and HLA-DR3 are small. More relevant, at least in Caucasians, is possession of the HLA class III allele *C4AQ0*. This is a silent allele encoding for the production of quantity 0 (Q0) of the A isotype of the C4 molecule, which belongs to the classical pathway of the complement system (see p. 13). This allele is part of an extended lupus-predisposing HLA haplotype *B8 DR3 DQ2 C4AQ0*. Normal levels of functioning C4 are essential in maintaining immune complexes in solution and in preventing their tissue deposition. It is not surprising, then, that possession of a C4A non-coding gene predisposes to an immune complex disease such as SLE. Intriguingly, well-defined clinical manifestations in lupus such as dermatitis, or possession of autoantibodies such as anticardiolipin antibody, also tend to be associated with HLA alleles, but these are different alleles from those actually predisposing to SLE, arguing in favour of heterogeneity of the disease. Amongst the predisposing factors, femaleness undoubtedly plays a major role (see box: 'Femaleness and SLE').

No definite environmental factors have been identified, with the exception of drugs known to provoke SLE (see below) and ultraviolet light, especially UV-B radiations. Three quarters of lupus patients are photosensitive. A role for a virus, frequently suggested but never actually demonstrated, as the cause of this autoantibody-dominated disease has received some recent support by the finding that the lupus-specific anti-Sm (Smith protein) autoantibody (see p. 169) reacts with the p24 gag protein of retroviruses and that anti-Ro, (Ro, Robert) another autoantibody typical of SLE, also recognises a nucleocapsid protein on vesicular stomatitis virus (see box: 'A man and his dog').

With these strong similarities between viruses and the targets of autoantibodies found in SLE, a process involving molecular mimicry between organisms and self (see p. 123) is one of the most frequent explanations for how the disease may arise. Autoantibodies found in SLE are produced by B lymphocytes that have undergone gene rearrangements and somatic mutations typical of an antigen-driven response. A generalised B lymphocyte dysregulation appears also to be involved, leading to vast amounts of autoantibodies being produced. These autoantibodies damage cells and tissues, either through direct binding to cell-surface membranes or by forming immune complexes that become deposited.

The damaging role of antiplatelet autoantibodies in the thrombocytopenia seen in SLE patients is well established, while antineuronal autoantibodies have been implicated in neurological manifestations of lupus. Antilymphocyte antibodies not only account for the generalised lymphopenia seen in lupus but also for a selective depletion of immunoregulatory T lymphocytes, whose role is to restrain autoimmune reactions. Therefore, a vicious circle of deficient immunoregulation, autoimmunity, antilymphocyte antibodies and further deficient immunoregulation is set up. Circulating anti-cardiolipin autoantibodies are additional pathogenic agents; they react with phospholipid moieties (one of the main ones being cardiolipin) and are involved in causing both arterial and venous thrombosis and in spontaneous abortion (see box: 'Antiphospholipid antibody syndrome'). Immune complexes of autoantibody and autoantigen lodge in highly vascularised tissues such as the renal glomerulus. Pathogenicity of these complexes increases with increasing ability of the antibody to fix complement: complex size, charge and clearance (dependent on functional C4 and complement receptors) are all of importance in influencing deposition in the tissues. As we have seen, C4 concen-

---

Femaleness and SLE

The F1 hybrid generated by crossing a New Zealand Black (NZB) with a New Zealand White (NZW) mouse is a very close animal model of human SLE. NZB/NZW females manifest the disease at an early age, have in their circulation anti-nuclear and anti-double stranded DNA antibodies (autoantibodies typical of SLE) and develop a lethal immune complex-mediated nephritis. Artificial control of sex hormones — by drug treatment or by castration — has a profound effect on the expression of the disease. Male hormones tend to suppress the disease, improve survival and decrease the severity of nephritis when they are administered to females. In contrast, female hormones accelerate the course of the disease.

A man and his dog

In the debate over the contribution of environmental factors to the aetiology of SLE it is worth noting that dogs owned by lupus patients have significantly higher levels of anti-dsDNA autoantibodies (*the* diagnostic test in SLE) compared with 'control' dogs. The sharing of this serological lupus hallmark has led to the suggestion that a common environmental factor, possibly a transmissible agent, is involved in causing SLE in the two species.

The debate has expanded as to the origin, human or canine, of this potential transmissible agent, and it has been concluded, with some reason, that a canine source was more likely in view of the higher chance of dogs biting and licking their owners than the reverse.

Antiphospholipid antibody syndrome

This syndrome, characterised by both venous and arterial thromboses, was described by G. R. V. Hughes in 1983 in a patient with SLE. It is now clear that it can occur in isolation as the **primary antiphospholipid antibody syndrome**. Venous thrombosis can manifest itself as deep-vein thrombosis and thrombosis of retinal, renal or hepatic veins (Budd–Chiari syndrome). Arterial thrombosis can induce limb ischaemia, strokes, amaurosis and myocardial infarction, and Addison's disease through adrenal thrombosis. Heart-valve disease is present in a quarter of patients and women have a much increased risk of spontaneous abortion. Thrombocytopenia is common (platelets have surface phospholipids). The serum of these patients contains antiphospholipid autoantibodies, deemed responsible for the clinical manifestations of the syndrome. The mechanisms through which these antibodies provoke damage, however, have not been clarified, even though reactivity to cell membranes — platelets, endothelial cells — and clotting factors has been documented.

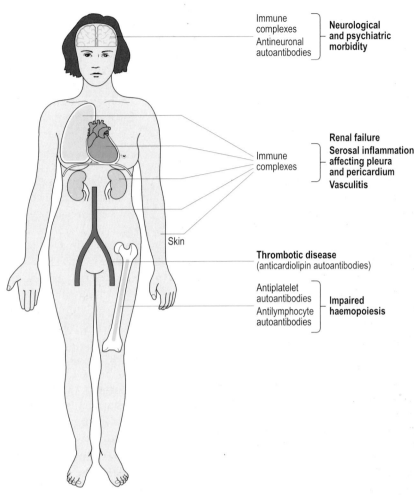

Fig. 12.1 **SLE clinical features.**

tration is often reduced. CR-1 (complement receptor 1) numbers are reduced on the erythrocyte surface of lupus patients: this defect, usually acquired but occasionally inherited in SLE, prevents delivery of the full immune complex load to the mononuclear phagocyte system within the liver and spleen. The cationic nature of DNA in immune complexes in lupus facilitates binding to capillary walls within the glomerulus (see Ch. 16).

Clinical features

SLE is a multisystem disease and can affect virtually all organs and systems (Fig. 12.1): whilst some manifestations are customary, others are rare. Therefore, joints, skin and blood are affected in 80–100% of patients, kidneys, CNS and cardiopulmonary system in over 50%; while thrombosis, a typical lupus manifestation associated with possession of the anticardiolipin antibody, is present in 10% of patients. The severity of clinical manifestations is variable and exacerbations typically alternate with periods of relative quiescence. Systemic manifestations, including fatigue, malaise, fever anorexia, nausea and weight loss, are present in the great majority of patients.

The diagnosis of SLE is made using the criteria set by the American Rheumatism Association (Table 12.1).

Musculoskeletal features. Arthralgias and arthritis, frequently migratory in nature, affect virtually all patients, with the degree of pain being disproportionate to the physical signs of synovitis. Joints in the hands (proximal interphalangeal and metacarpophalangeal) are affected, while the spine is spared. Erosions are rare.

Cutaneous features. A malar (butterfly) erythema over cheeks and bridge of the nose is typical but only occurs in one third of the patients (Fig. 12.2). More frequent is a maculopapular rash in sun-exposed areas (neck, extensor surfaces of arms and legs) that accompanies disease flare-ups. Alopecia, usually patchy but extensive at times, is also frequently seen (Fig. 12.3). A characteristic photosensitive, erythematous, papulosquamous rash, which becomes hypopigmented and leaves no scars, defines subacute cutaneous lupus (SCLE). Patients with this condition tend to have arthritis and fatigue but rarely renal or CNS involvement. Some such patients are negative for antinuclear antibody, while all tend to have anti-Ro (SS-A) antibody.

Table 12.1 **Diagnosis of SLE using the criteria set by the American Rheumatism Association[a]**

Criteria	Description
1. Malar rash	Fixed erythema, flat or raised over the malar eminences
2. Discoid rash	Erythematous raised patches with adherent keratotic scaling and follicular plugging; atrophic scarring may occur
3. Photosensitivity	
4. Oral ulcers	Includes oral and naso-pharyngeal, observed by physician
5. Arthritis	Non-erosive arthritis involving two or more peripheral joints, characterised by tenderness, swelling, or effusion
6. Serositis	Pleuritis or pericarditis documented by rub or ECG, or evidence of pericardial effusion
7. Renal disorder	Proteinuria greater than 0.5 g in 24 hours, or 3+, or cellular casts
8. Neurological disorders	Seizures without other cause or psychosis without other cause
9. Hematological disorders	Haemolytic anaemia or leukopenia (less than $4 \times 10^9/l$) or lymphopenia (less than $1.5 \times 10^9/l$) or thrombocytopenia (less than $100 \times 10^9/l$) in the absence of offending drugs
10. Immunological disorders	Anti-dsDNA or anti-Sm antibodies or positive LE cells or false positive serology for syphilis for at least 6 months
11. Antinuclear antibodies	An abnormal titre of antinuclear antibodies (ANAs) by immunofluorescence or an equivalent assay at any point in time in the absence of drugs known to induce ANAs

[a]If four of these criteria are present at any time during the course of disease, a diagnosis of systemic lupus can be made with 90% specificity and 97% sensitivity.

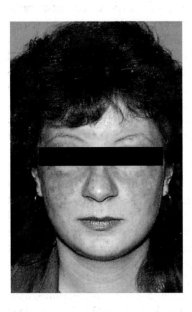

Fig. 12.2 **Butterfly rash.** A malar erythema over cheeks and bridge of the nose is typical of SLE. (Reproduced with permission of Grampion Health Board from McHardy K C et al 1997 Illustrated Signs in Clinical Medicine, Churchill Livingstone, Edinburgh.)

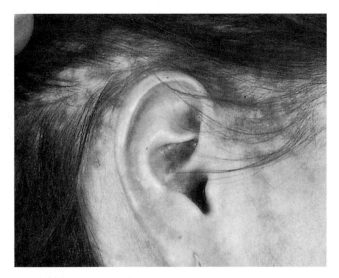

Fig. 12.3 **Alopecia is present in up to 50% of patients.**

are persistently abnormal urinalysis, elevated serum levels of antibodies to double-stranded (ds) DNA and low levels of complement factors, especially C4, all of which presage development of nephritis.

Neurological features. Any area of the central nervous system can be affected in SLE, with manifestations ranging from psychosis, through seizures to organic brain syndromes. A mild cognitive dysfunction is frequent, as are depression and anxiety. Microfocal scarring located in the subcortical white matter is associated with the presence of lupus neuropathy. These lesions are normally undetectable, or give non-specific alterations, even under magnetic resonance imaging. Some 50% of patients with neurological involvement have antineuronal autoantibodies in their serum and cerebrospinal fluid, but the pathogenicity of these is as yet unproved.

Cardiopulmonary features. Pericarditis is the most frequent cardiac manifestation of lupus. At times it is the presenting manifestation and is typically mild but can occasionally result in tamponade. Valvular abnormalities can be identified by ultrasound in a quarter of patients, probably representing the echocardiographic counterpart of the ovoid vegetations found at postmortem examination of lupus patients, known as Libman–Sacks verrucous endocarditis. Antiphospholipid antibodies are associated with this condition. Pleural effusion is also a common finding. A corticosteroid-responsive lupus pneumonitis, characterised by fleeting infiltrates, interstitial pneumonitis and pulmonary hypertension can occasionally occur in SLE.

Vascular features. These complications tend to be thrombotic in nature, affecting vessels of any size and are usually associated with antiphospholipid antibodies. Retinal vasculitis is a serious **ocular** manifestation, requiring aggressive immunosuppression. Up to 10% of lupus patients develop **Sjögren's syndrome** (see p. 178).

Renal features. Most patients have immunoglobulin deposits present in their glomeruli, and a clinically relevant glomerulonephritis is present in some 50% of patients, ranging from a mild focal proliferative disease to aggressive diffuse proliferative disease requiring vigorous treatment with corticosteroids and cytotoxic drugs. Urinalysis shows haematuria, proteinuria and renal casts. Of importance in monitoring renal disease

Table 12.2 **Antinuclear antibodies in connective tissue diseases**

Pattern	Antigen	Disease association
Homogeneous	DNA–histone complex	SLE; other rheumatic diseases
	Histones	Drug-induced SLE
Speckled	Sm (Smith) protein complexed to six small nuclear RNAs (U1 to U6)	SLE
	RNP (ribonucleoprotein) complexed to U1 RNA	Mixed connective tissue disease; SLE; Sjögren's syndrome
	Ro (Robert) (SS-A) protein complexed to RNAs Y1 to Y5	Sjögren's syndrome; SLE
	La (Lane) (SS-B) phosphoprotein complexed to RNA polymerase III transcripts	Sjögren's syndrome; SLE
	Jo-1, histidyl tRNA synthetase	Polymyositis; dermatomyositis
	Scl-70, DNA topoisomerase 1	Systemic sclerosis
	Centromere; proteins in kinetochore	CREST syndrome
Peripheral (membranous-rim-like)	Double-stranded DNA(?)	SLE
	Nuclear envelope proteins	
	Lamins A and C	SLE; systemic sclerosis
Nucleolar	RNA polymerase; PM-Scl; periribosomal particle	Systemic sclerosis
Crithidia luciliae kinetoplast	Double-stranded DNA	SLE

General laboratory findings

The most frequent laboratory alteration that is identified is normochromic normocytic anaemia of chronic disorders. Occasionally a Coombs-positive haemolytic anaemia is observed. Leukopenia (probably autoantibody mediated), especially lymphopenia, and thrombocytopenia are frequent. Urinalysis can show haematuria, proteinuria and renal casts in the presence of glomerulonephritis. The erythrocyte sedimentation rate is typically elevated, while C-reactive protein (CRP) tends to be normal. This last finding is intriguing, since CRP is usually elevated in inflammatory states.

Immunological laboratory findings

The sero-immunological hallmark of SLE is **antinuclear antibody** (ANA) (see Table 12.2). In the absence of ANA, the diagnosis of SLE is put into question, even though some 5% of patients may have an ANA-negative serology. It is safe to consider that, over time, all patients with SLE will have ANA in their serum. ANA is currently detected using the technique of indirect immunofluorescence (see box: 'Immunofluorescence'), where diluted patient's serum is applied to a tissue — or cell preparation — in which nuclei are prominent. Frozen tissue, especially liver, of rodent origin and cell lines of human origin, such as the HEp2 cell line derived from a laryngeal tumour, are used as substrate to detect ANA. Four ANA patterns (see Table 12.2) can be readily recognised in immunofluorescence: homogeneous, speckled, peripheral and nucleolar, the presence of the first three, alone or in association, being most relevant to the diagnosis of SLE. The homogeneous pattern is caused by an antibody directed against the DNA-related proteins called histones; the **speckled** pattern corresponds to a variety of antibodies directed against other antigens in the nucleus. These have become known collectively as the **extractable nuclear antigens** (ENA) and are normally detected by immunodiffusion (see box: 'Detection

of antibodies to extractable nuclear antigens (ENAs)') or ELISA (see p. 186) techniques. Anti-ENA antibodies are frequently named after the patient whose serum was used to identify them. Therefore, there is anti-Sm (Smith), found almost exclusively in SLE, and anti-RNP (ribonucleoprotein), more typically associated with mixed connective tissue disease (see below) than with SLE. Other antinuclear antibodies seen in SLE are anti-Ro (Robert) also called SS-A (for Sjögren's syndrome antigen A) and anti-La (Lane) or SS-B (Sjögren's syndrome antigen B). Other anti-ENA autoantibodies are anti-Jo-1, anti-Scl-70 and anti-centromere, which are associated mainly with polymyositis, systemic sclerosis and CREST syndrome, respectively (see below). The **peripheral** pattern of ANA staining is traditionally said to correspond to anti-dsDNA, but this is controversial. Antibodies to proteins of the nuclear envelope, such as lamins, are also responsible for the peripheral pattern. The **nucleolar** pattern is rare in SLE, being more associated with systemic sclerosis.

In summary, ANA is a very sensitive test for SLE, being present in virtually all patients and frequently at high titres; its disease specificity is relatively low since it is frequently found in other rheumatic diseases, as well as in autoimmune liver disease, during viral infections and, occasionally, at low titres, in normal subjects. It has a tendency to increase in prevalence with age in healthy adults. Transfer of autoantibodies from the mother to a fetus can occur (see box: 'Neonatal SLE').

While the disease specificity of ANA is low, that of anti-dsDNA autoantibodies is high. The DNA used in the assay must be double stranded: autoantibodies to single-stranded (ss) DNA exist in many diseases and are specific for none. The prevalence (70%) of anti-dsDNA autoantibodies is much higher in SLE, giving a higher diagnostic sensitivity (i.e. pick-up rate; see p. 188) than the similarly disease-specific anti-Sm autoantibodies (30%). Anti-dsDNA autoantibodies are

Immunofluorescence

The detection of antinuclear antibodies (ANAs) and their pattern definition is classically done by immunofluorescence. This technique permits the detection of antigens in tissues or on cell surfaces using antibodies specifically directed to these antigens. Alternatively, when a preparation is known to contain a given antigen, immunofluorescence can be used to identify its complementary antibody. To ascertain whether a lupus patient is 'ANA positive', serum is applied to nuclei-containing tissues, typically of rodent origin, or to a smear of a cell line culture characterised by large nuclei. The use of this latter substrate enables a good definition of the ANA pattern. If the patient is ANA positive, the autoantibody will bind to the nuclei. To reveal this binding, a second antibody is added. The second reagent has been raised in an animal against human immunoglobulin and is tagged with a fluorescent label. This second antibody will bind and ANA will then be seen by placing the preparation under a fluorescence microscope. This technique is known as **indirect immunofluorescence**, since the autoantibody is revealed through a two-step procedure (IFL; Fig. 12.4). Indirect immunofluorescence is the standard technique for the detection of a wide variety of autoantibodies.

In a patient with lupus nephritis, a kidney biopsy is frequently obtained for diagnostic reasons. The glomeruli of such bioptic renal material contain antigen–antibody complexes. By applying a fluorescent antibody directed against human immunoglobulin — similar to that used in the second step of ANA detection — to a frozen section of the kidney biopsy, it is possible to reveal glomerular immune complex. This one-step technique is known as **direct immunofluorescence** (DFL; Fig. 12.5).

Central to immunofluorescence are fluorochromes and the fluorescence microscope. Fluorochromes are substances emitting light of characteristic colour — green for fluorescein, red for rhodamine and phycoerythrin — at a wavelength lower than that used to excite them. They are used to label antibodies. The fluorescence microscope provides the light source to excite the fluorochromes and the optical devices to visualise the fluorescent image.

Immunofluorescence is also commonly used to identify cell types within a suspension using an antibody directed to a surface structure unique to that cell type (e.g. CD3 for total T lymphocytes, CD4 for helper T lymphocytes, CD8 for cytotoxic/suppressor T lymphocytes). Fluorescence microscopy has largely been replaced by cytofluorimetry (see p. 83) for cell counting and analysis.

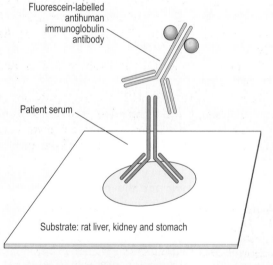

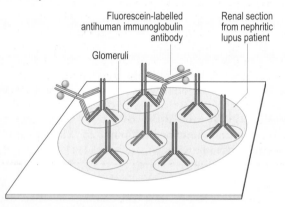

Fig. 12.5 **Direct immunofluorescence.**
A fluorescein-labelled antihuman immunoglobulin antiserum is applied to a frozen section of a kidney biopsy obtained from a lupus patient suffering from glomerulonephritis. (See Figure 16.9.)

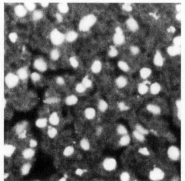
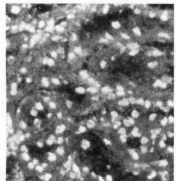
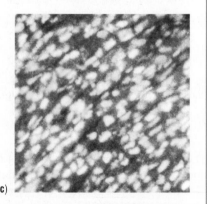

(a)   (b)   (c)

Fig. 12.4 **Indirect immunofluorescence.**
The patient's serum is applied to a frozen tissue section containing the relevant antigen. The method is described in the immunofluorescence box. In the insets, the appearance of antinuclear antibody on rat liver (**a**), kidney (**b**) and stomach (**c**) is shown.

Detection of antibodies to extractable nuclear antigens (ENAs)

Although the use of ELISAs (see page 186) has become widespread, in many laboratories ENAs are still detected using a technique developed some 3 decades ago. This is immunodiffusion in agarose gels. A gel is poured and wells cut into it as shown in Figure 12.6. The central well is filled with the extract containing the antigens, in this case a nuclear preparation. Test serum is placed in an outer well, adjacent to a serum known to contain the autoantibody of interest (in this case antibodies to the ENA called Sjögren's syndrome A, SSA). When the antigen and serum diffuse towards each other, antigen–antibody complexes form at the point of equivalence between the two, appearing as a white line. Certainty that the white line in the test sample represents anti-SSA comes from the fact that it joins that formed by the anti-SSA in the known serum sample (the so-called line of identity).

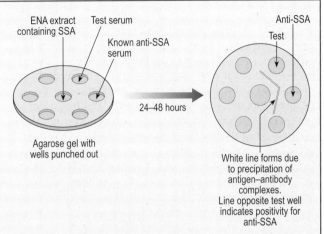

Fig. 12.6 **Detection of antibodies to extractable nuclear antigens (ENAs) by immunodiffusion in agarose gels.**

Neonatal SLE

This rare condition can affect babies born to women suffering from SLE. It is characterised by a cutaneous rash appearing shortly after birth, especially if there is exposure to UV light in the nursery. Another typical manifestation is congenital heart block, which can be fatal. The disease disappears within 6 month after birth, with the disappearance of maternal immunoglobulin from the newborn's circulation. Placental transfer of anti-Ro, one of the numerous autoantibodies characteristic of SLE, is pathogenic in this condition. Intriguingly, however, anti-Ro antibodies do not appear to cause cardiac dysfunction in adults.

usually detected by very analytically sensitive techniques, such as radioimmunoassay (RIA) or ELISA (see p. 186). They can also be detected by immunofluorescence staining of an organelle called a kinetoplast in the flagellate *Crithidia luciliae*, which contains dsDNA. Within SLE, dsDNA antibodies tend to associate with the presence of glomerulonephritis. Their levels are used by some clinicians to monitor disease activity.

The range of autoantibodies seen in SLE is outlined in Table 12.3.

Immune complexes (IC) are frequently present in the circulation, but no single test is available to measure their levels satisfactorily. Different tests measure immune complexes through their different properties:

Table 12.3 **Autoantibody spectrum in SLE**

Autoantibody	Prevalence (%)	Comments
Antinuclear (pattern: homogeneous, speckled or membranous)	95	The absence of this antibody questions the diagnosis of SLE
Anti-dsDNA	70	High specificity for SLE; high titres associated with low complement levels and glomerulonephritis
Anti-Sm	30	High specificity for SLE
Anti-RNP	30	More common in the so-called mixed connective tissue disease
Anti-SS-A(Ro)	20	More common in Sjögren's syndrome; associated with neonatal lupus
Anti-SS-B(La)	10	More common in Sjögren's syndrome; frequently associated with SS-A/Ro
Antiphospholipid	30	Anticardiolipin is the best defined amongst the antibodies of this group; responsible for thrombosis, recurrent abortions and for the antiphospholipid syndrome
Antierythrocyte	50	Directed to red cell-surface antigens; occasionally results in haemolytic anaemia
Antilymphocyte	50	Responsible for lymphocytopenia; up to 90% react also with neuronal cells
Antiplatelet	>10	Responsible for thrombocytopenia
Antineural cells	50	Possibly responsible for CNS manifestations
Rheumatoid factor	25	

such as their ability to fix complement, to bind Fc receptors, or according to their molecular weight. Tissue immune complexes, readily visualised by electron microscopy and by their characteristic granular pattern by light microscopy along the glomerular basement membrane, are presently of more value in diagnosis and management. **Antiphospholipid antibodies** are present in a minority of lupus patients (10–15%), but their presence is associated with defined clinical manifestations (see above). Anticardiolipin antibodies, detected in an ELISA, and lupus anticoagulant, identified by its ability to prolong the partial thromboplastin time, belong to the antiphospholipid antibody family and are both responsible for thrombosis. Antiphospholipid antibodies account for the false positive VDRL results (Venereal Disease Research Laboratory; a test for syphilis) observed at times in lupus patients. Assessment of the **complement** profile is of importance in management. Serial determinations of CH_{50}, a functional assay measuring complement haemolytic activity, and of the individual factors C3 (common pathway) and C4 (classical pathway), inform on how much immune complexes are consuming complement (for complement assays see p. 263).

Drug-induced lupus

A variety of drugs including procainamide, hydralazine, chlorpromazine, isoniazid, practolol, methyldopa and several others can cause manifestations closely mimicking SLE. ANA appears in over half of patients treated with procainamide and in a quarter of patients taking

hydralazine within months of commencement of treatment. Some 10–20% of ANA-positive individuals go on to experience systemic complaints and joint pain. The ANA is directed against histones; anti-dsDNA is usually absent and complement levels are normal. Other lupus manifestations may occur, even though renal and neurological manifestations are rare. Cessation of treatment is generally followed by abatement of symptoms; on occasional instances, corticosteroids may be temporarily required. ANA may remain present for years.

Treatment

Treatment is dictated by the type of manifestation. Non-steroidal anti-inflammatory drugs and aspirin should be used for arthritis, myalgias and mild serositis. Antimalarial drugs, such as hydrochloroquine, can be effective in cutaneous manifestations, with frequent checks for retinal toxicity. Corticosteroids alone or in association with cytotoxic drugs, such as cyclophosphamide and azathioprine, are used in case of severe, life-threatening manifestations. The addition of cytotoxic drugs is considered useful in controlling the rate of flare-ups and in decreasing the dose of steroids.

RHEUMATOID ARTHRITIS

Rheumatoid arthritis (RA) is a multisystem chronic inflammatory disease, principally affecting peripheral joints in a symmetric fashion and commonly leading to cartilage destruction, bone erosions and joint deformities. Its course is variable; extra-articular manifestations, such as vasculitis and subcutaneous nodules, are present in 20–25% of the patients. Women are affected more than men, with a female:male ratio of 3:1; the disease onset reaches its apex between 35–50 years. RA has a worldwide distribution, with a prevalence of approximately 1%.

Pathology

Hyperplasia and hypertrophy of the synovial lining are, with microvascular injury, early findings in the course of the disease. With time, the oedematous synovial tissue protrudes into the synovial cavity in what is known as pannus. A mononuclear infiltrate surrounds vessels and consists of T lymphocytes, macrophages and B lymphocytes. All these cells reveal their active involvement in the chronic inflammatory process through the expression of activation markers. Amongst T lymphocytes, CD4 cells vastly outnumber CD8 cells; with cells expressing the uncommon γδ T cell receptor being abundant. In contrast to the synovial membrane infiltrate, the inflammatory cells present in the exudate contained in the articular cavity are mainly polymorphonuclear leukocytes. The **rheumatoid nodule**, an extra-articular manifestation of RA (see below and Figs 12.7 and 12.8), contains a centre of fibrinoid

Systemic lupus erythematosus

- Antinuclear antibodies of homogeneous and/or speckled pattern are present in virtually all patients. These antibodies have high sensitivity but low specificity, being found almost invariably in SLE but also in several other connective tissue and autoimmune diseases.
- Anti-dsDNA and anti-Sm antibodies are specific for SLE but are not universally present, occurring in 70% and 30% of the patients, respectively.
- SLE is associated with the *HLA-DR3* (Caucasians) and *HLA-DR2* (Orientals) alleles within class II, and with the *C4AQ0* silent allele within class III *HLA* genes.
- Immunoglobulin, complement and dsDNA (immune complexes) gathered in a granular fashion are present in the glomerular basement membrane of patients with lupus nephritis.
- Immune complexes can derive from the circulation or originate from a 'planted' antigen (e.g. dsDNA).
- Active disease is characterised by decreased complement levels, especially those of C4, and by increased levels of anti-dsDNA.
- Antiphospholipid antibodies are associated with thromboembolic episodes and recurrent abortions.
- Autoantibodies against lymphocyte, platetelet, erythrocyte and neuronal cells may be directly involved in cell injury.

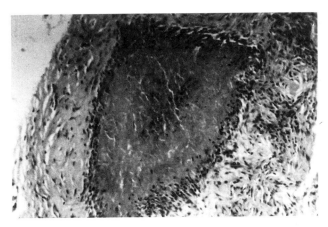

Fig. 12.7 **Rheumatoid nodule.**
A centre of fibrinoid necrosis is surrounded by palisading macrophages and an outer zone of granulation tissue.

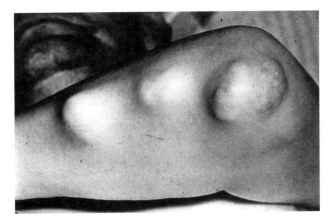

Fig. 12.8 **Rheumatoid nodule.**
On the extensor surfaces is a typical extra-articular manifestation of RA. (Courtesy of Dr J. Goodwill.)

necrosis, probably a remnant of focal vasculitis, surrounded by palisading macrophages and an outer zone of granulation tissue.

Pathogenesis

There is a clear genetic component to the pathogenesis of RA, as indicated by its familial clustering and by the higher concordance for the disease in monozygotic than in dizygotic twins. This genetic suceptibility is in part conferred by HLA class II alleles *DR4* and *DR1* (see box: 'HLA predisposition to rheumatoid arthritis: different alleles, same sequence'). In a pathogenic scenario (see p. 129), these class II molecules would present an arthritogenic (i.e. arthritis-inducing) peptide

Evidence for the involvement of IL-1 and TNF-α as mediators of joint tissue damage in rheumatoid arthritis

1. High levels of these cytokines, or their mRNA, are present in the rheumatoid synovium at sites of active tissue destruction.
2. Synovial fluids containing these cytokines are injurious to normal cartilage in vitro.
3. This damage can be prevented by specific cytokine inhibitors or antagonists.
4. Recombinant IL-1 and TNF-α produce damage to normal cartilage in vitro and in vivo.
5. Progression of tissue damage in patients with RA should be prevented by treatment with inhibitors of IL-1 and TNF-α. (This hypothesis is currently being tested.)

Adapted from Arend W P, Dayer J M 1995 Arthritis and Rheumatism 38: 156.

HLA predisposition to rheumatoid arthritis: different alleles, same sequence

Predisposition to rheumatoid arthritis is conferred by the class II HLA-DR4 and DR1 molecules. DR4 comprises five subtypes, according to variations in the polymorphic β chain, and while three subtypes predispose to the disease, two do not. The susceptibility DR types must contain the amino acid sequence LLEQKRAA in position 67–74 of the β chain, with only a possible conservative amino acid substitution of arginine for lysine in position 71. DR1 shares with the predisposing DR4 subtypes the same eight amino acid sequence on its β chain.

DR type by		Amino acid sequence								Association with RA
Serology	Beta chain	67	68	69	70	71	72	73	74	
DR4/D4	β1*0401	L	L	E	Q	K	R	A	A	Yes
DR4/D10	β1*0402	I	–	–	D	E	–	–	–	No
DR4/D13	β1*0403	–	–	–	–	R	–	–	E	No
DR4/D14	β1*0404	–	–	–	–	R	–	–	–	Yes
DR4/D15	β1*0405	–	–	–	–	R	–	–	–	Yes
DR1	β1*0101	–	–	–	–	R	–	–	–	Yes

These data indicate that a shared amino acid sequence present on different class II HLA molecules is responsible for conferring susceptibility to RA. Moreover, patients positive for both β1*0401 and β1*0404 tend to run a particularly severe course of the disease.

autoantigen to CD4⁺ T cells, which are particularly well represented and in a state of activation within the rheumatoid synovium. These helper T cells would in turn activate CD8 cytotoxic T cells, macrophages and B lymphocytes. Macrophage activation is indicated by elevated levels of monocyte-derived cytokines, such as TNF-α and IL-1, within the synovium, synovial fluid and circulation (see box: 'Evidence for involvement of IL-1 and TNF-α as mediators of joint tissue damage in rheumatoid arthritis').

A cytokine profile typical of T cell activation in RA has not yet been fully defined, and as yet there is no definite evidence for either of the two T helper cell subsets, T_H1 and T_H2, prevailing over the other. Intrasynovial B lymphocytes produce **rheumatoid factors**. These are autoantibodies directed against the Fc portion of IgG. These autoantibodies can belong to any of the three main Ig classes, G, A or M, but the 'classical' rheumatoid factor is a pentameric IgM. Rheumatoid factors react against IgG molecules that are abnormal in their carbohydrate moieties, a feature that probably renders them immunogenic. The resulting immune complex is likely to participate in the perpetuation of inflammatory processes. As a consequence, the level of complement is reduced through activation and consumption within the inflamed joint. C5a and C3a are released in abundance and exert their anaphylotoxic role, inducing the release of histamine; they also attract polymorphonuclear leukocytes towards the articular cavity. Here, polymorphs engulf immune complexes, release lysosomal enzymes, produce active oxygen metabolites and, in concert with locally generated leukotrienes and prostaglandins, participate in the destructive inflammatory process of the joint (see box: 'Does rheumatoid factor cause arthritis').

Does rheumatoid factor cause arthritis?

This question recurs frequently and remains usually unanswered. Some forgotten experiments conducted several decades ago have the answer to this question. At a rheumatological meeting held in the late 1950s, it was reported that the "transfusion of high-titre rheumatoid factor plasma into normal recipients was carried out. No symptoms appeared in the recipients. Simultaneous injection of high-titre rheumatoid plasma and living rheumatoid peripheral leukocytes did not change the recipient response pattern..." The authors concluded — with some reason — that under their experimental conditions, the rheumatoid factor was devoid of intrinsic pathogenicity. Two additional points are of note. First, that the 'volunteer' population included carcinoma patients, laboratory workers and prison inmates.... Second, that amongst the mainly technical and congratulatory debate following this presentation a discordant voice questioned who should be used as volunteers and whether this type of experiment is ever justified in human beings.

Mycobacterium tuberculosis and rheumatoid arthritis

M. tuberculosis has been the focus of recent interest in RA for a number of reasons. First, large sequences are shared in common between mycobacterial and human heat-shock proteins; second, mycobacterial heat-shock proteins are important in the induction of so-called 'adjuvant arthritis', an animal model of RA; third, the inflamed synovium is infiltrated by a relative abundace of γδ T cells. It appears that T cells bearing this less common form of the TCR have a great cytotoxic potential and also frequently react with heat-shock proteins. Since heat-shock proteins are expressed on stressed cells, it is possible that after an initial encounter with *M. tuberculosis* γδ T cells specific for its heat-shock proteins may expand and cross-react with stressed, endogenous cells expressing heat-shock proteins. How this inflammatory process becomes focused onto the synovium remains to be established.

Attempts at identifying environmental factors provoking RA have met with limited success. Mycoplasma, rubella virus, cytomegalovirus and herpes virus have been incriminated in turn as aetiological agents. Recently, parvovirus B19 has been added to the list of possible offenders, because of the anecdotal appearance of RA following infection with this organism in a few patients. Epstein–Barr virus (EBV) has long been associated with RA: renewed interest has been generated by the observation that the EBV glycoprotein gp110 shares five amino acid residues (QKRAA) with the HLA class II suceptibility gene products. A mechanism of molecular mimicry has been invoked, but how this would operate in the development of RA remains to be established.

In addition to IgG and heat-shock protein (see box: '*M. tuberculosis* and rheumatoid arthritis') as autoantigens, collagen type II could also be important: autoantibodies to this connective tissue protein are present in elevated titres in the serum of patients with RA.

Clinical features

The onset of this chronic polyarthritis is normally insidious with a symmetrical involvement of several joints, typically of the hands, wrists, knees and feet, though inflammation can affect any articulation involving two joint surfaces. The proximal interphalangeal and metacarpophalangeal joints (Fig. 12.9) are the most frequently affected. Pain is a major complaint and is aggravated by movement. On examination, swelling and warmth — both resulting from synovial inflammation — are evident. Morning stiffness lasting for longer than 1 hour is characteristic of RA. To minimise pain, patients tend to maximise the joint space by keeping the joints in flexion. With time, characteristic deformities develop, such as the swan-neck deformity (hyper-

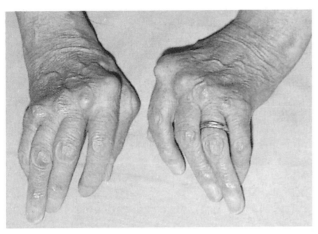

Fig. 12.9 **Symmetrical involvement of joints in RA.**
Advanced symmetrical involvement of joints of the hands (proximal interphalangeal and metacarpophalangeal joints) is typical of rheumatoid arthritis. Note the ulnar deviation. (Reproduced with permission of Grampion Health Board from McHardy K C et al 1997 Illustrated Signs in Clinical Medicine, Churchill Livingstone, Edinburgh; also Figs 12.10 & 12.11.)

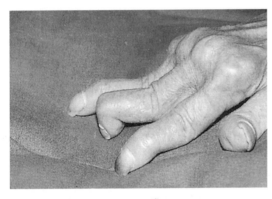

Fig. 12.10 **Swan-neck deformity.**
Hyperextension of the proximal interphalangeal joints with compensatory flexion of the distal interphalangeal joints.

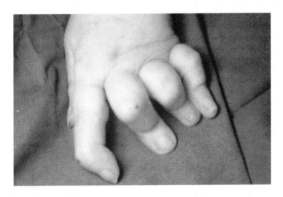

Fig. 12.11 **Boutonnière deformity.**
Flexion of the proximal interphalangeal joints and extension of the distal interphalangeal joints.

extension of the proximal interphalangeal joints with compensatory flexion of the distal interphalangeal joints (Fig. 12.10) and the boutonnière deformity (flexion of the proximal interphalangeal joints and extension of the distal interphalangeal joints (Fig. 12.11). The extent of cartilage loss and bone erosion is well documented by radiography (Fig. 12.12).

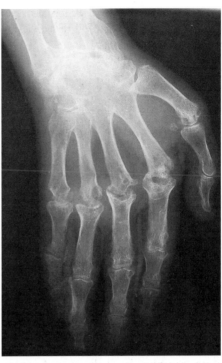

Fig. 12.12 **Radiogram of the hand of a patient with advanced RA.**
Cartilage loss and bone erosion are clearly documented. (Reproduced with permission from McRae R, Kinninmonth W G 1997 Orthopaedics and Trauma – An Illustrated Colour Text, Churchill Livingstone, Edinburgh.)

Extra-articular manifestations are associated with elevated levels of rheumatoid factor; rheumatoid nodules, usually asymptomatic, develop as tissue swellings in one third of the patients, usually on extensor surfaces and typically on the forearm (Fig. 12.8). Other sites for nodules include the pleura, sclera and myocardium. **Rheumatoid vasculitis** can affect almost every organ and in its most severe form produces polyneuropathy. Cutaneous vasculitis manifests itself with small brown lesions in the nail bed; ischaemic lesions leading to ulceration can also develop, especially on the legs. Pulmonary manifestations are more frequent in males and include pleuritis and pulmonary fibrosis. Pericarditis can occur and, like pleuritis, tends to be asymptomatic in life and a very common finding at autopsy. The presence in RA of splenomegaly, neutropenia and, at times, anaemia and thrombocytopenia define **Felty's syndrome.** This syndrome tends to affect patients with high titres of rheumatoid factor and other manifestations of extra-articular disease. Sjögren's syndrome (see p. 178) is present in 30% of the patients.

The guidelines used for classification of RA are given in Table 12.4.

Laboratory findings

Normochromic, normocytic anaemia is common. Both erythrocyte sedimentation rate and C reactive protein are elevated, reliably reflecting the severity of disease; for this reason they are commonly used to monitor disease progression. The rheumatoid factor (RF) measured routinely belongs to the IgM class and because of

Table 12.4 **Guidelines for classification of RA. Four of seven criteria are required to classify a patient as having rheumatoid arthritis**[a]

Criteria	Description
1. Morning stiffness	Stiffness in and around the joints lasting 1 hour before maximal improvement
2. Arthritis of three or more joint areas	At least three joint areas, observed by a physician, simultaneously have soft tissue swelling or joint effusions, not just bony overgrowth; the 14 possible joint areas involved are right or left proximal interphalangeal, metacarpophalangeal, wrist, elbow, knee, ankle and metatarsophalangeal joints
3. Arthritis of hand joints	Arthritis of wrist, metacarpophalangeal joint or proximal interphalangeal joint
4. Symmetric arthritis	Simultaneous involvement of the same joint areas on both sides of the body
5. Rheumatoid nodules	Subcutaneous nodules over bony prominences, extensor surfaces or juxta-articular regions, observed by a physician
6. Serum rheumatoid factor	Demonstration of abnormal amounts of serum rheumatoid factor by any method for which the result has been positive in less than 5% of normal control subjects
7. Radiographic changes	Typical changes of RA on posteroanterior hand and wrist radiographs, which must include erosions or unequivocal bony decalcification localised in or most marked adjacent to the involved joints

[a]Criteria 1–4 must be present for at least 6 weeks. Criteria 2–5 must be observed by a physician.

its pentameric structure is easily revealed in agglutination assays (see box: 'Agglutination').

IgM rheumatoid factor is present in three quarters of patients with RA (termed 'seropositive'). Virtually all patients seronegative by the conventional agglutination assays actually have monomeric rheumatoid factors of the IgG, IgA or IgM class. High titres of classical rheumatoid factor are particularly associated with extra-articular manifestations, and high titres at the onset of the disease tend to presage a poor prognosis. Antinuclear antibodies, usually at low titres, are frequently found in RA. Circulating levels of complement components (C3, C4) tend to be paradoxically elevated because of their behaviour as acute-phase reactants. Within affected joints, complement is always reduced, reflecting the local activation of the complement system induced by immune complexes.

Treatment

This is mainly empirical and follows a gradual approach. A first line of medication is represented by non-steroidal anti-inflammatory drugs, which tend to control symptoms by blocking cyclooxygenase and the production of prostaglandins, prostacyclins and thromboxanes. Gastrointestinal intolerance is a frequent side effect. To a second line of medications belong drugs thought to modify the disease course. They include agents such as anti-malarials, D-penicillamine and gold salts, with little anti-inflammatory activity but with the ability to ameliorate the course of the disease in a majority of patients. The use of corticosteroids, though symptomatically effective, is generally avoided, in view of the fact that they do not alter the course of the disease but are associated with important long-term side effects (although a recent study, yet to be confirmed by others, suggests that early introduction of steroids does alter the course of RA). Cytotoxic drugs — azathioprine and cyclophosphamide — are also usually avoided in view of their potential side effects, apart from in patients with severe extra-articular manifestations.

Rheumatoid arthritis

- RA is characteristically associated with the *HLA DR4* and *DR1* alleles.
- Pentameric IgM rheumatoid factor is the serological hallmark of RA.
- Rheumatoid factor levels are particularly elevated in the presence of extra-articular manifestations such as vasculitis.
- Mononuclear cells, especially CD4[+] T lymphocytes, predominate in the synovial infiltrate, while polymorphonuclear leukocytes are the dominant cells in the synovial fluid.
- Levels of complement factors (e.g. C3, C4) are low intra-articularly, reflecting complement consumption, and are high in the bloodstream, indicating an acute-phase reaction.
- Disease activity is monitored by the measure of erythrocyte sedimentation rate or C-reactive protein.

Agglutination

The detection of rheumatoid factor is conventionally carried out using an agglutination test. A range of inert particles including blood cells, latex or gelatin can be coated with antigen, which in the case of rheumatoid factor is IgG. Agglutination is a sensitive, semi-quantitative technique in which the reaction between antibody and antigen can be titrated to a visible end-point. The ability of pentameric IgM antibodies to agglutinate is some three orders of magnitude higher than that of IgG antibodies. Agglutination 'suffers' from the prozone phenomenon, in which very high titres of antibody can produce false-negative results: hence the need for the antibody under investigation to be tested at different dilutions. Antigenic determinants recognised by the rheumatoid factor are exposed on the particles and the addition of rheumatoid factor to the carriers results in agglutination (see Figs 12.13–12.15).

(a) Addition of IgG to particles

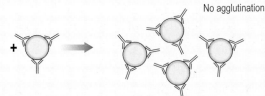

Sensitised particle

(b) RF-negative serum

No agglutination

(c) RF-positive serum

Agglutination

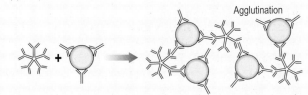

Fig. 12.13 **Basics of testing for rheumatoid factor.**
(**a**) IgG is adsorbed onto inert particles, such as latex or red blood cells. The addition of a negative-control serum results in no agglutination (**b**) while the addition of a rheumatoid factor-positive serum results in agglutination (**c**).

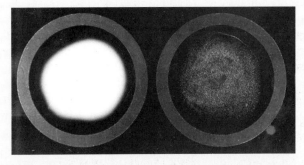

Fig. 12.14 **Detection of rheumatoid factor (RF) using sensitised latex beads.**
Left: RF-negative serum. Right: RF-positive serum.

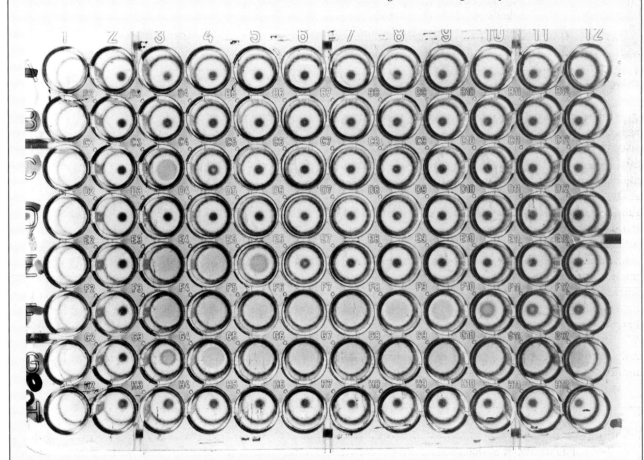

Fig. 12.15 **Titration of rheumatoid factor (RF) in a 96-well titration plate.**
Lane 1, diluent; lane 2, unsensitised gelatin particles; lanes 3–12, particles sensitised (i.e. coated) with IgG. The addition of sera in all the wells of lane 2 gives no agglutination and this negative reaction is seen as a tight button at the bottom of the wells. Wells in lane 3 receive patient sera diluted 1:20. The sera are then double-diluted so that in lane 12 all the sera are diluted 10, 240-fold. Rows A, B, D and H contain negative sera. Rows C, E, F and G contain RF-positive sera with titres of 1:20 (C), 1:40 (E), 1:1280 (F), 1:10 240 (G). In well G3 and to a lesser extent G4, it is possible to see a prozone phenomenon. This describes a suboptimal agglutination due to excess of antibody. To ascertain whether a given value is due to a low amount of antibody or to an excess of it, the serum must be tested at different dilutions against a fixed amount of antigen, in this case a fixed amount of antigen-coated particles. The prozone phenomenon can be seen in other immune reactions such as precipitation reactions.

JUVENILE CHRONIC ARTHRITIS

It is conventional to group under juvenile chronic arthritis (JCA) a series of distinct disorders that are only unified by having their onset below the age of 16.

Some 20% of children with JCA suffer from classical rheumatoid factor-positive rheumatoid arthritis, associated with HLA-DR4 and the least benign prognosis. The other conditions tend to remit in adult life and comprise Still's disease and arthritides with polyarticular or pauciarticular onsets. **Still's disease** is characterised by systemic manifestations, notably fever and hepatosplenomegaly, lymphadenopathy, leukocytosis and anaemia. The form of the disease with polyarticular (five or more joints) onset predominates in girls and tends to associate with DRw6, while the one with pauciarticular (four or less joints) onset can be further subdivided into two subsets. One affects girls below age 6, is associated with iridocyclitis, HLA-DR5 and antinuclear antibody of the speckled type. The other affects boys below 6 years of age and is associated with HLA-B27.

SERONEGATIVE SPONDYLARTHRITIDES

This group of disorders is collectively referred to as the seronegative spondylarthritides because of the absence of rheumatoid factor. They also share other features such as the involvement of sacroiliac and peripheral joints; the association with the HLA class I antigen B27; and the tendency to enthesitis (enthesis being the site of attachment of tendons to bone).

ANKYLOSING SPONDYLITIS

This condition typically affects the axial skeleton, but peripheral arthropathy can also occur. Men, usually below the age of 40, develop the disease three times more frequently than women (Fig. 12.16). Approximately 90% of the patients are HLA-B27 positive, while the prevalence of this antigen in the general population is 7%. Of all the adult HLA-B27-positive individuals, 1–2% have ankylosing spondylitis (AS). AS shows familial aggregation; the concordance in monozygotic twins is approximately 60%, indicating that both genetic and environmental factors must be involved.

Pathology

The lesion of sacroiliitis — first manifestation of the disease — is characterised by subchondral granulation tissue containing a mainly mononuclear cell inflammatory infiltrate. Inflammatory granulation is present also in the spine at the junction of the anulus fibrosus with the vertebral bone. Outer fibres are replaced by bone; these bony excrescences (syndesmophytes) ultimately join vertebral bodies, resulting in the radiological picture of the 'bamboo spine' (Fig. 12.17). In the

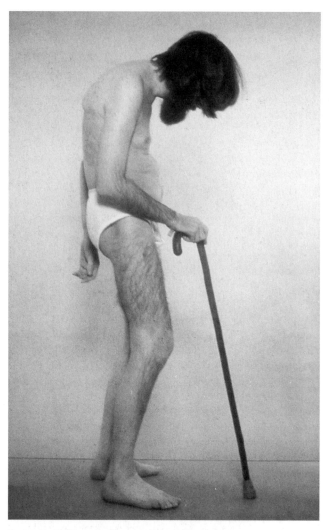

Fig. 12.16 **Patient suffering from ankylosing spondylitis.** (Reproduced with permission from McRae R, Kinninmonth W G 1997 Orthopaedics and Trauma – An Illustrated Colour Text, Churchill Livingstone, Edinburgh.)

peripheral joints the inflammation is similar to that of rheumatoid arthritis but less vigorous. Non-specific inflammatory changes are seen in the iris of those 20% of patients that suffer from uveitis.

Pathogenesis

It is believed that a form of molecular mimicry triggers the onset of AS (see box: 'The arthritogenic peptide molecule of ankylosing spondylitis').

Clinical features

The onset of AS tends to be insidious with a dull lumbar pain; this persists over 3 months and is accompanied by morning stiffness, relieved by exercise. Arthritis of the peripheral joints is seen in one third of the patients. Amongst extra-articular manifestations, iritis is the most troublesome: it tends to be unilateral and accompanied by photophobia and pain. Inflammation of the colon and ileum is frequent but usually asymptomatic. The course of the disease is very variable, the onset in adolescence being associated with poorer prognosis.

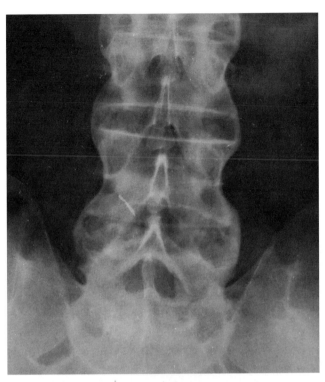

Fig. 12.17 **Spine radiogram showing the 'bamboo spine' typically seen in ankylosing spondylitis.**

The arthritogenic peptide model of ankylosing spondylitis

HLA-B27 is an HLA class I molecule and as such binds antigenic peptides and presents them to CD8$^+$ cytotoxic T cells (CTL). An 'arthritogenic peptide' model sees AS as being the result of a CTL-mediated response to a peptide only found in joint tissues and presented by HLA-B27 molecules. The theory suggests that under normal conditions the concentration of the self peptide is too low to trigger T cell recognition. Infection with microorganisms containing sequences shared by the arthritogenic peptide would activate T cells and lead them to recognise the arthritogenic peptide even at its normally low concentration (another example of molecular mimicry operating in autoimmune disease).

Laboratory findings

Patients with AS tend to have elevated levels of IgA and, when the disease is active, elevated erythrocyte sedimentation rates and levels of C-reactive protein. Rheumatoid factor and antinuclear antibody are consistently negative. The clinical need to assess the HLA-B27 status of a patient with symptoms and signs of AS is controversial. This HLA molecule is present in some 90% of Caucasoid patients and in a lesser proportion of patients of a different ethnic origin. Presence of B27 is neither pathognomonic of the disease nor necessary for making the diagnosis. In patients who have not yet developed clear radiological changes, however, it may be of diagnostic help.

OTHER SERONEGATIVE ARTHRITIDES

A large proportion of these conditions comprises reactive arthritides, the prototype of which is the **Reiter's syndrome**. The diagnostic triad of urethritis, conjunctivitis and arthritis defines this syndrome, even though the diagnosis can be made when just two of these are present, or when balanitis and buccal ulcerations are additional manifestations. The term 'reactive' in the description implies that they follow an infection, frequently unnoticed by the patient and also distant in time and space from the 'reactive' joints. Venereal and enteric infections are typically involved, with microorganisms such as *Chlamydia trachomatis* being the paradigm of venereal infection while a variety of *Shigella*, *Salmonella*, *Yersinia* and *Campylobacter* spp. may be responsible for the enteric infections. HLA-B27 is present in up to 85% of patients with reactive arthritis; the male/female ratio is 1:1 in post-enteric infection cases, while venereally acquired reactive arthritis is thought to be mainly a male disease, even though the disease in women can be underdiagnosed as a result of clinically inapparent urethritis and cervicitis.

Pathology and pathogenesis

The synovial histology is that of inflammatory arthritis with a mononuclear cell infiltrate where T lymphocytes and monocytes predominate. Enthesitis is common, as is the microscopic inflammatory involvement of colon and ileum. Almost all the elements to draw a pathogenic scenario are available. There are well-defined environmental factors: the microorganisms (which, interestingly, are mainly intracellular parasites) responsible for the initial infection. There is a well-defined genetic factor: the HLA-B27 molecule. As for AS, the assumption must be that cells harbouring the infectious agent process and present it as small peptides in the B27 peptide-binding groove as the target of harmful CD8$^+$ cytotoxic T lymphocytes. The unanswered question is why the immune reaction should just be confined to the joints, and only some of them at that, in view of the fact that HLA class I molecules are present on virtually all nucleated cells. Intriguingly, though, there is now evidence to show that antigens from *Chlamydia*, *Yersinia* and *Salmonella* spp. can actually be found in the joints in reactive arthritis, possibly accounting for the localisation of the injurious immune response. Moreover, there is the pivotal observation that synovial T lymphocytes can proliferate in response to antigens of the triggering microorganism. A critique to the above pathogenic scenario has been that not all the patients have HLA-B27; however, a number of HLA-B27-negative patients are HLA-B7 positive, and these two HLA molecules have much of their amino acid sequences in common. Lastly, the importance of the *HLA-B27* gene in the causation of these arthritides and AS is emphasised by a B27-transgenic rat model (see box: 'More on HLA-B27 and seronegative spondylarthritides'). This animal develops inflammatory disease of the axial

More on HLA-B27 and seronegative spondylarthritides

Recent studies show that HLA-B27 transgenic rats with up to 10 copies of the transgene per cell do not develop arthritis-like disease; however, they do so if the copies are 50 per cell. Moreover, arthritis develops only in those animals that are not raised in germ-free conditions, indicating the need for 'germs' for the disease to manifest itself.

At a molecular level, the characteristics of the peptides occupying the HLA-B27 groove have been delineated. These peptides tend to be composed of nine amino acid residues and have a number of motifs in common. Reading the nonamers left to right (with the N terminal as left), one finds arginine invariably in position 2, position 3 occupied by a hydrophobic or aromatic amino acid, and the C-terminus having a polar or hydrophobic side chain. Positions 2 and 9 anchor the peptide to the HLA-B27 groove, positions 1, 4 and 8 are crucial for the binding to the T cell receptor. Intriguingly, all the peptides so far isolated from the HLA-B27 groove belong to normal cytosolic proteins, not to microorganisms.

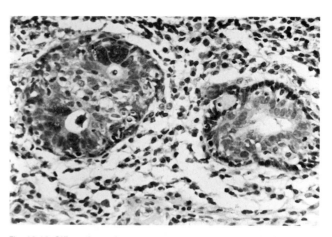

Fig. 12.18 **Sjögren's syndrome.**
The histology of the parotid gland reveals a dense mononuclear cell infiltrate. (Courtesy of Dr J. Salisbury)

rate during acute phases of the disease, mild anaemia, the presence of HLA-B27 in 80% of patients and, in some, increased levels of antibodies against the triggering infection. The infection has usually subsided by the time arthritis appears. The treatment is based on non-steroidal anti-inflammatory drugs, occasionally on the local use of corticosteroids for tendinitis and enthesitis. In the case of uveitis, treatment involves vigorous systemic use of corticosteroids.

joints, gut and male genital tract. Any triggering microorganism remains to be defined.

Clinical features

The manifestations can vary from a transient monoarthritis to an asymmetrical additive polyarthritis with prominent constitutional symptoms like fever, malaise, fatigue and weight loss. An infection preceding the onset of arthritis can be found by taking a careful history in the majority of patients, but not in a considerable minority, even though a history of a new sexual partner is at times elicited. Dactylitis, also referred to as 'sausage digit' is typical of reactive arthritis and is caused by diffuse swelling. Urogenital ulcers can occur any time during the course of the disease and ocular manifestations can range from conjunctivitis to the much more severe anterior uveitis. The laboratory findings are few: elevated erythrocyte sedimentation

SJÖGREN'S SYNDROME

Sjögren's syndrome (SS) is a chronic inflammatory condition affecting lacrimal and salivary glands, leading to dry eyes and mouth (also referred to as keratoconjunctivitis sicca and xerostomia). There are two forms: primary, when the disease occurs alone, and secondary, when it is associated with rheumatoid arthritis, SLE and, less frequently, with systemic sclerosis. SS affects middle-aged women (nine females for one male) and has a strong association with the *HLA-B8 DR3* haplotype. The histology of lacrimal and salivary glands reveals a mononuclear cell infiltrate (Fig. 12.18), mainly composed of T and B lymphocytes, with a predominance of CD4[+] T lymphocytes, all expressing markers of activation. Hypergammaglobulinaemia is frequent and usually polyclonal. Rheumatoid factors of the pentameric IgM type are present in 90% of the patients. Antinuclear antibodies of the speckled and homogeneous type are found in two thirds of patients. More specific to SS are autoantibodies to the extractable nuclear antigens, anti-SS-A (anti-Ro; see above) and anti-SS-B (anti-La), which are present in at least half of the SS patients, in a small proportion of lupus patients (frequently with symptoms of SS) and in virtually no other condition. The production of SS-associated autoantibodies is controlled from genes within the HLA region: possession of specific amino acid sequences in the second hypervariable region of the HLA-DQα and

---

Ankylosing spondylitis and other seronegative arthritides

- AS is characteristically associated with HLA-B27, being present in ~90% of patients.
- Elevated IgA levels are common; antinuclear antibodies and rheumatoid factor are usually absent.
- Reactive arthritis is also characteristically associated with HLA-B27 (~80% of patients).
- An enteric or venereal infection precedes joint manifestations.
- Increased levels of antibodies against the triggering infection are found.

Retroviruses and connective tissue diseases

A growing body of evidence indicates a role for retroviruses in the development of Sjögren's syndrome and other immune-mediated inflammatory diseases. In a Japanese study, the prevalence of antibodies to human T lymphotrophic virus type 1 (HTLV-1) was eight times higher in patients with SS than in blood donors. Again from Japan came the demonstration that the transactivator gene of HTLV-1 is expressed in the labial salivary glands of a proportion of SS patients. In another study, the sequence of retroviral reverse transcriptase has been documented in tissues obtained from SS patients. Antibodies to the major group antigen (gag) of retroviruses, including p24 of HIV, have been repeatedly found in the sera of a significant proportion of patients with SS, SLE, systemic sclerosis and juvenile arthritis. Last in this compendium of incriminating evidence is the finding that the SS-B/La and Sm antigens share limited sequence homologies with retroviral gag proteins.

Sjögren's syndrome

- Anti-SS-A(Ro) and anti-SS-B(La) autoantibodies are typically present in the serum of SS patients.
- Inflammation of lacrimal and salivary glands leads to dry eyes and mouth; the glands have a mononuclear cell infiltrate.
- Retroviruses may be involved in the development of SS.

HLA-DQβ chain gene products promotes both SS-A and SS-B autoantibody production. The molecular targets of these autoantibodies have also been identified. SS-A recognises polypeptides complexed with Y_1–Y_5 RNAs. SS-B is a phosphorylated protein complexed with small RNA polymerase transcripts. The pathogenesis of SS is open to conjecture. Whether activation of B lymphocytes, as suggested by the production of a variety of autoantibodies and the presence of hypergammaglobulinaemia, is a key defect is not established. However, in favour of this view is the tendency for the disease to culminate in monoclonal gammopathy, and the fact that patients with SS have a 40-fold increase in the incidence of lymphoma. However, CD4$^+$ T cells predominate in the inflammatory infiltrate, and culture of these from SS patients has led to the isolation of an A-type retrovirus (see box: 'Retroviruses and connective tissue diseases'), indicating the possibility that infection of regulatory T cells could be an important disease trigger.

The **clinical features** of SS include dry eyes with a gritty feeling under the eyelids, symptomatically treated with artificial tears. A reduction in tear flow is documented through the Schirmer's test, while the detection of punctate corneal ulcerations by slit lamp examination after Bengal staining is highly diagnostic. Dry mouth, accompanied by a high incidence of caries, requires fastidious oral hygiene; dysphagia for dry food is the result of involvement of glands of the gastrointestinal tract; dryness of the vagina is accompanied by dyspareunia. Extraglandular manifestations include fatigue, low-grade fever, arthralgias and myalgias. The erythocyte sedimentation rate is frequently elevated, and mild anaemia can be observed.

SYSTEMIC SCLEROSIS

Systemic sclerosis (scleroderma) is a chronic, disabling condition of unknown aetiology, characterised by fibrosis of the skin, blood vessels and internal organs, including lung, heart, gastrointestinal tract and kidney. It is subdivided into (1) a more severe diffuse cutaneous form that rapidly involves the skin extensively and the internal organs; and (2) a limited cutaneous form, in which the skin thickening is limited to the distal extremities and face. This form can be part of the so-called **CREST syndrome**, the acronym standing for calcinosis, Raynaud's phenomenon, oesophageal involvement, sclerodactyly and telangiectasia. Systemic sclerosis can also affect the visceral organs alone, sparing the skin (systemic sclerosis without scleroderma). Females are affected three times more frequently than males, with a peak incidence in the third to fifth decade. Occurrence of multiple familial cases and a loose association with the HLA antigens DR1, DR3 and DR5 have been described.

Pathology

Bundles of collagen bind the skin to the underlying tissue. In early lesions of systemic sclerosis, a mononuclear cell infiltrate consisting of T cells, monocytes, plasma cells and mast cells is seen. The epidermis is thin. In the oesophagus, a thin mucosa, frequently ulcerated, covers abundant collagen deposition in the lamina propria, submucosa and serosa. Similar changes can be seen in other gastrointestinal tract segments, with accompanying mononuclear cell infiltrate. In the lung, a thickening of the alveolar membrane characterises alveolar fibrosis. The alterations of the synovial membrane are similar to those of other inflammatory arthritides, with oedema and an infiltrate of mononuclear cells. Interstitial fibrosis is seen in muscles and myocardium, the fibrosis at times involving the conduction system resulting in conduction defects. The lesions of primary biliary cirrhosis can be noted in the liver, when systemic sclerosis is associated with this liver disease. IgM, complement and fibrinogen can be detected by immunofluorescence in affected renal vessels. These vessels show thickening of the intima of interlobular arteries and fibrinoid necrosis of the intima and media of afferent arterioles.

Pathogenesis

The pathogenic process can be divided into two phases. The first phase, characterised by endothelial injury, is followed by a second phase where fibrosis predominates.

In the early phase, it is thought that activated T cells release a serine protease that is toxic to endothelial cells; endothelial cells are also targeted by antibodies that mediate damage by antibody-dependent cellular cytotoxicity (see p. 109). TNF-α derived from activated macrophages can also induce endothelial damage. The binding of the von Willebrand factor released by damaged endothelium leads to activation of platelets, with the consequent release of platelet-derived growth factor (PDGF; a factor mitogenic for fibroblasts) and TGF-β, which stimulates collagen production by fibroblasts. Both these 'fibrogenic' cytokines are also secreted by activated macrophages and fibroblasts, while activated T lymphocytes produce TGF-β. The state of activation of T cells is demonstrated by elevated circulating levels of soluble IL-2 receptor and IL-2. Lymphocytes from patients proliferate in the presence of laminin and type IV collagen, components of the endothelial cell membrane. Fibroblasts in the skin lesions express elevated levels of messenger RNA for collagen I and III; when fibroblasts are isolated from affected skin, they continue to produce an abundance of collagen.

Clinical features

Raynaud's phenomenon is usually the first manifestation of systemic sclerosis, frequently preceding other symptoms by months or years. It is typically triggered by cold and reveals itself as pallor and/or cyanosis of the fingers followed by rubor (redness) on rewarming. This phenomenon is present in virtually all patients with systemic sclerosis and may remain a solitary manifestation. The initial skin lesions are characterised by oedema, either localised to the hands or diffuse in character, followed by an indurative phase when the skin becomes firm and bound to the subcutaneous tissue. This can limit extension of digits, leading to flexion contractures. The involvement of the face results in effacing of wrinkles and microstomia, which can interfere with eating (Fig. 12.19). The skin tends to lose hair and become dry and coarse. In a third stage, the skin undergoes softening. Arthritic symptoms, at times resembling those of RA, and an inflammatory myopathy are frequent manifestations affecting the musculoskeletal apparatus. Pulmonary fibrosis is frequent, but it is also frequently asymptomatic. Pulmonary hypertension develops in 10% of patients. Pleuritis, pericarditis and cardiac fibrosis are frequent post-mortem findings.

Renal involvement is somewhat unusual but can be fatal. SS can be superimposed onto systemic sclerosis.

Laboratory findings

Laboratory tests reveal elevated erythrocyte sedimentation, anaemia and hypergammaglobulinaemia. Low titres of rheumatoid factor are present in a quarter

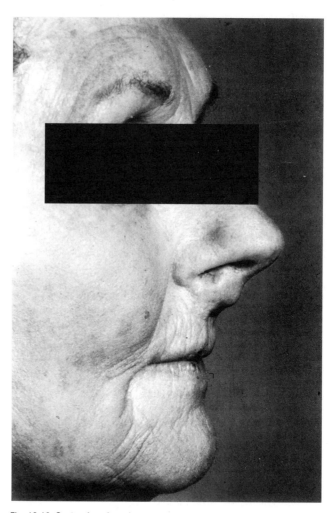

Fig. 12.19 **Systemic sclerosis.**
Typical facies with tight skin, partial effacing of wrinkles and microstomia. (Courtesy of Dr J. Goodwill.)

of the patients and antinuclear antibodies are usually present. A speckled pattern is frequently seen, the target antigen being the nuclear enzyme DNA topoisomerase 1 (also known as Scl-70). Antitopoisomerase 1 autoantibodies are present in 20% of the patients and tend to be associated with the diffuse cutaneous form of the disease and with pulmonary interstitial fibrosis. Anticentromere autoantibodies, however, are associated with the localised form of the disease or with the CREST syndrome. Antinucleolar autoantibodies are considered to be specific for systemic sclerosis, above all when they are an isolated finding. Their targets comprise RNA polymerase I, the peri-ribosomal particle and an antigen referred to as PM-Scl. Antibodies to PM-Scl give a homogeneous nucleolar pattern and are associated with polymyositis and renal involvement.

Treatment

The treatment of systemic sclerosis is symptomatic. Raynaud's phenomenon is treated by keeping warm and controlling stress. The renal hypertensive crises are successfully treated with drugs blocking the renin–angiotensin system (captopril, enalapril). Oesophageal and intestinal hypomotility can be improved with metoclopramide.

POLYMYOSITIS AND DERMATOMYOSITIS

The unifying feature of this group of diseases is an inflammatory process involving the skeletal — typically proximal — muscles and skin, in which a mononuclear cell infiltration is prominent. The following classification into five subgroups is currently adopted:

I. primary idiopathic polymyositis
II. primary idiopathic dermatomyositis
III. polymyositis or dermatomyositis associated with neoplasia
IV. polymyositis or dermatomyositis of childhood associated with vasculitis
V. polymyositis or dermatomyositis associated with connective tissue disorders.

A sixth group, polymyositis or dermatomyositis associated with infections, has been added by some taxonomy-crazed authors. There is a familial occurrence of this group of diseases, indicating a genetic influence.

Pathology

The histological examination of a skeletal muscle biopsy, required for diagnosis in a majority of patients, shows an inflammatory infiltrate, consisting of lymphocytes, macrophages, plasma cells and occasional eosinophils and neutrophils, associated with local or diffuse degeneration of muscle fibres. The inflammatory infiltrate can also be observed around vessels, while signs of muscle fibre degeneration tend to co-exist with signs of regeneration.

Pathogenesis

The disease is associated with the class II HLA alleles *DR3* and *DR52*; electron microscopic examination has repeatedly suggested the presence of viral particles within muscle fibres, though no virus has ever been isolated. A polymyositis-like condition can be induced in animals by coxsackie virus, and a mild form of myopathy can accompany human infections with coxsackie and influenza viruses. The presence of antibodies to ribonucleoprotein in the serum of these patients has suggested their origin in cross-reactivity with viral antigens. In animals, it is possible to induce allergic experimental myositis, a close model of the human disorder, by immunising animals with muscle antigens in Freund's adjuvant. The muscle injury appears to derive mainly from a cellular immune attack on the muscle fibre. Lymphocytes isolated from patients with polymyositis and cultured in the presence of autologous (i.e. their own) unaffected muscle release a soluble factor toxic to cultures of normal human fetal muscle cells. A possible damaging role for humoral immunity is suggested by the finding of IgG, IgM and the membrane attack complex of the complement system (C5b-9) in vessels of the skin and muscle in dermatomyositis.

Clinical features

Primary idiopathic polymyositis affects twice as many women as men, usually has an insidious onset and is characterised by weakness in proximal limb muscles, manifesting itself as difficulty in climbing or descending stairs, rising from a chair or from the squatting position, or combing hair. The additional cutaneous lesions of primary idiopathic dermatomyositis may precede or follow muscular symptomatology, and typically include a lilac (heliotrope) rash either limited to eyelids and knuckles or occasionally extending to large areas of the body. Polymyositis or dermatomyositis associated with neoplasia can precede or follow its diagnosis. The most frequently associated malignancies are those of the lung, ovary, breast, stomach and myeloproliferative disorders. The paediatric forms are associated with vasculitis of skin, muscles and gastrointestinal tract, while those associated with connective tissue disorders are most frequently linked to SLE, RA and mixed connective tissue disease (see below). The diagnosis is supported by increased levels of the muscle enzymes creatine kinase and transaminases and by typical electromyographical and histological changes.

Laboratory findings

In addition to the characteristic enzymatic profile, erythrocyte sedimentation rate is normally increased, rheumatoid factor is found in half and antinuclear antibody in up to three-quarters of the patients, frequently showing a speckled pattern. An antigenic target for this antibody has been identified as tRNA synthetase or Jo-1, which is typically found in polymyositis when there is an interstitial pulmonary involvement. Other antinuclear autoantibodies are seen when polymyositis is associated with other connective tissue diseases. The treatment is based on the vigorous use of corticosteroids, at least in the severe cases, with decreasing levels of creatine kinase reflecting the effectiveness of the treatment. Cytotoxic drugs (azathioprine, cyclophosphamide and methotrexate) are used to spare corticosteroids and/or supplement their action. Leukapheresis (removal of leukocytes from the blood) and intravenous immunoglobulin have also been used with anecdotal reports of success.

> **Polymyositis and dermatomyositis**
>
> - Lymphocytes, macrophages and plasma cells infiltrate degenerating muscle fibres.
> - Class II HLA alleles *DR3* and *DR52* are frequently present.
> - Antinuclear autoantibody, often speckled, is present in three-quarters of the patients; rheumatoid factor in half.
> - An antigenic target for the antinuclear autoantibody is tRNA synthetase, also called Jo-1.
> - Anti-Jo-1 is typically found in patients with polymyositis who also have interstitial pulmonary involvement.

MIXED CONNECTIVE TISSUE DISEASE

Mixed connective tissue disease (MCTD) is described as an 'overlap' syndrome, which borrows elements from several other connective tissue diseases. Elevated titres of a speckled pattern antinuclear antibody directed against ribonucleoprotein (anti-RNP) is the distinguishing feature that makes MCTD a separate diagnostic and a pathological entity. The majority of the patients are female and typically experience the Raynaud's phenomenon. The cutaneous manifestations can be those of lupus, or those of dermatomyositis (typically the heliotrope rash). The arthritis tends to be non-deforming, even though it may acquire the features of RA. The skeletal muscle involvement is that of polymyositis, with mononuclear cell inflammatory infiltrate and increase in the circulating levels of creatine kinase. The oesophageal dysmotility and impaired diffusing capacity of the lung are those of systemic sclerosis, as indeed is the renal involvement. Constitutional symptoms such as fever and lymphadenopathy and an association with Sjögren's syndrome have been occasionally reported.

> **Connective tissue diseases and HIV**
>
> In trying to understand the pathogeneses of 'immune-mediated' diseases such as the rheumatic disorders, it is useful to observe their course during infection with HIV, when the CD4 lymphocytes — key regulatory cells in immune homeostasis — are gradually being removed (see Ch. 20). Patients with RA who acquire HIV infection suffer from a much milder form of the disease, strengthening the notion that CD4 lymphocytes play a key role in the pathogenesis of RA. Patients with reactive arthritis such as Reiter's syndrome, however, who contract HIV infection see the course of their disease worsen significantly. Why the depletion of CD4$^+$ T cells should exacerbate the course of reactive arthritis is far from clear. What this does tell us is that the pathogenesis of these two types of arthritis is likely to be different.

> **Mixed connective tissue disease**
>
> - Antinuclear antibody with a speckled pattern is typically found in this condition.
> - This antinuclear antibody is directed against ribonucleoprotein (anti-RNP).

Endocrine autoimmune disease

The autoimmune disorders affecting the endocrine glands are an example of organ-specific autoimmune diseases (see Ch. 9); other diseases within this classification include pernicious anaemia and autoimmune hepatitis (see Ch. 15). Tissue damage is cell specific and the resulting organ failure or dysfunction gives rise to the clinical syndrome. Research into the pathogenesis of these diseases has concentrated on two areas: the immune *effectors* (antibody, T lymphocytes, cytokines) that damage tissues or interfere with cell function and the nature of the *targets* (cell-specific autoantigens) against which the immune response is directed. An exciting future lies ahead for manipulation of such components to cure these disorders.

Endocrine autoimmune diseases are typically more common in women, strongly implying a hormonal influence on their development. These disorders are also influenced by two other main factors: genes and environment. The disorders frequently 'run' in families and have an association with certain HLA types. However, simply having the predisposing genes is not enough; factors in the environment are also at play. One of the other main features of the organ-specific autoimmune diseases is the presence in the serum of autoantibodies directed against a variety of components of the target organ or cell. Similar, complementary reactions by T cells also exist but are currently less well defined. Broadly speaking, the targets may be within the cell and are often enzymes; targets may also be on the cell surface, such as molecules with receptor function; or they may be the secreted products of the cell, such as hormones.

TYPE 1 (INSULIN-DEPENDENT) DIABETES MELLITUS

Type 1, or insulin-dependent, diabetes mellitus is a state of hyperglycaemia resulting from lack of insulin secretion by the β cells in the islets of Langerhans of the pancreas, and patients require exogenous insulin to sustain life. Glucose is usually present in the urine at diagnosis (glycosuria), which is often associated with prodromal symptoms of weight loss, thirst, polydypsia and polyuria. Patients may occasionally present in a state of severe metabolic disturbance known as keto-acidotic coma. The diagnosis of diabetes is confirmed by an overnight fasted whole blood glucose level in excess of 6.7 mM. An oral glucose tolerance test may also be performed after overnight fasting, in which 75 g glucose (adult dose) is given in 200 ml of fluid and a 2-hour glucose level above 10.0 mM is diagnostic of diabetes. Although it is true to say that the advent of injected insulin earlier in the nineteenth century restored health in what had always been an acutely fatal disease, this treatment does not hold all the answers. Diabetes is still associated with high mortality rates resulting from its complications, the most important being arterial disease, blindness and renal failure.

Type 1 diabetes has a peak onset around puberty and the incidence within Europe ranges from 5 to 43 cases per 100 000 of the population per year, along a north–south gradient from Finland to Greece. There are occasional 'blips' along the gradient: so-called 'hot-spots' such as Sardinia, which has the second highest incidence in Europe; and 'cold-spots' such as Poland, with only six cases per 100 000 per year even though it is on the same latitude as Scandinavia, which has the highest incidence. In the UK and USA, the incidence is estimated at some 16 cases per 100 000 per year and appears to be rising. The prevalence of the disease is approximately 0.3%. Unlike other autoimmune diseases, type 1 diabetes affects the sexes equally.

Type 1 diabetes arises on a distinct genetic background. Some 90% of cases are sporadic, whilst the remainder occur within families that already have a diabetic member. Much of this genetic susceptibility maps to the HLA system, although other genes also have a role. Between 5 and 8% of siblings of type 1 diabetic children develop the disease themselves, the risk being higher the more class II genes that are shared with the diabetic brother or sister. The chance of an individual carrying a gene or other characteristic acquiring a disease is expressed as the **relative risk** (Table 13.1). Some 95% of UK patients with type 1 diabetes have *HLA-DR3* or *HLA-DR4* alleles, and even stronger associations are being identified by sequencing the *DQ* genes.

Table 13.1 **Calculation of relative risk, and its implications for type 1 diabetes**

Relative risk (RR) of carrying gene A	=	$\dfrac{\text{patients with A} \times \text{controls lacking A}}{\text{patients without A} \times \text{controls with A}}$

Characteristic	Relative risk of developing type 1 diabetes
Background population	1.0[a]
HLA-DR3	5.0
HLA-DR4	6.8
HLA-DR2[b]	0.1
HLA DR3/4 heterozygote	25.4
HLA identical sibling of diabetic	44.0
DQB1*0302 genotype[c]	4.2
Identical twin of diabetic	230.0

[a]Population risk of developing type 1 diabetes is 1/400
[b]Protective HLA DR type
[c]Non-aspartate residue at position 57 on DQβ chain (susceptibility allele)

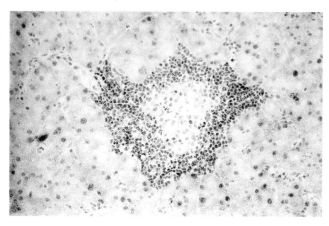

Fig. 13.1 **Insulitis.**
Histological section of a pancreas, demonstrating lymphocytic infiltration in the NOD mouse model of autoimmune diabetes. A similar appearance is seen in human diabetes. (Haematoxylin and eosin; original magnification ×25.)

Pathology

Since the early 1970s, the medical management of ketoacidosis has improved vastly, such that mortality from this complication is extremely rare. In the 1960s, however, post-mortem samples from patients dying at diagnosis of type 1 diabetes were still available for histological analysis. The availability in more recent years of frozen pancreatic tissue from three children dying in ketoacidotic coma at diagnosis of diabetes has enabled histological findings to be extended by the use of monoclonal antibodies to identify specific cell subsets in the inflammatory infiltrate.

Healthy human islets of Langerhans are composed of a core of some 80% β cells, with a mantle of other endocrine cell types, producing glucagon (α cells), somatostatin (δ cells) and pancreatic polypeptide (PP cells) making up the remainder. Histologically, the islets of Langerhans at diagnosis of type 1 diabetes have a mixture of appearances. A proportion are small, completely devoid of β cells and have no inflammatory infiltrate. Others, with numerous intact β cells, are surrounded by a layer of chronic inflammatory cells, with occasional infiltrating cells within the islet. A third group lie somewhere between these extremes, with few β cells remaining and few inflammatory cells. The exocrine pancreas and non-β cells of the islets are unaffected by this infiltrative process, which has been termed **insulitis** (Fig. 13.1).

The cells involved in the insulitis are predominantly lymphocytes. Of these, the most prominent are CD8+ T lymphocytes, though CD4+ T cells, B lymphocytes and macrophages are also found. Many of the cells show evidence of activation, with increased surface expression of HLA class II molecules and the IL-2 receptor on T lymphocytes. Although preliminary evidence suggested class II HLA molecules are aberrantly expressed on the remaining β cells, this finding remains controversial.

Pathogenesis and immunological features

On the basis of the features of the insulitis, several hypotheses regarding the mechanism of β cell death have been proposed. Currently, two of these have centre stage (Fig. 13.2). In the first, the presence of T lymphocytes and selective loss of insulin-producing cells suggests targeting by T cell receptors of a β cell-specific autoantigen. The predominance of CD8+ T lymphocytes in the insulitis supports the proposal that β cells may be damaged in a cell-mediated cytotoxic reaction. However, it is clear from animal models of type 1 diabetes that to transfer the disease from a diabetic to a naive (virgin) recipient requires both CD4+ and CD8+ T cells. It, therefore, seems likely that a recognition event involving CD4+ T lymphocytes is needed. Since this would require presentation of autoantigens by class II HLA molecules, it is in keeping with the strong association between type 1 diabetes and class II HLA genes.

The alternative model proposes that the inflammatory process within the islet is not directed specifically against a β cell target. The insulitis could be initiated by a viral infection, for example, which results in the production of cytokines. Some of these, such as IL-1, are cytotoxic, and in vitro studies suggest that the β cell is exquisitely sensitive to its toxic effects (see p. 130). There is also support for this proposal from animal models of type 1 diabetes, in which macrophages, which secrete IL-1, are the first cells to be seen in numbers in the islet. In the same models, if macrophage function is inhibited, by treatment with silica for example, diabetes does not develop.

Because of the inaccessibility of the target organ in humans, the major immunological features of type 1 diabetes have been sought in the peripheral blood, with studies centring on the identification of autoantibodies and T cell reactions. In general, the autoantibodies (Table 13.2) seem of greatest relevance in the diagnosis and prediction of the disease. The inability to transfer the disease to animals using serum from diabetic

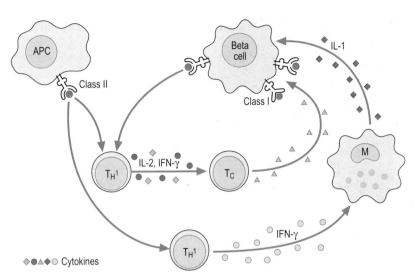

Fig. 13.2 **Possible mechanisms of immune damage to the islet β cells in type 1 diabetes.**
Beta cell autoantigens presented by class II MHC molecules on APCs or possibly by
the β cell itself, stimulate CD4$^+$ T helper cells. T$_H$1 cells release IL-2 and IFN-γ to
induce CD8$^+$ cytotoxic T cells, which damage β cells following identification of
autoantigens presented by class I molecules. IFN-γ may also induce macrophage
release of IL-1 leading to β cell damage.

Table 13.2 **Principal autoantibodies found at diagnosis of type 1 diabetes**

Autoantibody	Antigen	Beta cell specific?	Prevalence at diagnosis (%)	Role in disease
Islet cell antibody (ICA)	Unknown	No	75	Prediction in at-risk groups
Islet cell surface antibody	Unknown	Possibly	40	To be defined
Insulin autoantibody (IAA)	Insulin	Yes	40	Prediction in at-risk groups
Anti-glutamic acid decarboxylase (GAD) antibody	Glutamic acid decarboxylase	No	75–80	Prediction in at-risk groups
Anti-phogrin and anti-IA-2 antibodies	Related tyrosine phosphatases	No (CNS)	75–80	Prediction in at-risk groups

patients, the lack of β cell specificity in some of the
autoantibodies described and the lack of β cell dysfunction in babies born to diabetic mothers (when placental
transfer of IgG class autoantibodies can occur) has
meant that autoantibodies are largely discounted as
having a major role in the pathogenesis of the disease
(Table 13.3). One thing that studying the autoantibodies has told us is that type 1 diabetes has a long,
asymptomatic prodromal period. This is suggested by
the fact that in many cases islet-specific autoantibodies,
as indicators of ongoing β cell damage, are present for
several years before hyperglycaemia is apparent.

In several of the organ-specific autoimmune diseases, autoantibodies were first described using indirect
immunofluorescence techniques (see p. 168). Using
sections of human pancreas, an autoantibody binding
to the islet cell cytoplasm (**islet cell antibody**, ICA) is
detectable in some 75% of patients at diagnosis (Table
13.3, Fig. 13.3). ICA is the best studied autoantibody
in diabetes and binds to all islet cell types (α, β, γ
and PP cells) although its molecular target remains
unknown. **Insulin autoantibodies** (IAA) are defined
as those appearing before treatment with insulin (not
to be confused with insulin antibodies which appear

Table 13.3 **Criteria for deciding whether autoantibodies may be pathogenic in the organ-specific autoimmune disorders**

Criterion	Indicates pathogenic role	Against pathogenic role
Nature of autoantigen/antibody	Autoantigen exposed and accessible on cell surface; only found on target cells	Autoantigen cytosolic and inaccessible to antibody; found in cells not affected by disease
Prevalence of autoantibody	Only found in patients with disease; found in all patients with disease; titres relate to disease activity	Found in healthy individuals
Animal transfer	Serum from patients passively transfers disease to recipient animal	No passive transfer
Placental transfer	Fetus or baby affected by disease associated with autoantibody	Fetus or baby not affected

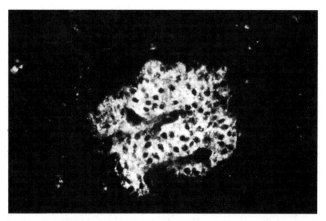

Fig. 13.3 Detection of islet cell antibody by indirect immunofluorescence on a section of normal human pancreas using serum from a patient with type 1 diabetes.
Note cytoplasmic fluorescence in all islet cells. (Original magnification ×40.)

after treatment with insulin). They are present at low titre and are best detected by sensitive radioimmunoassays (see box: 'Antibody-based assays'), with a prevalence of 40% in patients tested at diagnosis. Antibodies directed against components of the islet cell surface (**islet cell surface antibodies**) have been identified using intact islet cells of several species, including humans, but their role in the disease is unclear as yet.

An autoantibody recently identified binds the enzyme **glutamic acid decarboxylase** (GAD) (see box: 'Identification of GAD as an autoantigen: serendipity in medical research'), which catalyses the conversion of glutamic acid to the neurotransmitter gamma-aminobutyric acid (GABA). GABA is probably involved in controlling the release of insulin from secretory granules and GAD is present in the cytoplasm of the human

---

Antibody-based assays

The antibody has become the scientist's 'flexible friend'! For example, antibodies raised against hormones, serum proteins, cell constituents, cytokines, or even immunoglobulins themselves, allow these parameters to be measured in immunoassays.

Radioimmunoassay (RIA)

Radioimmunassays are widely used for the detection of molecules (often termed analytes) in the circulation. The principle relies upon the availability of an antibody that specifically recognises the analyte (Fig. 13.4). In a common design (the so-called competitive assay) a fixed amount of antibody is added and competes for analyte, either in the sample or added to the sample in a radiolabelled form (e.g. bound to ^{125}I). Analyte–antibody complexes form and are precipitated by physicochemical means. The radioactivity in the precipitate is then measured. High levels of radioactivity reflect a low concentration of analyte in the serum sample; low radioactive counts indicate a high level of analyte.

Enzyme-linked immunosorbent assay (ELISA)

The ELISA relies upon a 'capture' antibody fixed to a plastic plate (see Fig. 13.4b). This immobilises analyte in the sample. A second antibody, recognising a different part of the analyte molecule, is then added. This second, 'revealing' antibody has been linked to an enzyme. Now the substrate for the enzyme can be added, and a coloured product is generated that can be quantified photometrically. The intensity of the colour is proportional to the amount of revealing antibody bound in the assay, which itself depends on the concentration of analyte.

(a)

Serum sample containing unknown amount of analyte ×

Analyte labelled radioactively

Fixed quantity of antibody

Mix and precipitate complexes

Low serum levels of analyte

High serum levels of analyte

Precipitate contains high counts

Precipitate contains low counts

(b)

Low level of analyte

High level of analyte

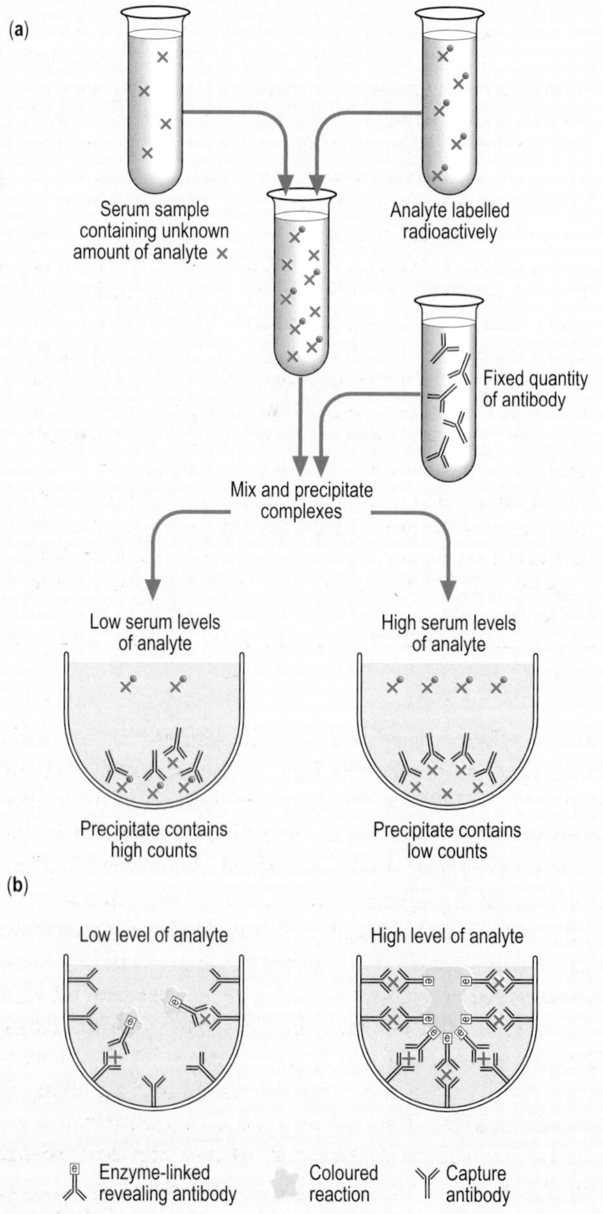

Fig. 13.4 Antibody-based assays.
(**a**) Radioimmunoassay (RIA). (**b**) Enzyme-linked immunosorbent assay (ELISA).

Enzyme-linked revealing antibody

Coloured reaction

Capture antibody

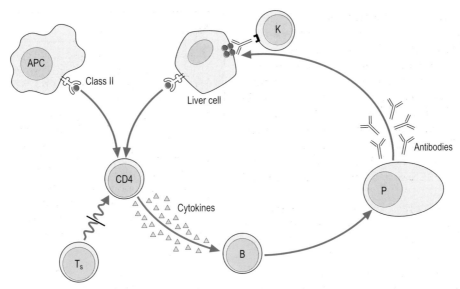

Fig. 14.3 Model of immune attack on the liver cell in autoimmune hepatitis.
A normal component of the liver cell — possibly the ASGPR — is presented to CD4 T lymphocytes either directly or by an APC in the context of class II HLA antigens. Impaired T suppressor lymphocytes permit the CD4 lymphocyte to direct autoantibody production by B lymphocytes with engagement of Fc-receptor expressing killer (K) lymphocytes.

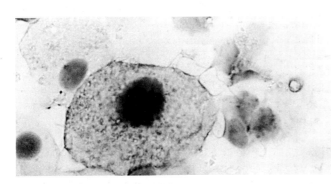

Fig. 14.4 Direct immunoperoxidase staining of a hepatocyte isolated from a patient with AIH with anti-HLA class II antibody.
The positive peripheral staining indicates that HLA class II molecules — absent from the hepatocytes of healthy individuals — are present on the membrane of the cells of this patient enabling them to present autoantigens to the immune system.

- hepatocytes from patients with active AIH express class II HLA antigens (Fig. 14.4), not normally expressed on liver cells and can, therefore, present autoantigenic peptides
- CD4⁺ and activated lymphocytes are present in areas of piecemeal necrosis
- liver-specific autoantibodies are present in the circulation of these patients in high titres and coat their liver cells, which then become susceptible to damage by killer lymphocytes
- T suppressor cell number and function are impaired.

Clinical features

The onset of disease tends to be insidious in most cases, although the presentation may be that of an acute, even fulminant, hepatitis. Fatigue, jaundice,

malaise, anorexia and low grade fever are common. At times, the disease presents with the complications of cirrhosis, including ascites, bleeding from oesophageal varices, encephalopathy or coagulopathy. The course is variable, but the disease is usually controlled by a life-long treatment with immunosuppressive drugs. Alterations of liver function tests do not necessarily reflect the extent of the histological lesion. An increase of aspartate aminotransferase (AST) is common, as is an elevation of globulins and in particular of IgG with values frequently exceeding 20 g/l (normal upper limit 15 g/l). Diagnostic autoantibodies (ANA, SMA, LKM-1) are present at titres of ≥1/40 in adults (Fig. 14.5). The condition is treated with a combination of cortico-steroids and azathioprine, the dosages of which are guided by the levels of AST.

Autoimmune hepatitis

- Two forms of the disease are defined by the presence of anti-smooth-muscle and/or antinuclear antibody (type I AIH) or by the presence of anti-liver/kidney microsomal antibody (type II).
- Class II HLA genes confer susceptibility to the disease.
- Asialoglycoprotein receptor, a transmembrane protein exclusively found on the liver cell membrane, is the likely target of the immune attack.
- Autoimmune hepatitis is characterised by the histological picture of chronic aggressive hepatitis.
- Hepatocytes are coated with IgG in vivo probably produced under the direction of autoantigen-specific CD4⁺ lymphocytes.

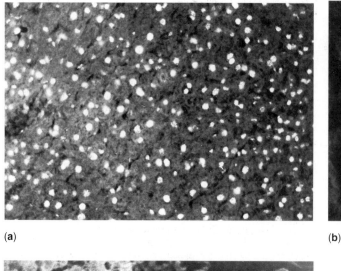

(a)

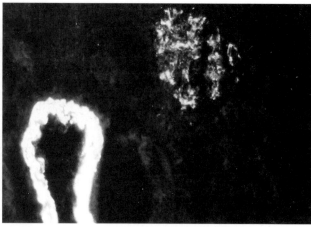

(b)

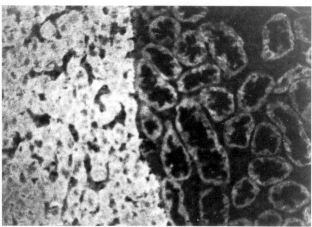

(c)

Fig. 14.5 **Indirect immunofluorescence pattern of ANA, SMA and LKM-1 autoantibodies.**
This is of diagnostic value in AIH. (**a**) ANA stains the nuclei of hepatocytes homogeneously. (**b**) SMA stains the smooth muscle structures contained in the wall of a renal artery. Frequently the glomeruli are also stained by SMA. (**c**) LKM-1 reacts with renal tubules, mainly proximal, and the cytoplasm of hepatocytes. (Substrate: rat liver and kidney, original magnification ×40)

AUTOIMMUNE SCLEROSING CHOLANGITIS

Autoimmune sclerosing cholangitis (ASC) is a rare disorder of unknown aetiology, characterised by chronic inflammation and fibrosis leading to narrowing and dilatation of the intrahepatic or extrahepatic bile ducts, or both. The condition is associated in the majority of cases with chronic inflammatory bowel disease, particularly ulcerative colitis.

Patients are normally children or young adults and may present with clinical, biochemical, immunological and histological features indistinguishable from those of type I autoimmune hepatitis and can, therefore, be erroneously diagnosed. In both conditions, there is an increase in the levels of IgG and circulating non-organ-specific autoantibodies, in particular ANA, SMA and peri-nuclear anti-neutrophil cytoplasmic antibody (pANCA; see p. 229). Histological features common to both conditions are a portal tract infiltrate and peri-portal hepatitis. In some cases, the correct diagnosis can be made only by demonstrating the characteristic bile duct abnormalities by endoscopic retrograde cholangio-pancreatography (ERCP) (Fig. 14.6).

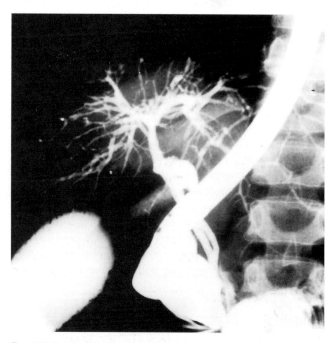

Fig. 14.6 **Endoscopic retrograde cholangiopancreatographic picture showing the bile duct alterations (narrowing, dilatations and beading) of sclerosing cholangitis.**

Pathogenesis

Akin to AIH, liver-specific autoantibodies, including antibodies to LSP and ASGPR are found in the autoimmune form of sclerosing cholangitis (Table 14.1). Autologous microcytotoxicity assays have shown that also in ASC liver cell damage is likely to be mediated by an antibody-dependent cell-mediated mechanism. In contrast to AIH, T suppressor cell number and non-antigen-specific suppressor function tend to be normal in patients with ASC. It appears, therefore, that although liver-damaging effector mechanisms are similar in the two conditions, there are differences in the behaviour of the immunomodulatory cells.

Clinical features

The course and management of this condition are similar to those of AIH.

Autoimmune sclerosing cholangitis

- Rare disorder characterised by chronic inflammation and fibrosis.
- Often associated with chronic inflammatory bowel disease.
- Indistinguishable from type I autoimmune hepatitis unless endoscopic retrograde cholangiopancreatography is performed.

PRIMARY BILIARY CIRRHOSIS

Primary biliary cirrhosis (PBC) is a chronic liver disease of unknown aetiology characterised by slowly progressive intrahepatic cholestasis caused by an inflammatory destruction of small intrahepatic bile ducts. It is 10 times more common in women than in men and is most common in women over the age of 50. The clinical course of PBC is variable ranging from a few years, in rapidly progressive cases, to a normal life-expectancy in a proportion of asymptomatic cases. It has long been recognised that the disease is characterised by the presence of high-titre antimitochondrial antibodies (AMA) in over 90% of the patients (Fig. 14.7) and elevated serum IgM (Table 14.1). This, in addition to the observation that these patients often have associated autoimmune disorders (rheumatoid arthritis, sicca syndrome, thyroiditis, scleroderma), has led to the concept that PBC is an autoimmune disease. The predisposing role of the HLA system to the disease has not been fully clarified, although an association with HLA-DR8 has been reported.

Pathology

The histological picture is characterised by lymphocyte infiltration and destruction of small and medium size bile ducts, ductular proliferation, periductular granu-

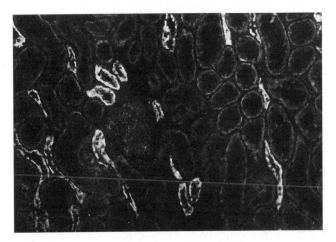

Fig. 14.7 **Indirect immunofluorescence pattern of AMA.** Note the staining of the distal tubules (smaller than the proximal), which are particularly rich in mitochondria. (Substrate: rat kidney)

lomas, fibrosis and ultimately cirrhosis. The histological alterations are frequently patchy and for this reason the result of a liver biopsy is considered consistent with, rather than diagnostic of, PBC.

Pathogenesis

Several types of **antimitochondrial autoantibodies** (AMA) have been described in PBC including M2, M4, M8 and M9. The AMA which serves as the diagnostic marker for PBC, is the subtype anti-M2, while anti-M4, anti-M8 and anti-M9 have been proposed as markers for particular subsets or stages of PBC. For example, anti-M4 (with anti-M2) would identify an autoimmune hepatitis–PBC overlap syndrome, and anti-M9 cases with a benign clinical course. In a recent workshop, however, in which the diagnostic ability of different AMAs was evaluated critically, it became clear that only AMA-M2 maintains its undeniable diagnostic power. The identification of the molecular targets of AMA-M2 is well under way (see box: 'Mitochondrial autoantigens') and their use for classification and staging of PBC is in progress.

The few available histochemical studies agree that in PBC T lymphocytes in the portal lymphoid infiltrates greatly outnumber other lymphoid cells, and these T cells exhibit markers of activation. CD4 helper T cells predominate overall but are localised more in the portal infiltrates, whereas the T cells around and in the walls of bile ducts, which may be the actual effectors, are of the cytotoxic (CD8$^+$) phenotype. Immunohistochemistry has also been applied to the identification of HLA-encoded molecules on hepatocytes and bile duct cells, since this may give clues to the pathogenesis. Bile duct epithelium normally expresses HLA class I molecules; in PBC, HLA class II molecules also become expressed on biliary epithelial cells, presumably under the influence of lymphokines, including INF-γ. Bile duct damage may derive from different effector mechanisms. Given that HLA class I molecules are constitutively expressed on biliary epithelial cells and that CD8$^+$ T cells are identifiable histochemically at sites of damage,

Mitochondrial autoantigens

Gel electrophoresis and Western blotting, using human mitochondrial preparations, disclosed that anti-M2 sera react with up to six polypeptides of molecular weights ranging from 74 to 36 kDa. The M2 autoantigens have been identified as components of the mitochondrial multienzymatic complex comprising pyruvate dehydrogenase (PDH), branched chain 2-oxacid dehydrogenase and 2-oxo-glutarate dehydrogenase. Each of these enzymes has three subunits, E1 to E3. For PDH, an autoepitope has been identified as a decapeptide containing the attachment site of lipoic acid, an essential co-factor for enzyme activity. Current questions include the degree to which antibodies to PDH, and related enzymes, account for the mitochondrial reactivity defined by immunofluorescence, the cell-surface expression of M2 autoantigens, and the significance of the occurrence of non-mitochondrial (such as anti-centromere) autoantibodies in PBC. The reasons for the localisation of the lesions of PBC to intrahepatic biliary ductules is unclear since mitochondrial auto-antigens are not tissue specific. Based on available evidence the following suggestions have been proposed to explain hepatobiliary localisation of the injury: (1) there are allelic forms of PDH specific to the hepatobiliary cells, (2) bile favours penetrance of immune effector agents such as antibodies or T cells, and (3) the biliary tract is colonised by a microorganism displaying epitopes, cross-reactive with human dehydrogenase enzymes.

Man or mouse?

Severe combined immunodeficiency disease (SCID) mice have a defect in a recombinase necessary for the generation of antigen receptors on T and B cells; and as a result, they lack mature B and T cells. These mice can be repopulated with human lymphocytes, to give SCID-hu mice. The lymphocytes not only survive in this adoptive host but are even able to function. Gershwin and collaborators transferred human peripheral blood lymphocytes from patients with PBC to SCID mice. By 8 weeks after the injection of up to 40 million cells, human lymphocytes were detected in the spleen and human IgG was present in the serum of these mice. Moreover the serum contained human AMA. Histologically, a human mononuclear cell infiltrate was present in the portal areas of the liver and inflammation, bile duct atypia and necrosis of bile duct cells were observed. This evidence suggests a role for lymphocytes in causing tissue damage in PBC.

a cytotoxic T-cell response to a mitochondrial peptide, associated with a class I HLA molecule, on the biliary epithelial surface is one possibility. An alternative (or co-existing) process would be an induction of CD4+ helper T lymphocytes, with release by activated cells of lymphokines with tissue-damaging potential (see box: 'Man or mouse').

Clinical features

PBC is often asymptomatic, the earliest symptom usually being pruritus. Jaundice, darkening of the skin in exposed areas and manifestations resulting from impaired bile excretion follow. The latter range from steatorrhoea to impaired absorption of lipid-soluble vitamins, leading to osteomalacia (from vitamin D malabsorption), bruising (vitamin K) and occasionally night blindness (vitamin A). Elevation of serum lipids leads to the formation of xanthelasmata and xanthomata (lipid accumulation under the eyes and over joints/tendons, respectively). Whilst the physical examination can be rather unremarkable, laboratory investigations tend to be informative. Alkaline phosphatase is elevated early in the course of the disease, and AMA at a titre >1:40 is present in over 90% of patients. Serum bilirubin rises over time, an increase in AST levels is frequently seen but it is never dramatic, hyperlipidaemia is common.

Treatment

No treatment is able to alter the natural history of the disease: corticosteroids are contraindicated and the claims for D-penicillamine, colchicine and azathioprine in slowing the progression of the disease remain unsubstantiated. Trials are currently under way with cyclosporin, ursodeoxycholic acid, chlorambucil and methotrexate. The symptomatic treatment is directed at alleviating pruritus, steatorrhoea and at replacing fat-soluble vitamins. End stage disease is treated with liver transplantation.

Primary biliary cirrhosis

- Antimitochondrial antibody is present in over 90% of patients.
- A multienzymatic complex comprising pyruvate dehydrogenase, branched chain 2-oxacid dehydrogenase and 2-oxoglutarate dehydrogenase contains the target antigens of antimitochondrial (M2) antibody.
- Serum IgM is typically elevated.
- Bile ducts are infiltrated by lymphocytes and destroyed.

VIRAL HEPATITIS

This section will deal with the immunological aspects of viral hepatitis; the virological and clinical features are comprehensively discussed in other texts. The list of hepatitis viruses grows steadily and currently extends from A to G. We will concentrate on those types of viral hepatitis in which the immune system is thought to cause or contribute to the liver damage.

HEPATITIS B

The liver damage caused by the hepatitis B virus (HBV) (Fig. 14.8) varies greatly in severity: it can be mild and transient, severe and prolonged, or fulminant. The mechanisms responsible for determining the course and outcome of hepatitis B are not known. However, many investigations have suggested that HBV is not directly cytopathic, but that liver damage derives from the host immune response to the virus-infected hepatocytes. A normal immune response would lead to self-limiting acute hepatitis, an impaired immune response to chronic hepatitis, and a hyperactive response to fulminant hepatic failure. During viral infections, T lymphocytes recognise viral antigens on the surface of the infected cell in association with HLA molecules. Following infection of the liver cell, viral peptides can bind to HLA class I molecules, which carry the viral antigens to the cell surface where the complex becomes a target for CD8+ cytotoxic T lymphocytes.

It is not clear why certain patients progress to chronic infection while others clear HBV after acute infection (see box: 'Elimination of HBV in acute hepatitis'). That is, why do some individuals get chronic and others acute hepatitis? Probably a combination of host, infective agent and environmental factors determine the outcome of the infection, but there are several clear possibilities that, acting in isolation or in combination, may explain the persistence of HBV infection.

- HLA molecules or viral determinants on the infected cells may be 'hidden' by an excessive production of antiviral antibody and escape immune clearance.
- Lymphocytes infected and functionally impaired by the HBV may be unable to mount a normal immune response.
- A genetic or acquired deficiency in IFN production may lead to impaired display of hepatocyte surface HLA class I molecules and reduced presentation of viral peptides to the immune system.
- HBsAg-specific T suppressor cells may play a role in the maintenance of non-responsiveness to HBsAg in chronic HBV carriers.
- Viral replication and viral antigen production may occur by a change in transcription and translation of the viral genes. This mechanism underlies persistence of viruses that produce defective interfering particles or generate a great number of mutants.

In chronic hepatitis B, defective viral particles are produced in great numbers, and recent data indicate that spontaneous mutations in the genome are associated

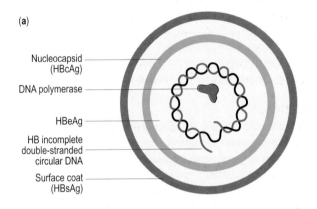

(a)

Nucleocapsid (HBcAg)

DNA polymerase

HBeAg

HB incomplete double-stranded circular DNA

Surface coat (HBsAg)

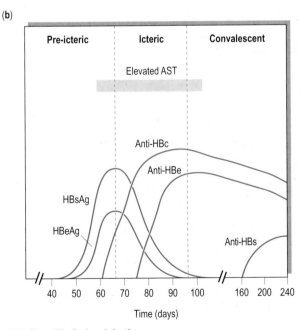

(b)

| Pre-icteric | Icteric | Convalescent |

Elevated AST

Anti-HBc

Anti-HBe

HBsAg

HBeAg

Anti-HBs

Time (days)

Fig. 14.8 Hepatitis B virus infection.
(a) The constituents of the hepatitis B virion. This DNA virus is composed of a surface coat and of a core. Other key components are DNA and DNA polymerase. (b) The dynamics of HBV serological markers during acute hepatitis. Serum hepatitis B surface antigen (HBsAg) and hepatitis e antigen (HBeAg) precede jaundice and AST increase. Antibodies against core (anti-HBc) are the first to appear, belonging to the IgM class first and then the IgG. Anti-HBe appears later followed by production of anti-HBs. This last is deemed to be protective and is a marker of acquired immune status.

Elimination of HBV in acute hepatitis

Recently, HLA class I restricted cytotoxic T cells reacting with the amino-terminal end of the hepatitis B virus core molecule have been demonstrated in the peripheral blood of patients with acute hepatitis B. CD4+ lymphocytes also play a key role in virus elimination by recognising viral antigens, ingested and processed by APCs and expressed on the APC surface within the groove of HLA class II molecules. HLA class II-restricted CD4+ T lymphocytes recognising an immunodominant 20 amino acid sequence located within the amino-terminal part of the core molecule have been identified in the peripheral blood of patients with self-limiting acute hepatitis B. Moreover, CD4+ lymphocytes, obtained from liver biopsies and cloned in vitro, are capable of providing help to B cells for anti-HBc production. It is conceivable that the virus-specific CD4+ and CD8+ cell responses just described act in concert in the elimination of HBV during acute hepatitis B.

with the development of particularly aggressive forms of chronic hepatitis or fulminant hepatic failure.

HEPATITIS A

The liver damage in acute hepatitis A has long been thought to derive from a direct cytopathic effect of the virus. However, it is now believed that a T cell-mediated immune attack on virus-infected cells plays a major additional pathogenic role, similar to that in hepatitis B. Infection with hepatitis A virus (HAV), however, does not become chronic, suggesting that the interaction between virus and host is different from that observed in HBV infection, and that the immune system is generally very efficient in eliminating HAV.

HEPATITIS C

Like hepatitis B, hepatitis caused by the C virus (HCV) can be acute and self-limiting or progress to chronic liver damage. The mechanisms leading to hepatocyte injury remain to be elucidated. There is great interest in findings suggesting a connection between HCV and autoimmune hepatitis. LKM-1 — the diagnostic marker of AIH type II — has been found in the serum of several patients chronically infected with HCV; this has led to the proposal that the virus is the trigger of 'autoimmune hepatitis'. The additional finding that HCV and the target of LKM-1 (the cytochrome P4502D6) share a sequence in common, appeared to sanction beyond doubt a link between virus and autoimmune disease, the autoimmune response being triggered through molecular mimicry. The enthusiasm generated by the above observations was tempered by the finding that no sign of infection with HCV is present in patients suffering from the classical AIH type II. In summary, it appears that a proportion of patients with HCV infection develop LKM-1; but LKM-1 is present, without signs of HCV infection, in most patients with type II AIH.

Viral hepatitis

- Liver damage may result from host immune responses to virus-infected hepatocytes.
- Defective interfering particles (HBV) or frequent mutation (HCV) may allow persistence of infection and lead to aggressive hepatitis.
- HAV infection is eliminated by the immune system and does not become chronic.
- HCV may trigger autoimmune reactions.

DRUG-INDUCED HEPATITIS

Probably the best documented example of drug-induced liver damage with an immune pathogenesis is severe hepatitis after halothane exposure.

Halothane-induced hepatitis

The spectrum of liver damage that may follow halothane exposure varies from minor increases in concentration of serum AST to the rarer instances of fulminant hepatic failure. It is not clear whether they represent two different forms of liver damage or extreme ends of a spectrum.

The severe form of halothane hepatitis is very uncommon and more frequent in patients exposed to halothane on more than one occasion. Many of the clinical and serological features of patients who develop halothane hepatitis suggest that the severe form of liver damage is an immune-mediated adverse reaction. The disease is rare, affects mainly females and is often associated with features of immunological disturbance, such as circulating immune complexes, peripheral eosinophilia and non-organ-specific autoantibodies (particularly anti-LKM). Studies have shown that such patients also have a high incidence of antibodies to both normal liver components and, specifically, to halothane-related antigens. These antigens, which have not yet been fully defined, are associated with metabolism of halothane by the oxidative route and occur in both laboratory animals and in humans. It remains to be established whether these halothane antibodies are involved in the pathogenesis of halothane hepatitis. In vitro studies showing that lymphocytes from patients with severe halothane hepatitis are cytotoxic to hepatocytes prepared from rabbits following halothane anaesthesia, but not to hepatocytes from normal rabbits, and that halothane antibody-coated liver cells become susceptible to damage by lymphocytes prepared from normal individuals, suggest that these antibodies are likely to be involved in the pathogenesis of the disease.

Gastrointestinal diseases

The gastrointestinal tract presents a number of immunologically perplexing conditions. These range from **food intolerance**, in which immune mechanisms account for only a small fraction of the disorders gathered under that label, to **coeliac disease** in which there is equal support for both toxic and immune pathogenesis models. The exception may be **pernicious anaemia**, which is considered a typical organ-specific autoimmune disease. This chapter also deals with **ulcerative colitis** and **Crohn's disease**, which are collectively referred to as **inflammatory bowel disease**. This tendency to constrain under a single name what are two distinct diseases gives a hint to the uncertainty as to whether they are different manifestations of the same disease or different diseases sharing similar pathogeneses and clinical manifestations.

THE MUCOSAL IMMUNE SYSTEM OF THE GASTROINTESTINAL TRACT

There are two major factors at play when considering the lymphoid system of the gastrointestinal tract as distinctive. The first is functional, the second anatomical. Antigens ingested orally tend to elicit qualitatively different immune responses to antigens arriving by other routes. Most strikingly, mucosal tissues are associated with high levels of production of IgA, the major externally secreted immunoglobulin. There is also a tendency for antigens administered orally to induce tolerance rather than active immune responses. This may be an important protective mechanism: many foreign animal and vegetable proteins will be encountered in the gut, along with antigens deriving from colonising bacteria, and it would be dangerous to the host to mount massive immune responses to these. The distinctive anatomy of the lymphoid system of the gastrointestinal tract is revealed by histological analysis, which shows lymphocytes scattered in the lamina propria, in Peyer's patches (p. 6), and also within the epithelial layer of the luminal surface (Fig. 15.1).

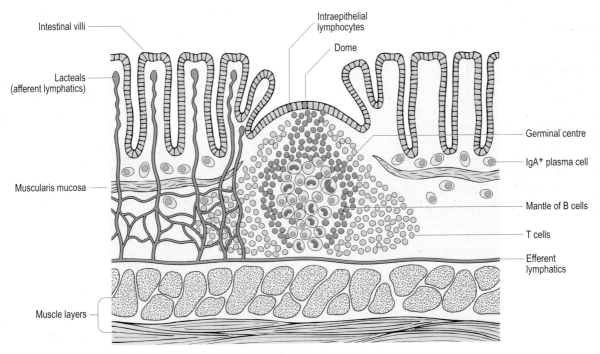

Fig. 15.1 **Anatomical structure of the mucosal lymphoid tissue found in the gut.**
Note the presence of intraepithelial T and B lymphocytes abutting the mucosal surface, the high density of plasma cells, particularly IgA$^+$ ones, the open, unencapsulated architecture of the Peyer's patch lymphoid follicle, and the rich draining lymphatics.

Peyer's patches are collections of lymphoid tissue organised into follicles similar to those found in other lymphoid sites but lacking a capsule or afferent lymphatics. One other difference is that the germinal centre B lymphocytes are more frequently surface IgA-positive, indicating a preferential maturation/migration at this site. Lamina propria lymphocytes are mainly CD4$^+$ T lymphocytes, and frequently bear markers of activation (CD25, HLA-DR). Many B cells and plasma cells are also found at this site. The intra-epithelial lymphocytes are predominantly T cells, and are better characterised in mice than in man. In mice, up to half of the T cells bear the more unconventional γδ TCR (p. 49), but in man the figure is more like 10% although still higher than the peripheral blood. The diversity of TCR chain usage in the intraepithelial T cells appears less than in other sites, and it has been speculated that the gut could be a site of extra-thymic T cell maturation.

PERNICIOUS ANAEMIA

Pernicious anaemia is a megaloblastic anaemia caused by a deficiency of vitamin B_{12} resulting from mal-absorption, thought to be due to autoimmune reactions to gastric parietal cells and their products. Impaired absorption is the result of defective **intrinsic factor** (IF) secretion, which in turn results from atrophy of the gastric mucosa. Vitamin B_{12}, with a minimum daily requirement of 2.5 μg, derives from animal products only. It combines in the duodenum with intrinsic factor, a glycoprotein of 50 kDa produced in the gastric parietal cells of the stomach. In this complexed form it is absorbed in the distal ileum. Were absorption to cease abruptly, 3–6 years would be required for a normal individual to become deficient. The long time over which the condition develops, therefore, helps explain why the severe anaemia that results is singularly well tolerated.

Pernicious anaemia is the most common form of vitamin B_{12} deficiency in temperate climates; it affects both sexes equally, is more common in individuals of northern European descent and is rare under the age of 30, the average presenting age being 60 years.

It shows family clustering and is frequently associated with other organ-specific autoimmune diseases, such as Graves' disease, myxoedema, Addison's disease (idiopathic adrenocortical insufficiency), vitiligo and hypoparathyroidism. Pernicious anaemia is also frequently present in patients with common variable immunodeficiency. A genetic predisposition, indicated by familial occurrence of the disease, is not accounted for by *HLA* genes, since the reported associations are weak and inconstant.

Pathology

The most characteristic abnormality in pernicious anaemia is gastric atrophy affecting the acid- and pepsin-secreting portion of the stomach; the antrum is unaffected.

Pathogenesis

A variety of immunological abnormalities are seen in pernicious anaemia, some of which indicate an immune pathogenesis for the disease. **Gastric parietal cell antibody** is detected, using an indirect immunofluorescence assay, in virtually all patients, in 20–30% of first-degree relatives and in 5% of the normal population. This antibody stains in the cytoplasm of gastric parietal cells (Fig. 15.2) targeting antigens in the secretory canaliculi, which are the intracellular channels carrying hydrochloric acid into the gastric lumen (Fig. 15.3). A major target of this antibody has been identified as the β subunit of the gastric proton pump (H$^+$, K$^+$, ATPase), an enzyme composed of two transmembrane components, the α and β subunits. Auto-epitopes may also be present on the α subunit. The pathogenicity of antigastric parietal cell antibody is unresolved, since it is unclear how readily accessible the proton pump is to circulating antibodies.

A different type of autoantibody has been described directed against a gastric parietal cell surface component, but the nature of the antigen remains to be elucidated. The ability of this antibody to induce complement-mediated cytotoxicity suggests a role in parietal cell destruction. In addition, there are at least two types of antibody against intrinsic factor: **blocking** and **binding** antibodies (Fig. 15.4); the blocking type reacts with the combining site for vitamin B_{12} on IF and is found in most patients (over 70%), while the binding antibody reacts with other epitopes on IF (whether this is free or complexed to vitamin B_{12}) and is present in some 60% of patients. Both inhibit absorption of vitamin B_{12} and are more frequently found in gastric juices than in serum, although they are more conveniently measured in serum. The decline of antigastric parietal cell antibody titres with the loss of gastric parietal cells has suggested that this immune response is antigen

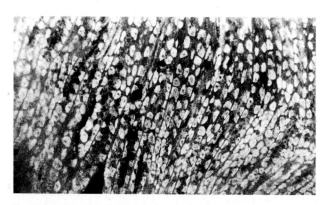

Fig. 15.2 **Indirect immunofluorescence pattern of antigastric parietal cell antibody.**
The staining in parietal cells is intracytoplasmic. This reflects the intracellular distribution of canaliculi containing the gastric proton pump. (Rat stomach, ×400.)

(a)

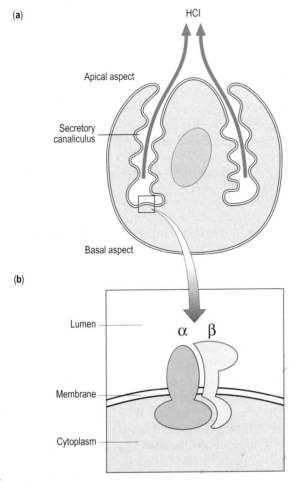

Fig. 15.3 Gastric parietal cells.
(**a**) Stimulated gastric parietal cell displaying the secretory canaliculus. (**b**) Within this structure resides the gastric proton pump whose β and possibly α subunits contain the targets of antigastric parietal cell antibody.

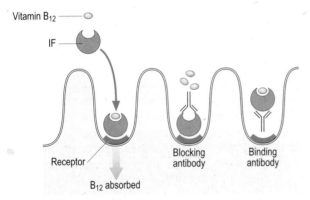

Fig. 15.4 Absorption of vitamin B$_{12}$.
Vitamin B$_{12}$ binds to intrinsic factor (IF) and is absorbed after binding to a receptor in the ileal mucosa. Anti-IF **blocking** antibody prevents vitamin B$_{12}$ from binding to IF, whilst the **binding** type prevents vitamin B$_{12}$–IF complex from binding to its receptor. Both prevent vitamin B$_{12}$ absorption.

driven and T cell dependent. The nature and specificity of T cell responses, however, remain to be clarified.

The observations that (1) antigastric parietal cell antibodies can be found in normal individuals, and (2) anti-IF antibodies are present in the unaffected rela-

tives of patients, both suggest that the disease may not be antibody mediated. On balance, however, the evidence for a role of the immune system in the pathogenesis of pernicious anaemia is stronger than that against it.

Clinical features

The main symptoms of pernicious anaemia are those of severe anaemia. The patient is pale and slightly jaundiced, reflecting an increase in indirect bilirubin resulting from ineffective erythropoiesis. Gastrointestinal manifestations are the results of vitamin B$_{12}$ deficiency acting on the rapidly proliferating gastrointestinal epithelium; a typical example is a sore tongue that on inspection appears as beef red. Neurological manifestations, albeit relatively rare, are serious since they do not fully remit with treatment. Demyelination, followed by axonal degeneration and eventual neuronal death, affects peripheral nerves and the posterior and lateral columns in the spine. Paraesthesiae, numbness and ataxia are the ensuing clinical manifestations.

Laboratory findings

The laboratory findings show macrocytosis (mean corpuscular volume (MCV) greater than 100 fl), and a low reticulocyte count. In the blood film, haemoglobinised macro-ovalocytes are seen, and the neutrophils are typically oversegmented: finding six nuclear lobes is highly suggestive of megaloblastic anaemia. The bone marrow is hypercellular with a decreased myeloid:erythroid ratio and the red cell precursors are abnormally large, with immature nuclei. Measurement of vitamin B$_{12}$ will demonstrate a deficiency and a Schilling test will pinpoint the diagnosis. This test consists of two parts. In the first part, the patient is given radioactive vitamin B$_{12}$ orally and the absorption measured as radioactivity present in the urine of the next 24 hours. This part of the test is abnormal in pernicious anaemia where absorption is impaired. The test returns to normal in the second part when radio-labelled B$_{12}$ is given with intrinsic factor, a manoeuvre that overcomes defective absorption.

Treatment

Vitamin B$_{12}$ replacement therapy corrects all but the neurological abnormalities. Patients with pernicious

Pernicious anaemia

- Pernicious anaemia is a megaloblastic anaemia caused by vitamin B$_{12}$ malabsorption.
- Antigastric parietal cell antibodies are present in virtually all the patients and target the gastric proton pump.
- Blocking and binding antibodies to intrinsic factor prevent absorption of vitamin B$_{12}$. They are of diagnostic importance in pernicious anaemia but are not found in all patients.

anaemia develop gastric polyps very frequently and have an increased incidence of gastric malignancy.

COELIAC DISEASE

Coeliac disease is a disorder of the small intestine characterised by malabsorption, villous atrophy (Fig. 15.5) and intolerance to gluten, a protein found in wheat, barley and oats. It is also called **gluten-induced enteropathy** since the disease improves when treated with a gluten-free diet but relapses if gluten is reintroduced. It is either limited to the intestine or associated with a vesicular skin disease known as **dermatitis herpetiformis**.

The incidence of coeliac disease in siblings is many times higher than in the general population: 3–20% of first-degree relatives are affected by the condition. This strong genetic predisposition is in part accounted for by the association of the disorder with the haplotype *HLA-B8*, *HLA-DR3* or *HLA-DR7*, and by the

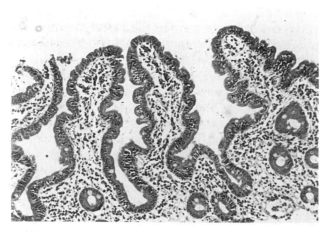

(a)

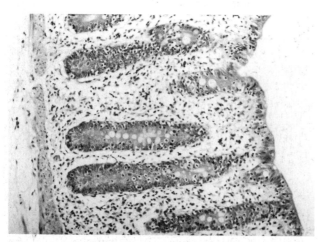

(b)

Fig. 15.5 **Coeliac disease.**
(a) Histology of normal jejunal mucosa. (b) Jejunal mucosa in coeliac disease: note the virtual absence of villi, elongated crypts and mononuclear cell infiltrate. (Courtesy of Dr J. Salisbury.)

even closer association with the *HLA-DQ2* allele (HLA-DQA1*0501, DQB1*0201) (see box: 'HLA-DQα/β heterodimer') (Fig. 15.6). It is possible that a **disease-susceptibility gene** is in linkage disequilibrium with the DR/DQ locus, and that this gene controls an individual's reaction to a gluten antigenic fraction.

The fact that 70% — and not 100% — of monozygotic twins are concordant for coeliac disease implies that non-genetic (environmental) factors are involved in the pathogenesis of the disease. A role for adenovirus serotype 12 (Ad12) has been suggested by the shared sequence between the virus and the gluten-related protein gliadin, and by the much higher frequency of antibodies to Ad12 in untreated patients (90%) when compared with treated patients or normal controls (20%). It has been proposed that infection with adenovirus sensitises the genetically predisposed host to gluten by molecular mimicry.

Pathology

Jejunal biopsy specimens (Fig. 15.5) show the classical lesion characterised by blunting and flattening of the mucosal surface, with villi either absent or broad and short. The crypts are elongated, a sign of a marked increase in epithelial cell turnover, and the lamina propria is infiltrated by a variety of mononuclear cells including plasma cells, CD4$^+$ T lymphocytes, macrophages, mast cells and basophils. IgA plasma cells are increased in number and predominate, but there is also a disproportionate increase in IgG plasma cells. The surface epithelium is altered, with sparse brush border, cuboidal rather than columnar cells and an increase in intraepithelial T lymphocytes. The histological lesions, including the infiltrate, regress with a gluten-free diet.

Pathogenesis

There are two main pathogenetic theories: toxic and immunological. According to the **toxic** theory, patients with coeliac disease lack specific mucosal peptidases. The ingestion of the high-molecular-weight gluten and its related substance gliadin would lead to accumulation of poorly digested toxic peptides within the mucosa. This would damage the absorptive cells, which are shed in the gut lumen, and stimulate cell proliferation, crypt hypertrophy and produce an overall increase in cell turnover. This accelerated cell renewal is halted by a gluten-free diet. A number of enzymatic alterations, including decreased levels of disaccharidases, alkaline phosphatase and peptide hydrolases, have been found in the intestinal mucosa of these patients but disappear with successful treatment. The toxic theory is questioned by the fact that to-date no persistent, primary specific peptidase deficiency has been demonstrated in coeliac disease.

The **immunological** theory rests on the presence of a mononuclear cell infiltrate in the lamina propria, increase in intraepithelial T lymphocytes and evidence in the mucosa and serum of gliadin-specific reactivity.

HLA-DQα/β heterodimer

The strongest predisposition to coeliac disease is conferred by possession of the haplotype *HLA-DR3,DQ2* (DQA1*0501, DQB1*0201). Patients with the disease who are negative for this are frequently heterozygous *HLA-DR7DQ2/DR5DQ7* (DQA1*0501, DQB1*0301). Therefore, as shown in Figure 15.6, the same *DQA1* and *DQB1* genes can be present in individuals with coeliac disease who have different HLA haplotypes. If the patient is *DR3DQ2* positive, *DQA1* and *DQB1* are in the *cis* position while they are *in trans* if the patient is *DR5DQ7/DR7DQ2* heterozygous. Therefore, most patients may express the same HLA-DQα/β heterodimer, *cis*-encoded in *DR3DQ2*-positive individuals and *trans*-encoded in *DR5DQ7/DR7DQ2* heterozygotes (*trans*-complementation). Binding of gliadin peptides to this heterodimer may be crucial to the pathogenesis of coeliac disease.

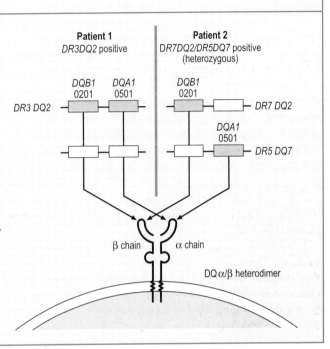

Fig. 15.6 **Expression of the DQα/β heterodimer.**
The DQα/β heterodimer can be encoded by the haplotype *DR3DQ2* or by the heterozygous *DR7DQ2/DR5DQ7* status.

These patients have antigliadin antibodies in their serum detected by ELISA, mostly belonging to the IgA class. Approximately 60% of the serum IgA antigliadin antibody is dimeric, suggesting its origin is in the intestinal mucosa. Anti-endomysium and antireticulin antibodies, typically belonging to the IgA class, are also found in the majority of coeliac patients (Fig. 15.7) and in those first-degree relatives who — with or without mucosal atrophy — share the same HLA antigens as the patient's, indicating that antireticulin antibody production is under genetic control. These antibodies give a 'reticular' pattern on rodent tissue when examined by indirect immunofluorescence: this corresponds to the pattern of reticulin fibres obtained by silver impregnation. A third autoantibody of diagnostic importance is antiendomysium, which also belongs to the IgA class. The density of intraepithelial lymphocytes is strikingly increased.

About 70% of the T lymphocytes express the memory marker CD45R0, suggesting that they are antigen-primed memory cells. In addition, there is a two-fold to six-fold increase in γ/δ-positive T lymphocytes, negative for both CD4 and CD8 markers. Since γδ T cells are usually cytotoxic it has been suggested that they may be involved in causing damage to the intestinal epithelium. Favourable response to glucocorticosteroids has been used as additional evidence implicating an immune pathogenesis. To-date, however, there is no conclusive proof that immune mechanisms are central to initiation or perpetuation of the disorder.

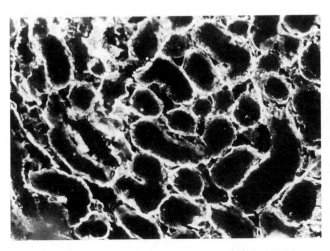

(a)

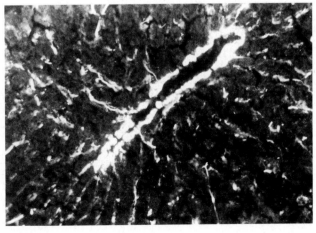

(b)

Fig. 15.7 **Antireticulin antibody detected by indirect immunofluorescence staining of the connective structures of the renal tubules (a) and the portal tract in the liver (b).** (Rat kidney and liver, ×400.)

Clinical features

Most patients with coeliac disease present with the typical picture of a malabsorption syndrome characterised by failure to thrive when gluten is introduced in the diet, weight loss, abdominal distention and bloating, diarrhoea, steatorrhoea and abnormal tests of absorption function. Patients can present, however, with isolated abnormalities: iron-deficiency anaemia or a metabolic bone disease can be the initial features in the absence of overt diarrhoea and steatorrhoea.

In the absence of a specific diagnostic test, the diagnosis rests on:

- evidence of malabsorption,
- typical histological picture of the jejunal mucosa with blunting and flattening of the villi
- clinical and histological improvement on a gluten-free diet.

In ambiguous cases, the patient may be challenged with oral administration of gluten. The diagnosis is settled if this manoeuvre promptly results in diarrhoea and steatorrhoea.

Management and prognosis

Treatment with a gluten-free diet is effective in about 80% of patients, but this may take up to 24 months to work. Patients resistant to this treatment can benefit from treatment with glucocorticosteroids. Although normal health and life expectancy is usually restored by a gluten-free diet, it is of note that coeliac disease is associated with an increased incidence of intestinal carcinoma and lymphoma.

Coeliac disease

- Coeliac disease is a disorder of the small intestine with malabsorption and intolerance to gluten.
- High serum levels of antigliadin, antireticulin and antiendomysium antibodies, all belonging to the IgA class, are present.
- Mononuclear cell infiltrate is seen in the lamina propria.
- The heterodimer HLA-DQB1*0201/DQA1*0501 is present in the vast majority of patients.
- Association is also seen with dermatitis herpetiformis.

INFLAMMATORY BOWEL DISEASE

Inflammatory bowel disease (IBD) may be divided into two major groups:

- ulcerative colitis
- Crohn's disease.

Ulcerative colitis is confined to the colon and affects the mucosal layer only, whilst Crohn's disease may affect any part of the gastrointestinal tract, classically the ileocaecal region, with a transmural inflammation. Clinically these disorders are characterised by recurrent inflammation of intestinal segments with diverse clinical manifestations, often resulting in a chronic, unpredictable course. Although it is usually possible to tell the two conditions apart on the basis of clinical, pathological, radiological and laboratory findings, the two processes appear to share common pathogenetic mechanisms.

Both conditions affect the sexes similarly but are more common in whites than blacks and more frequently seen in Ashkenazi Jews. In most populations, there is no clear association with the genes of the HLA region. Both appear to be more common in industrialised nations, to be steadily rising in their incidence and to share a peak occurrence between 15 and 35 years of age. Family clustering and high concordance in monozygotic twins suggest genetic components for both disorders. A role for an infective agent has not been established, although the atypical mycobacterium *Mycobacterium paratuberculosis* has been incriminated in Crohn's disease, having been isolated from patients after prolonged culture.

Pathology

The inflammatory reaction of **ulcerative colitis** involves principally the colonic mucosa leading to the macroscopic appearance of an ulcerated, hyperaemic, usually haemorrhagic colon. The surface mucosa is destroyed and the submucosa is heavily infiltrated with polymorphonuclear neutrophils. Small crypt abscesses are characteristic, though not specific. Recurrent inflammation leads to chronic lesions characterised by fibrosis, longitudinal retraction, with the attendant loss of haustral pattern radiologically, and formation of pseudopolyps. Dysplasia is also present in long-standing ulcerative colitis.

The earliest pathological manifestations of **Crohn's disease** — a hyperaemic ileum with swollen and reddened mesentery and mesenteric lymph nodes — are not unique to Crohn's disease, being found in other forms of ileitis, most notably that caused by *Yersinia enterocolitica*. Typical alterations such as leathery, stenotic bowel are found as the disease progresses. In contrast to ulcerative colitis, the mucosa can have a normal appearance or, in more advanced cases, assume a cobblestone pattern. Ulcerations penetrate the submucosa and muscularis, resulting in fissures and fistulae.

The inflammatory process is continuous in ulcerative colitis but is frequently discontinuous in Crohn's disease, with skip areas interrupting the affected segments. Granulomas are not found in ulcerative colitis but are present in Crohn's disease, albeit in only 50–60% of the cases.

Pathogenesis

The issues regarding the pathogenesis of inflammatory bowel disease have been exemplified by the following question: does the chronic, recurring inflammatory activity in the disease reflect an appropriate response to a persistently abnormal stimulus (e.g. a structural alteration of the intestine or a causative agent in the environment) or an abnormally prolonged response to a normal stimulus (i.e. an aberrant immune response) (Fig. 15.8).

A number of alterations suggest a pathogenic role for the immune system in ulcerative colitis and Crohn's disease. Changes in the relative proportions of macrophages, T and B lymphocytes, increases in the number of mucosal IgG-bearing cells and IgG production have been described. In addition, deposition of complement components in the mucosa of patients with inflammatory bowel disease has also been demonstrated. An IgG antibody directed against a 40 kDa protein present in both diseased and normal colonic tissue has been eluted from the tissue of patients with ulcerative colitis.

Inappropriate expression of MHC class II antigens has been found on intestinal epithelial cells of patients with inflammatory bowel disease, suggesting that these cells are presenting antigens (possibly autoantigens) to an activated immune system. Other features indicative of immune activation include increased production of the cytokines IL-1 and IL-6, produced by macrophages, and high levels of soluble IL-2 receptors, released by activated T lymphocytes, in both tissue and circulation. Pathological and clinical features of inflammatory bowel disease could reflect the effects of cytokines, and manoeuvres intended to restrain their action may be of use in treatment. Thus, an IL-1 receptor antagonist has been reported to reduce the severity of inflammation in a rabbit model of colitis.

Several prostaglandin and thromboxane products are also increased during episodes of active inflammatory bowel disease. A possible damaging role of oxygen free-radicals generated by neutrophils and macrophages has been suggested recently.

Although the relative role of different components is far from clear, there is little doubt that soluble mediators and cellular and humoral immune responses are involved in generating the initial signs and sustaining the long-term manifestations of inflammatory bowel disease.

Clinical features

In **ulcerative colitis**, bloody diarrhoea and abdominal pain with fever and weight loss in the more severe cases are the main symptoms. Constipation, instead of diarrhoea, and tenesmus may be the major complaints in case of rectal involvement. Non-specific physical signs include abdominal distention and tenderness along the course of the colon. The laboratory findings are also mostly non-specific and reflect blood loss and inflammation. They include anaemia (iron deficiency, chronic disease), leukocytosis with left shift (i.e. appearance of immature forms) and elevated sedimentation rate, hypokalaemia and hypoalbuminaemia. The measurement of C-reactive protein and possibly orosomucoid is believed to reflect disease activity. Seventy percent of patients with ulcerative colitis, but not with Crohn's disease, have been reported to have in their sera an antineutrophil cytoplasmic antibody (ANCA) that gives a characteristic perinuclear staining (pANCA; see p. 230). This autoantibody differs from that found in Wegener's granulomatosis (see p. 228) and can also be

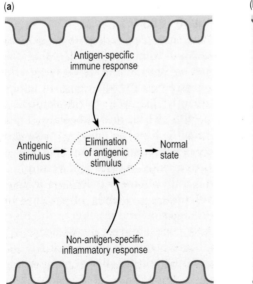

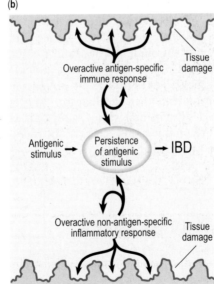

Fig. 15.8 **Possible mechanisms leading to inflammatory bowel disease.**
In the normal state (**a**), an intraluminal antigenic stimulus (dietary, microbial) is dealt with by the concerted action of antigen-specific immune responses and inflammatory reactions, which are down-regulated following the elimination of the stimulus. In inflammatory bowel disease (**b**), either the stimulus persists (chronic infection) or the immune and inflammatory responses are dysregulated. In either case the result is a persistently heightened immune response that causes tissue damage.

seen in primary sclerosing cholangitis, a hepatobiliary disease with a probable immune pathogenesis and frequently associated with ulcerative colitis.

In **Crohn's disease** the major clinical manifestations include fever, abdominal pain, diarrhoea (often without blood) and fatigability. Typical laboratory findings include anaemia (chronic disease, iron deficiency, vitamin B_{12} deficiency, folate deficiency) leukocytosis, thrombocytosis, elevation of the sedimentation rate, hypoalbuminaemia and electrolyte imbalance in the presence of severe diarrhoea. The measurement of C-reactive protein appears to be of use in monitoring the progress of the disease.

Diagnosis

In both inflammatory bowel diseases, the key diagnostic procedures are radiologic, endoscopic and histologic. In ulcerative colitis, a double-contrast barium enema gives precise mucosal detail, revealing granularity, ulceration, inflammatory pseudopolyps, loss of haustral pattern and shortening of the bowel. Careful X-ray examination of the small bowel in Crohn's disease may initially show loss of mucosal detail and rigidity, with the appearance later on of the characteristic cobblestoned pattern and fistulae. Endoscopy in ulcerative colitis — and in Crohn's disease when affected areas are accessible — has the advantage of providing a direct evaluation of disease activity and allows bioptic material to be collected.

Management and prognosis

Treatment of both conditions is similar. The anti-inflammatory agent sulphasalazine is given to control less severe cases, while corticosteroids are used in more severe disease. Mesalazine and osalazine are sometimes preferred to sulphasalazine, from which they are derived, in the treatment of ulcerative colitis. Azathioprine, although ineffective when given alone, is used as a steroid-sparing drug. Metronidazole has similar efficacy to sulphasalazine in Crohn's disease: it is not clear whether the drug is effective through its antibacterial properties or through another mechanism. Approximately two thirds of patients with Crohn's disease require surgery for complications, such as obstruction, abscess, fistula or haemorrhage.

Inflammatory bowel disease

- Mucosal inflammation of the colon occurs in ulcerative colitis and transmural inflammation of the intestinal wall in Crohn's disease.
- Levels of C-reactive protein reflect disease activity.
- Monocyte/macrophage-produced IL-1 and IL-6 may be important in the pathogenesis of both conditions.
- Antineutrophil cytoplasmic antibody (perinuclear pattern) is found in 70% of patients with ulcerative colitis.

The disease almost invariably relapses after surgery. Patients with Crohn's disease have an increased risk of intestinal carcinoma. Intractable ulcerative colitis may require colectomy, which usually eliminates the disease. The risk of developing carcinoma of the colon is significantly increased in patients with long-standing disease.

ALLERGIC FOOD REACTIONS

The topic of allergic food reactions is undoubtedly one of the most confused of clinical immunology. The term 'allergic' is frequently used inappropriately to describe all conditions where reproducible reactions are triggered by food ingestion, disappear on an elimination diet and recur on a blind challenge. 'Food intolerance' is the appropriate term to define the entirety of these conditions.

Pathogenesis

Allergic food reactions should be confined to those cases where an immune mechanism can be demonstrated. Most instances of food intolerance are not explained by a clear immunological mechanism, being caused by toxic (spices, sulphites) and pharmacological (caffeine, sodium nitrite) stimuli or by enzymatic deficiencies (lactose deficiency in some cases of milk intolerance). In these non-immune food reactions, however, many of the manifestations may be accounted for by activation of the alternative complement pathway. It is postulated that this pathway is triggered by non-immune stimuli such as food contaminants, leading to formation of anaphylotoxins such as C5a.

Clinical features

In the first year of life, food intolerance is relatively common, with cow's milk being the most frequent initiating stimulus. It appears as gastrointestinal symptoms and possibly wheezing. In adults the foods most frequently involved in intolerance are milk, eggs, fish, nuts, wheat and chocolate. These food reactions frequently have an allergic pathogenesis. Symptoms include urticaria, angioedema, asthma, anaphylaxis and, less frequently, nausea and vomiting. Such manifestations, but even more those comprising the **oral allergy syndrome** — swelling of the lips within minutes of food ingestion and tingling in the mouth and throat — closely correlate with the presence of specific IgE and implicate a type I hypersensitivity as the mechanism responsible for the clinical manifestations.

Diagnosis

Involvement of type I hypersensitivity can be documented by the detection of specific IgE using the RAST or, less expensively, with a skin prick test (see p. 136). The prick test, unfortunately, is only as good as the test antigen it uses. Therefore, while antigenic preparations from eggs, milk or shellfish may provoke a positive skin reaction in sensitised individuals, highly purified preparations from apple rarely do, even if a hypersensitive subject gives strikingly positive reactions when challenged with cruder preparations from apple juice or apple peel. The main diagnostic procedure in food intolerance is an elimination diet from which suspect foods are gradually removed until symptoms disappear. A positive diagnosis is made when symptoms reappear upon reintroducing a specific food. This challenge should be done in a double-blind manner using placebo controls. The challenge should be avoided, however, if the food is suspected to have caused systemic anaphylaxis in the past.

Management

The management of food intolerance consists of avoidance of the offending food.

Allergic food reactions

- Food intolerance occurs where reproducible symptoms are triggered by food ingestion.
- There are some IgE-mediated food reactions appropriately termed food allergies.
- Some cases of non-immune food intolerance may be caused by activation of the complement alternative pathway.
- Elimination of the offending food 'cures' both allergic and non-allergic food reactions.

HLA studies have revealed no consistent, marked associations with class I or class II alleles.

Clinical features

Patients usually present with haematuria, frequently macroscopic and recurrent, and this is sometimes accompanied by proteinuria. Renal failure may develop slowly in a small proportion (10–20%) over 10–20 years. In therapeutic terms, it appears that neither cure nor prevention are yet possible in IgA nephropathy. Since many of the cases pursue a benign course, treatment protocols are dependent upon the severity of the GN. Corticosteroids are of some benefit if crescentic nephritis is present. Other treatments, which need further evaluation, include plasma exchange, tonsillectomy and phenytoin, all as approaches to reducing systemic IgA circulation.

GLOMERULONEPHRITIS IN SLE

SLE is a multisystem inflammatory disease of connective tissue, characterised by autoantibody reactions to a range of tissue components (see Ch. 12). Glomerulonephritis represents a common and life-threatening complication of the disease. Some 50–60% of patients have proteinuria; 90% have abnormalities on conventional histological analysis of renal biopsies; and almost 100% have abnormalities by electron microscopy and immunofluorescence. It appears that most of the different histological patterns of GN we have discussed may be seen in SLE (Table 16.1), and that the pattern can be different even in sequential biopsies from the same patient. Equally, the clinical presentation is varied with hypertension, proteinuria, haematuria, nephrotic syndrome or end-stage renal failure.

Pathology

In general terms, deposition of IgG, IgM and IgA, along with C3, C4 and C1q and the membrane attack complex, is seen in the subendothelial part of the GBM and in the mesangium. The typical granular appearance on immunofluorescence is shown in Figure 16.9. The variable pattern of abnormalities seen in SLE has invoked the use of a classification system, which is a useful index of the degree of damage (Table 16.2).

Table 16.1 **Renal immunofluorescence patterns seen in glomerulonephritis associated with SLE**

Pathology	Direct immunofluorescence
Little or no change by light microscopy	GBM and mesangial deposits of IgG, IgA, IgM and C3
Focal or diffuse proliferative GN	GBM and mesangial deposits of IgG, IgA, IgM and C3
Membranous GN	GBM and mesangial deposits of IgG, IgA, IgM and C3
Tubulointerstitial nephritis	IgG, IgA, IgM and C3 deposits in tubular basement membrane

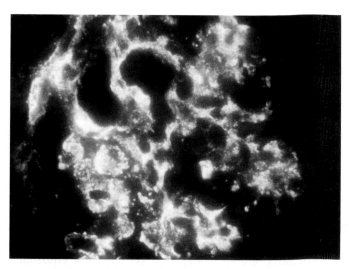

Fig. 16.9 **Systemic lupus erythematosus.**
Direct immunofluorescence examination of a renal biopsy from a patient with SLE using fluorescein-conjugated antiserum raised in rabbits against human complement component C1q. The staining pattern is granular along the GBM and within the mesangium. (Courtesy of Dr F. Dische and M. Norman.)

Table 16.2 **Pathological glomerular changes in SLE**

Class	Renal pathology
I	Normal glomeruli, no deposits by EM or IFL
II	Mesangial changes only; immune deposits seen by EM and IFL, with or without LM changes
III and IV	Changes seen in II plus: capillary wall deposits, usually subendothelial, by EM and IFL; changes may be proliferative, necrotising or sclerosing and may involve crescents; class III affects <50% of glomeruli, class IV > 50%
V	Changes similar to membranous nephropathy, with mesangial deposits

LM, light microscopy; EM, electron microscopy; IFL, immunofluorescence

Pathogenesis and immunological features

Elution of immune deposits from diseased kidneys shows that a proportion of the complexes are made of DNA–anti-DNA, but these form a minority. The titres of anti-nuclear and anti-DNA antibodies, levels of circulating immune complexes and the degree of complement activation show only rough correlations with the degree of nephritis, arguing against them being the single pathogenic mechanism. In addition, there is evidence that nephritis typical of SLE can present years before the serological abnormalities typical of the disease are detectable. However, complement levels and erythrocyte complement receptors (CR-1) are reduced, contributing to potential immune complex disease.

An attractive theory at present is that autoantigens are 'planted' in the glomeruli and that the critical damaging antigen–antibody interactions take place there. DNA is an example of a cationic molecule that binds to the GBM, and to its collagen V components in particular.

Clinical features

Mild forms of GN associated with SLE are usually managed with corticosteroids, while more severe disease requires the addition of azathioprine or cyclophosphamide. Surprisingly, the long-term survival of renal function appears to be associated with the degree of interstitial scarring, rather than with the severity of glomerular damage.

> **Glomerulonephritis associated with immune complexes**
>
> - Inflammation of the glomerulus may arise after deposition of immune complexes on or in the GBM, or after in situ formation of immune complexes involving fixed antigens.
> - The renal damage is associated with recruitment of complement and inflammatory cells into the glomerulus.
> - There are a variety of pathological processes that can result in this form of GN, involving bacterial antigens, autoantigens, possibly tumour antigens and also unidentified antigens. Different antigen–antibody complexes have distinct characteristics in terms of where they are deposited in the GBM and mesangium.

RENAL DISEASE ASSOCIATED WITH VASCULITIS

Systemic vasculitis is a manifestation of several disorders and involves a necrotising (i.e. necrosis-inducing) inflammatory process taking place within blood vessel walls. This leads to organ damage through loss of the blood supply. Any organ may be affected, and the distribution of the disease may be influenced by the size of the vessels involved. The best working classification of vasculitic disorders is that based on the size of the vessels affected. The kidney is typically damaged when small (e.g. **Wegener's granulomatosis** and **micropolyarteritis**) or intermediate (e.g. **polyarteritis nodosa**) vessels are targeted in the vasculitis. Vasculitis is also a manifestation of **cryoglobulinaemia**.

GLOMERULONEPHRITIS ASSOCIATED WITH CRYOGLOBULINAEMIA

Cryoglobulins are immunoglobulins that form precipitates at low temperatures. The condition of cryoglobulinaemia may be primary, or it may be secondary to disorders including lymphoproliferative disease, the connective tissue diseases and viral infection. Perhaps the most important practical consideration is that cryoglobulins can precipitate at room temperature. When this happens in a blood sample, the precipitate will be removed with the cells and clot on centrifugation. Therefore, under normal blood-taking conditions, cryoglobulins will not be detectable in a serum sample: blood must be collected at 37°C and maintained at this temperature until serum has been separated. Serum is then exposed to lower temperatures to establish whether a precipitate forms.

Cryoglobulins are classified according to their properties (Table 16.3), with 50% of cases involving type III cryoglobulins and the remainder equally divided amongst types I and II.

Pathology

The most typical pathological lesion is that of mesangiocapillary GN. Immunofluorescence shows granular staining of cryoglobulin along the capillary wall, and deposits seen on electron micrographs are typically subendothelial.

Pathogenesis and immunological features

The reason for the generation of immunglobulins with the property of precipitating at low temperature is not known. Analysis of the immunoglobulin genes in B cells producing cryoglobulins indicates that the germline configurations have frequently been maintained without recombinations. The possibility that this represents a somewhat primordial type of defence system has been put forward. The association with chronic infection suggests that chronic antigen stimulation may be one factor in exposing such responses. One area of great interest is the development of cryoglobulins in relation to chronic infection with the hepatitis C virus, and the exact prevalence of this remains to be established.

Once present, cryoglobulins have the capacity to precipitate in the cold extremities, lodging in vessel walls

Table 16.3 **Classification of cryoglobulins**

Type	Components	Activity	Disease association	Other features
I	Usually monoclonal IgM	None	Lymphoproliferative disease (Waldenström's macroglobulinaemia, lymphoma, myeloma)	Hyperviscosity syndrome, vasculitis, Raynaud's phenomenon (only rarely associated with GN)
II	Usually monoclonal IgM, complexed to IgG	Rheumatoid factor	Lymphoproliferative disease (lymphoma, chronic lymphocytic leukaemia, Waldenström's macroglobulinaemia, myeloma, viral hepatitis)	Typical features of 'immune-complex disease': vasculitis, arthritis and glomerulonephritis
III	Polyclonal IgM, complexed to IgG	Rheumatoid factor	30% of cases are primary (**mixed essential cryoglobulinaemia**); others are associated with connective tissue disease (rheumatoid arthritis, SLE, polyarteritis nodosa) and viral hepatitis	Typical features of 'immune-complex disease': vasculitis, arthritis and glomerulonephritis

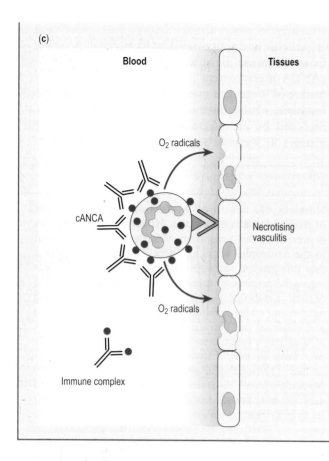

(c)

Blood

Tissues

O₂ radicals

cANCA

Necrotising
vasculitis

O₂ radicals

Immune complex

agammaglobulinaemia who regularly received immunoglobulin-replacement therapy developed uveitis and vasculitic lesions in the retina, associated with cANCA in the serum. Given the unlikelihood of a patient with his form of immunodeficiency being able to generate any antibody-mediated immune response, the batch of immunoglobulin that he had most recently received was also checked for cANCA — and was positive. The other apparent co-factor in Wegener's granulomatosis, infection with activation of neutrophils, would certainly have been an ever present complication of this boy's immunodeficiency. Therefore, it appears that cANCA in association with infection is sufficient to induce vasculitic lesions.

Fig. 16.12 **Schematic representation of a possible pathogenic scenario for the role of ANCA in Wegener's granulomatosis.**
(c) In the presence of ANCA, adherent neutrophils expressing surface PR3 become further activated by autoantibody binding, releasing toxic oxygen metabolites and causing vessel damage. Immune complexes composed of cANCA and PR3 may establish secondary inflammatory foci at a distance from this site by an immune complex-mediated mechanism.

may be beneficial. Constitutional symptoms (fever, malaise and weight loss) reflect the systemic nature of the illness.

Aggressive use of corticosteroids with cyclophosphamide, has led to a considerable improvement in the outcome of a disease associated with an 80% 1-year mortality rate in early series in the 1950s. The titre of cANCA appears to be a useful guide to the management of the disease, with rising titres closely correlated with relapse.

MICROSCOPIC POLYARTERITIS

This condition is a small-vessel vasculitis, and the histological appearance of the vessels affected is the same as that seen in Wegener's granulomatosis. There is a related condition, **idiopathic rapidly progressive GN** (IRPGN) in which the vasculitic lesions appear localised to the kidney and there is a rapid onset of severe nephritis. Both microscopic polyarteritis and IRPGN are associated with the presence of ANCA, but of a different type to that seen in Wegener's granulomatosis.

Pathology

Focal necrotising GN is seen, with crescent formation. Necrotising vasculitis is seen systemically in microscopic polyarteritis. Granulomata are not seen. Vessel lesions may be associated with immune deposits containing IgG and C3, but occasionally the evidence for immunological involvement in the vasculitis is lacking, with few or no immune deposits, and this may be described as 'pauci-immune'.

Pathogenesis and immunological features

The distinctive immunological feature of microscopic polyarteritis and IRPGN is a form of ANCA, present in some 60% of patients. This gives a different pattern to the cANCA associated with Wegener's granulomatosis, since the staining is concentrated around the nucleus, so-called perinuclear or **pANCA**. In fact the main pANCA target autoantigen, myeloperoxidase, is cytoplasmic and its perinuclear localisation in the immunofluorescence test used is an artefact of the alcohol fixation.

Clinical features

Response to treatment involving immunosuppression with corticosteroids and cyclophosphamide is very dramatic in these disorders.

POLYARTERITIS NODOSA

Polyarteritis nodosa (PAN) is a disease characterised by swelling of the media of medium-sized vessels, associated with fibrinoid necrosis and an inflammatory infiltrate. The vessel walls tend to weaken and there is aneurysm development and vessel occlusion.

Table 16.4 **Summary of the characteristics of the nephritic disorders**

Disorder	Glomerular pathology	Direct immunofluorescence	GBM deposits seen by EM	Immunopathology	Other features
Antibody mediated					
Anti-GBM nephritis	Diffuse proliferative ± crescents	Linear IgG, C3 along GBM	None	Circulating antibody to NC1 domain of α3 chain of type IV collagen	Association with HLA-DR2 and haemoptysis (Goodpasture's syndrome)
Associated with immune complexes					
Post-streptococcal GN	Diffuse proliferative ± crescents	Granular IgG, C3 along GBM	Subepithelial	? Circulating immune complexes or cross-reactive antibacterial antibodies	
Membranous GN	Thickened GBM	Granular IgG, C3 along GBM	Subepithelial	? Circulating autoantibodies to fixed renal antigen	Association with HLA-DR3
Minimal change GN	Minimal (foot process effacement)	Negative	Negative	? Soluble 'immunological factor' causes damages	
Mesangiocapillary GN (I and II)	Mesangial proliferation and capillary thickening	Granular C3 and IgG along GBM	Subendothelial (type I) and intramembranous (type II)	? Immune complex mediated	Type II associated with partial lipodystrophy and C3Nef
IgA nephropathy	Mesangial proliferation	IgA, C3 and properdin, ± IgG in mesangium	Negative	? Immune complexes or antibodies to fibronectin, laminin	
SLE nephritis	Variable	Granular IgG, IgM, C3, C4 along GBM	Subendothelial and/or subepithelial	? Immune complexes deposited or 'planted'	
Associated with vasculitis					
Cryoglobulinaemia	Similar to mesangio-capillary GN	IgG, IgM, C3 along capillary wall	Subendothelial	Immune complexes deposited	
Wegener's granulomatosis	Focal proliferative GN with crescents	Negative	Negative	Immune damage to vessel walls ± immune complex involvement	cANCA
Microscopic polyarteritis	Focal necrotising GN with crescents	Negative	Negative	? Immune damage to vessel walls ± immune complex involvement	pANCA; idiopathic rapidly progressive GN is similar but restricted to kidney
Poyarteritis nodosa	Fibrinoid necrosis of renal vessels	Negative	Negative	Unknown; ? immune complex mediated	pANCA; associated with hepatitis B virus infection

Pathology

In affected vessels, fibrinoid necrosis of the vessel wall with intense neutrophil infiltration is seen in association with aneurysms.

Pathogenesis and immunological features

The pathogenesis of this condition is not known. There is an important association, however, with hepatitis B infection, with some 40% of patients having serological evidence of infection.

Clinical features

Aneurysms are visible by renal angiography and the other diagnostic test of value is a muscle biopsy to look for vessel changes. Other evidence of an inflammatory condition is commonly seen, with raised ESR, C-reactive protein and immunoglobulin levels. A minority of patients have pANCA. PAN is a life-threatening condition, with end-stage renal failure in 30%, and other complications such as malignant hypertension and cerebrovascular accidents.

Aggressive therapy with corticosteroids and cytotoxic agents is needed to control the disease, giving a 5-year survival in excess of 60%.

Renal vasculitis

- The kidney is particularly sensitive to inflammatory processes involving damage to blood vessels.
- In some cases of vasculitis associated with renal damage, the mechanisms are well defined (e.g. cryoglobulinaemia, Wegener's granulomatosis). In the diagnosis of both of these conditions, the immunology laboratory is prominent. Measurement of ANCA, which may be involved in disease process or generated secondarily, is important.
- In the small and middle-sized vessel vasculitic disorders, the immune processes precipitating vessel inflammation are still to be fully defined.

CHAPTER 17

Immune-mediated skin disease

NORMAL AND DISEASED SKIN

IMMUNOBIOLOGY OF THE SKIN

The skin is an important homeostatic organ, regulating amongst other things body temperature and salt and water content. In immunological terms, it forms a major, innate, physical barrier to infection. In recent years it has become clear that the skin also has a specialised contingent of immune cells. The Langerhans cell plays an important role in immune surveillance within the skin and, in addition, it now appears that the major epidermal constituent, the keratinocyte, is capable of cytokine secretion and may also present antigen to T lymphocytes.

To understand the role of the skin and its immune system in disease, it is necessary to revise the histology and physiology of the organ, with particular attention to the site and function of the immune cells. By convention, skin has three layers, the epidermis, dermis and fat (Fig. 17.1). The epidermis is a stratified layer of squamous epithelial cells, the predominant member being the keratinocyte. These cells arise from the basal layer of the epidermis, which abuts onto the basal lamina, or basement membrane zone (BMZ). The keratinocyte migrates upwards from the basal layer, gradually acquiring increasing amounts of the fibrous protein keratin and gradually becoming more flattened in shape. At the surface, keratinocytes have become a dead envelope of keratin, the so-called 'horny layer' (stratum corneum), with important barrier functions. At intervals throughout the epidermis, occasional

Langerhans cells may be seen. The BMZ is composed predominantly of laminin, fibronectin and collagen type IV and divides the epidermis from the dermis. Within the dermis lie the blood and lymphatic vessels, as well as the skin adnexal structures (sweat and sebaceous glands, hair follicles).

Immune cells are found predominantly in the dermis, particularly around the post-capillary vessels in what has been termed the **dermal perivascular unit** (Fig. 17.1). Here, in close proximity to the endothelium lie mast cells, macrophages, T cells and dendritic cells, some of which are similar to Langerhans cells. At this site, immune cells are perfectly poised to respond to signals arising from epidermal injury or infection, and to regulate post-capillary endothelial adhesion molecules. Some 10^9–10^{10} T lymphocytes are found in the skin of an adult, and 90% of these are in the dermal perivascular units.

Examination of the epidermis in inflammatory skin conditions has shown that the **keratinocyte** expresses class II MHC molecules and ICAM-1 under stress. The keratinocyte is also capable of phagocytosis, since this is the process involved in the acquisition of melanin pigment from melanocytes. Following stimulation of healthy skin keratinocytes in vitro, several cytokines may be produced: IL-1, IL-6, IL-8, IFN-α and IFN-β, TNF-α and colony-stimulating factors for myeloid cells (G-CSF, GM-CSF). It is, therefore, possible to envisage roles for keratinocytes in attracting and anchoring immune cells (IL-8, CSFs, ICAM-1); cell activation (IL-1, IL-8, TNF-α); in exerting cytotoxicity against microbial organisms (IFN-α/β, TNF-α); and even in antigen processing and presentation (class II MHC molecules).

Langerhans cells are bone-marrow derived and constitute the skin component of the mononuclear phagocyte system. They have a dendritic morphology (i.e. have many processes to provide an extensive area of contact) and are derived from the bone marrow as a member of the mononuclear phagocyte system. Langerhans cells have a high level of constitutive expression of class II MHC molecules, and a current view on their life cycle suggests that they trap and process antigen within the skin and then migrate to the local lymph node to present peptide antigens to T lymphocytes.

T lymphocytes in the skin bear the $\alpha\beta$ or $\gamma\delta$ TCRs in roughly the same proportions as in blood. The CD4:CD8 ratio within the skin approximates one, with most CD4$^+$ T lymphocytes bearing the CD45R0 memory phenotype and a high proportion expressing the activation markers HLA-DR or CD25.

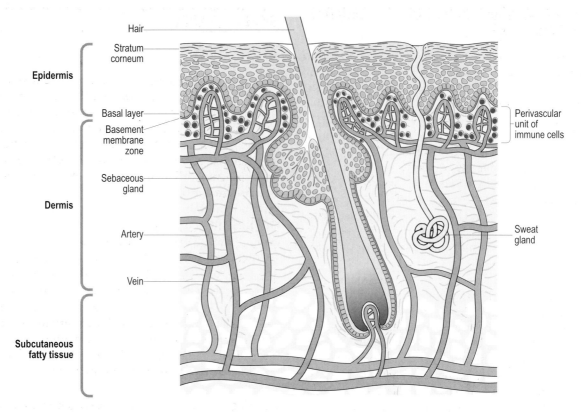

Fig. 17.1 **The structure of skin.**

CELL ADHESION IN THE SKIN

Adhesion between cells and between cells and the extracellular matrix is critical to the maintenance of an intact skin barrier. Recent advances in skin biology have identified the mechanisms and structures used to maintain skin integrity.

Cell–cell junctional organelles in the skin, which may be viewed by electron microscopy, are termed **desmosomes**. Recently, several of these glycoprotein molecules have been identified at the structural and DNA level. From the information acquired, it is apparent that desmosomes are part of the **cadherin** family of cell–cell adhesion structures, and they are generally now termed **desmosomal cadherins**. Cadherins are calcium-dependent transmembrane cell adhesion molecules that operate in a process termed 'homophilic adhesion' (i.e. one cadherin on a cell binds to the same molecule on another cell).

Structures involved in the adherence of basal layer keratinocytes to the BMZ and thence to the dermis are shown in Figure 17.2. The hemidesmosomes are analogous to the desmosomal cadherins in function and serve to anchor the basal layer keratinocytes to the lamina densa of the BMZ.

TERMINOLOGY IN SKIN DISEASE

The classics scholar *cum* physician is ideally placed to become a dermatologist. The descriptive terms used to define skin lesions and the diseases associated with them are best addressed ahead of the immunology (Table 17.1).

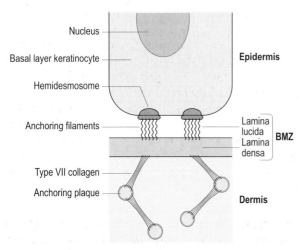

Fig. 17.2 **Cell adhesion in the skin.**

Table 17.1 **Terms used in the description and diagnosis of skin disease**

Term	Definition
Plaque	Elevated lesion with larger surface area in relation to height
Wheal	Elevation of skin caused by dermal oedema
Angio-oedema	Oedematous reaction in dermis, covering large skin area
Vesicle	Blister (< 0.5 cm)
Bulla	Blister (> 0.5 cm)
Erythema	Redness caused by vasodilatation

SKIN DISEASES AND IMMUNOLOGY: GENERAL CONSIDERATIONS

Skin diseases in which there is an immune component to the pathogenesis fall into several categories. There are the allergic type I hypersensitivity diseases, such as eczema, urticaria and angio-oedema; there is also the eczema generated as a result of a type IV hypersensitivity reaction (contact dermatitis). In addition, skin disease may be a consequence of vasculitis. These disorders are discussed in other chapters (see Chs 12 and 16). The other main category of immune-mediated skin disease is termed the **vesiculo-bullous disorders**. In these diseases, fluid-filled vesicles and bullae appear as a result of damage to the mechanisms involved in the maintenance of cell–cell and cell–structure adhesion within the skin.

The main diagnostic tool for the diagnosis of immune-mediated skin disease is analysis by immunofluorescence (p. 168). Direct immunofluorescence on biopsies demonstrates immunoglobulin or complement deposition in the skin of the patient. Skin biopsies should be peri-lesional, since the skin components and architecture within a blister are disrupted. Indirect immunofluorescence on an appropriate skin substrate (e.g. normal human skin, or monkey oesophageal mucosa) demonstrates the presence of circulating autoantibodies against skin components. The pattern of the fluorescence is of considerable diagnostic help, and in some of the vesiculo-bullous diseases it is generally agreed that the autoantibody itself is responsible for the tissue damage. In some disorders, antibodies are directed against components of the BMZ, at the dermal–epidermal junction. It can be of diagnostic help to establish whether the antibodies identify targets on the dermal or epidermal side of the BMZ. To investigate this, the skin biopsy can be split at the dermal–epidermal junction by treatment with a concentrated salt solution, and fluorescence studies then carried out to identify whether the site of antibody binding is on the dermal or epidermal side of the BMZ.

Psoriasis and vitiligo are also discussed. These diseases undoubtedly have an immune component, although the pathogenesis of psoriasis remains enigmatic.

Normal and diseased skin

- Skin has important homeostatic functions, including the control of infection, and contains a specialised immune system.
- Immune cells are found predominantly in the dermis (dermal perivascular units) and include Langerhans cells, keratinocytes and T cells.
- Cell–cell junctional organelles, called desmosomal cadherins, are important in maintaining an intact skin barrier.

SKIN DISEASES

PEMPHIGUS

Pemphigus is a group of disorders characterised by blister formation within the epidermis in association with autoantibodies directed against constituents on the surface of squamous epithelial cells. There are two major types of pemphigus, divided according to whether the blisters form in the superficial epidermis (**pemphigus foliaceus**) or in the deep epidermis (**pemphigus vulgaris**).

Pemphigus vulgaris

Although pemphigus vulgaris is rare in Europe and North America, this is the most common form of pemphigus; it principally affects the 40–60 year-old age group. Although pemphigus vulgaris (PV) may affect members of all races, it is characteristically seen in people of Mediterranean or Jewish origin. There is a strong association between PV and possession of the HLA genotype *DQA1*0101, DQB1*0503*, which in Israelis carries a relative risk of over 100.

Pathology. Direct immunofluorescence reveals deposition of IgG, as well as the complement component C3, on the keratinocyte surface at all levels in the epidermis (Fig. 17.3). In indirect immunofluorescence, circulating IgG that binds to the surface of normal stratified squamous epithelium in the skin can be demonstrated in almost all untreated patients, and titres of the autoantibody correlate with disease severity. Skin histology reveals acantholysis (separation of keratinocytes from each other). Typically, there is little in the way of inflammatory infiltrate and the dermis is intact. The antigen recognised by sera from patients with PV has recently been identified. It has a molecular mass of 130 kDa and is a desmosomal cadherin known as **desmoglein 3** (Dsg 3) a member of the desmoglein subfamily of the cadherin family of cell adhesion molecules.

Clinical features. Blisters typically appear first in the mouth and are also seen on the skin. Blisters are thin, flaccid and form on a base of normal or erythematous skin. Since the blisters form in the epidermis and have a thin ceiling, they are frequently ruptured and replaced by large, superficial skin erosions. By the time a patient reaches the dermatologist, true blisters may be few and far between. There is increased skin fragility, such that rubbing apparently unaffected skin leads to removal of the epidermis (Nikolsky's sign). There is little tendency for PV to resolve spontaneously, and it is fatal without treatment as skin function is lost.

Treatment. Therapy consists of high-dose systemic steroids, frequently supplemented with azathioprine and cyclophosphamide. Treatment must be maintained

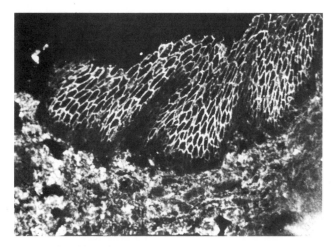

Fig. 17.3 **Pemphigus vulgaris.**
Indirect immunofluorescence analysis of a section of monkey oesophagus incubated with serum from a patient with pemphigus vulgaris, followed by a fluorescein-conjugated antihuman IgG antiserum raised in rabbits. Positive staining is seen as linear fluorescence around the perimeter of the keratinocytes in the intercellular space, producing a 'chicken wire' effect. The dermal–epidermal junction is not stained; this patient has circulating skin autoantibodies.

for lengthy periods, and PV remains a potentially fatal disease with up to 25% of patients dying from the disease or the consequences of the therapy.

Pemphigus foliaceus

Pemphigus foliaceus (PF) is less common in temperate climes, but is relatively common on the Indian sub-continent. It is more benign than PV.

Pathology. Immunofluorescence studies and histology are identical to those with PV. The antigen recognised by sera from patients with PF has also been identified recently. It is the desmosomal cadherin **desmoglein 1** (Dsg 1), a 160 kDa member of the desmoglein sub-family of cadherins.

Clinical features. PF is less severe than PV with oral lesions being rare and the disease controllable with topical steroid therapy. Drug-induced lesions similar to PF have been described, and an endemic form of the disease, termed fogo selvagem, is seen in Brazil (see box: 'Endemic pemphigus foliaceus'). Separation between the keratinocytes takes place high in the epidermis and blisters rupture quickly leaving erosive surfaces.

Pathogenesis of pemphigus

A consensus view in dermatological circles is that the autoantibodies generated in pemphigus are pathogenic and cause the blistering. The accumulated body of evidence for this is given in Table 17.2.

The precise mechanism of tissue damage is not clear, however, and neither is there any explanation for the different patterns of superficial and deep blisters in PF and PV. Recruitment of complement as the damaging component is a strong possibility, though several stud-

Endemic pemphigus foliaceus

Endemic pemphigus foliaceus (EPF), or fogo selvagem, is an autoimmune blistering disorder. Clinically it is identical to pemphigus foliaceus. The autoantibodies generated are of the IgG4 subclass and transfer the disease to neonatal mice. The major autoantigenic target of EPF serum, like that of PF serum, is desmoglein 1. What makes EPF of great interest is that the epidemiology of this autoimmune disease strongly suggests involvement of insect bites. Descriptions of EPF first appeared in Brazil at the turn of this century. During the 1980s, it became clear that the majority of cases occur within 15 km of several large rivers inland from Rio de Janeiro. This is the maximum flying distance of insects such as mosquitoes and the black flies known as simulium, which have the rivers as their main habitat. Of these two potential vectors, the link with the black flies appears the strongest. One of the anecdotal pieces of evidence supporting simulium as the vector regards a local farmer moving to an area within the endemic zone of EPF. The people already in this locality complained bitterly of the constant irritation of bites from the black flies and had themselves already made the link between these and EPF. The newly arrived farmer decided to purchase a flock of canaries to try to reduce the number of black flies in the area. Amazingly, both the number of simulium and the incidence of EPF in his locality declined dramatically! What remains to be established in EPF is the nature of the stimulus for generating pathogenic antibodies to Dsg 1. A possible cross-reactive epitope in the insect's secretions, or in an organism carried by the vector, seems the most likely explanation.

Table 17.2 **Evidence that antidesmoglein autoantibodies cause pemphigus**

	Observations
Clinical studies	Antidesmoglein antibodies are detected in almost all patients Titres of autoantibodies reflect disease severity, response to therapy and relapse
Animal studies	IgG from patients with PV, or from rabbits immunised with PV antigen, recreates clinical, histological and immunological features of PV after injection into neonatal mice Severe combined immunodeficient mice reconstituted with lymphocytes from patients with PV deposit human IgG in the skin and suffer PV-like lesions (see box)
In vitro studies	IgG from PV patients causes loss of cell–cell adhesion in skin organ culture

ies have now shown that the autoantibodies in PV are of the IgG4 subclass, which fixes complement poorly. In vitro, the effect of IgG from PV patients in reducing cell–cell adhesion in skin organ culture does not require complement. However, keratinocyte intercellular C3 deposition is seen in affected human skin but not in the murine passive transfer model. An alternative possibility is that PV autoantibody binding activates plasminogen activator. Plasminogen activator converts plasminogen to the active proteolytic enzyme plasmin, which could in turn digest the cadherins. In animal models of PV (see box: 'SCID mice: a new model for autoimmune disease'), disruption of cell–cell adhesion can be prevented by antibody that inhibits plasminogen activator.

SCID mice: a new model for autoimmune disease

These mice have recently become a much studied model of human disease, since their immune system can be artificially reconstituted with peripheral blood lymphocytes (PBLs) from a human as discussed elsewhere (see p. 202). The SCID mouse is incapable of rejecting the human lymphocytes, and, for their part, the human immune cells do not appear to generate a graft-versus-host disease. The SCID mouse, thus, becomes a living vessel for the study of human immunology. The human PBLs appear reasonably healthy and functional, since human IgG is produced and begins to circulate in the mouse blood. This provides an ideal opportunity for studying the role of autoantibodies in disease. In a recent report, some 50 mice were reconstituted with PBLs from patients with pemphigus vulgaris. Approximately two thirds of the mice developed circulating PV antibodies of the IgG class, and half had deposits of IgG in the skin. In some mice, human skin had been grafted on before reconstitution. In almost all of these mice, PV-like blistering lesions containing human IgG developed in the human skin grafts. The SCID mouse, therefore, appears to be a powerful model for studying autoimmune diseases in which a circulating autoantibody has a pathogenetic role.

Before the identification of the BMZ antigens recognised by sera from patients with BP, evidence from careful light and electron microscopic studies suggested that more than one autoantibody-binding site might exist. In direct immune studies, IgG deposition appeared in the lamina lucida layer of the BMZ, directly below the basal keratinocyte layer. However, in indirect studies, in which sections cut through the skin laid open the cytoplasm of the cells in this region, binding also took place within the cells of the basal layer. It is now established that there are two BP antigens. One of 180 kDa is an extracellular hemidesmosomal protein in the lamina lucida. The other 230 kDa protein is a hemidesmosomal protein found within keratinocytes

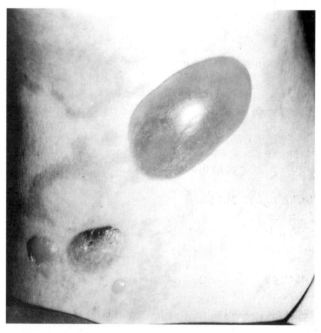

Fig. 17.4 **Bullous skin disease.**
Tense, fluid-filled blister in the skin of a patient with a bullous skin disease. In this case, the patient had bullous pemphigoid. (Courtesy of Dr E. Higgins.)

BULLOUS PEMPHIGOID

Bullous pemphigoid (BP) is a fairly common blistering disorder (Fig. 17.4) in which bullae arise from the subepidermis in association with autoantibodies directed against constituents in the BMZ.

Pathology

Direct immunofluorescence reveals deposition of IgG and C3 in almost all patients, and the pattern is characteristically linear along the epidermal BMZ (Fig. 17.5). Circulating autoantibodies of the IgG class are found in the majority (approximately 80%) of patients on indirect immunofluorescence, but titres of the autoantibody correlate poorly with disease severity. Skin histology reveals blister formation in the BMZ and although there may be little inflammation, in some cases an extensive infiltrate including lymphocytes, macrophages and eosinophils is seen.

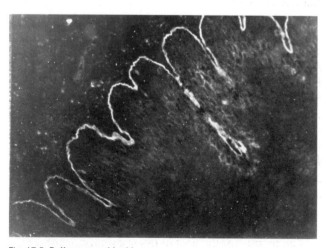

Fig. 17.5 **Bullous pemphigoid.**
Direct immunofluorescence analysis of a skin biopsy from a patient with bullous pemphigoid. The biopsy has been stained with a fluorescein-labelled antiserum raised in rabbits against human IgG. There is a linear fluorescence pattern along the dermal–epidermal junction, indicating deposition of IgG on the basement membrane.

and not normally exposed in vivo. These antigens appear to have structural homology to the **desmoplakins**, a family of proteins involved in cell adhesion. Whilst almost all BP sera can be demonstrated to react to the 230 kDa antigen, only half show reactivity to the 180 kDa protein.

Pathogenesis

The presence of lymphocytes, as well as mast cells, eosinophils and neutrophils around the BMZ in the skin of some patients argues for an immune pathogenesis to the blisters in BP. However, the evidence that BP is an antibody-mediated disease is much less clear cut than for PV (Table 17.3). One of the major pieces of evidence against BP sera being pathogenic has been the inability to reproduce the disease by passive transfer of patient IgG into neonatal mice, and this has led to a general consensus over the years that BP autoantibodies do not cause disease. Recently, an explanation for this failure has been put forward. Sequence analysis of the human and murine 180 kDa hemidesmosomal proteins demonstrates that they differ at a critical 14 amino acid residue stretch that is the immunodominant epitope recognised by BP sera. If this is the case, it is not surprising that human sera from patients with BP do not bind the murine basement membrane and cause disease. To test this hypothesis, antibodies have been generated in rabbits against the murine form of the dominant epitope. When injected into neonatal mice, these antisera reproduce BP lesions very accurately. Therefore, it appears that the history of the role of BP sera in causing the disease may yet need rewriting.

Clinical and immunological features

This is the most common bullous disorder, principally affecting those aged 50–80 years. Unlike PV, there is no characteristic racial or HLA association with BP. Blisters may be generalised or localised on the skin (Fig. 17.4) and are also found on the mucous membrane in approximately one third of cases. The blisters, which are tense and typically occur on a base of erythematous skin, are often preceded by intense pruritus. The thicker

Table 17.3 **Evidence for and against circulating autoantibodies as the cause of bullous pemphigoid**

For	Against
In vitro, on skin sections, complement-fixing BP antibodies mediate attachment of neutrophils to the BMZ	Titres of BP autoantibodies do not reflect disease severity or response to treatment
Subepidermal blisters inducible in guinea-pigs after intradermal injection of BP sera	Other researchers have failed to reproduce the guinea-pig studies; no passive transfer of disease with neonatal mice (but see text)
Terminal attack complexes of complement demonstrable in BMZ	
Evidence of complement activation in blister fluid	

capsule to these blisters means that they are usually intact and present on examination. There is a tendency for BP to resolve spontaneously and it is rarely fatal. Therapy is similar to pemphigus but requires less intensity and shorter maintenance.

Occasionally pemphigoid lesions are confined to the mucous membrane (**mucous membrane** or **cicatricial pemphigoid**). This may have serious consequences when the conjunctiva is involved (blindness secondary to scarring) and can also lead to hair loss when the scalp is affected.

PEMPHIGOID GESTATIONIS

Previously termed 'herpes gestationis', pemphigoid gestationis (PG) is a rare bullous disorder associated with pregnancy (1 case in every 20 000 pregnancies). It is not related to herpes, but the small vesicles are very similar to those seen in herpetic infections.

Pathology

Direct immunofluorescence is positive in approximately half the cases diagnosed clinically, revealing linear BMZ deposition of IgG and complement, though in some cases only heavy complement deposition is seen. Indirect immunofluorescence is positive in only 20% of patients, although a recent study claims 100% may be positive if a specific anti-IgG1 antibody is used to reveal IgG1 deposited in the BMZ. Patients with PG have reactivity to the same 180 kDa antigen as that recognised by some sera from patients with BP, and both sera appear to recognise the same immunodominant 14 amino acid residue sequence in the non-collagenous part of the molecule.

Clinical features and pathogenesis

The disorder is characterised by an intense burning itchiness, with the appearance of blisters, usually in the second or third trimester of pregnancy. It usually resolves after delivery, although exacerbations associated with the menses and the oral contraceptive pill have been reported. PG also has a tendency to recur, at an earlier stage, with each subsequent pregnancy by the same partner. An association with possession of *HLA-DR3* and *HLA-DR4* has been described. There are also rare reports of the newborn infant having transient skin blisters caused by placental transfer of maternal antibodies. Treatment is aimed at alleviating symptoms with oral corticosteroids, whilst avoiding suppression of fetal adrenal function.

The rarity of this syndrome, and the fact that circulating antibodies tend to be of lower titre, have precluded extensive studies on the pathogenesis of PG. There is some speculation that the disease is initiated as part of an allogeneic immune response to paternal HLA antigens exposed in the placenta. This could spread to include normal placental basement membrane antigens, which cross-react with antigens in normal skin BMZ. Some support for this proposal derives from the demonstration that mothers with PG are more likely to have circulating antibodies to paternal HLA antigens.

DERMATITIS HERPETIFORMIS

In dermatitis herpetiformis (DH), small tense vesicles on an erythematous base are seen, typically on the extensor surfaces (e.g. elbows and buttocks), and occur in association with intense burning and itching. Oral lesions are rare.

Pathology

Direct skin immunofluorescence in DH reveals a characteristic deposition of IgA and complement in the dermal papillae (Fig. 17.6). Indirect immunofluorescence analysis tends to be negative, although circulating antibodies to gliadin, reticulin and the endomysium are seen, strengthening the proposed association with coeliac disease.

Clinical features and pathogenesis

The most striking clinical feature of DH is its association with pathology of the gastrointestinal tract. Although overt symptoms of gastrointestinal disease such as malabsorption are rare, jejunal biopsies from patients with DH reveal a patchy villous atrophy indistinguishable from that seen in coeliac disease (see Ch. 15). In addition, there is a strong association (95–100% of patients) with the HLA genotype *DQA1*0501*, *DQB1*0201* (serologically identified as DQ2), the same susceptibility genes as found in coeliac disease. In fact, the HLA-DQ2 phenotype in DH and coeliac disease is usually inherited as part of an extended HLA haplotype, most frequently *HLA-B8, DR3* or *HLA-B44, DR7*, both of which have distinctive complement genes, including the null allele for *C4, C4A*Q0*. A recent study of extended haplotypes carried out by HLA typing patients with DH and coeliac disease

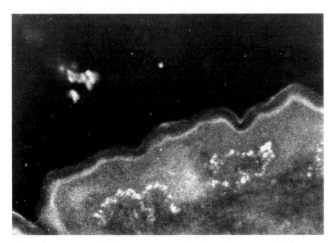

Fig. 17.6 **Dermatitis herpetiformis.**
Direct immunofluorescence analysis of a skin biopsy from a patient with dermatitis herpetiformis. The biopsy has been stained with a fluorescein-labelled antiserum raised in rabbits against human IgA. There is patchy, granular staining in the dermal papillae, indicating deposition of IgA at these sites.

and their family members has shed more light on the contribution of HLA genes to these diseases. It was noted that in coeliac disease, the genetic susceptibility is closely linked to the *DR, DQ* regions, whilst in DH, the linkage is much stronger with the complement genes. The disease becomes even more intriguing when one considers that the same gluten-free diets used to treat coeliac disease cause the skin IgA deposits in DH to disappear, though they recur if gluten is reintroduced. Dapsone will also control the skin lesions, but the skin immunofluorescence appearances do not change.

The pathogenesis of this skin disease remains a mystery. Neither circulating nor deposited IgA-containing immune complexes contain gliadin, and although there is a strong link between adenovirus 12 and coeliac disease (see Chs 9 and 15), there is as yet no link with the skin manifestations.

OTHER VESICULO-BULLOUS SKIN DISEASES

The main and best characterised bullous disorders are pemphigus, pemphigoid, herpes gestationis and dermatitis herpetiformis. Other diseases can cause bullae and have some diagnostic overlap, and will be discussed briefly.

Epidermolysis bullosa. This defines a heterogeneous group of inherited and acquired bullous diseases, the hallmark of which is that the bullae are trauma induced. In acquired epidermolysis bullosa (**epidermolysis bullosa acquisita**, EBA) there is no family history of blistering and the disease runs a chronic relapsing/remitting course, for which long-term immunosuppressive therapy with gold, dapsone, or azathioprine is required. The blisters are subepidermal and an infiltrate of mononuclear cells and neutrophils is present. Linear IgG and C3 deposition along the BMZ indistinguishable from that in BP is seen on direct immunofluorescence, and circulating antibodies are found in roughly half the patients. However, split skin analysis shows that EBA sera bind to the dermal side of the BMZ, whilst BP sera bind to the epidermal side. The antigenic target of EBA sera appears to be type VII collagen, important in anchoring the epidermis (Fig. 17.7).

Linear IgA bullous dermatosis (LABD). This disease may have several features in common with BP and DH, yet it is probably a separate entity. Subepidermal blisters forming in young adults and frequently associated with mucosal involvement may mimic BP and DH clinically. The lesions respond to dapsone and sulphonamides. On skin direct immunofluorescence, linear deposition of IgA is seen at the BMZ, with complement in about one third of cases, and circulating antibodies in one fifth. The disorder is distinguished from DH by the lack of association with *DQA1*0501, DQB1*0201* or gluten enteropathy, and lack of circulating antibodies to gliadin. However, occasional diagnostic con-

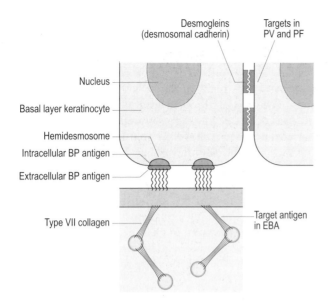

Fig. 17.7 Targets of skin autoantibodies.
BP, bullous pemphigoid; EBA, epidermolysis bullosa; PV, pemphigus vulgaris; PF, pemphigus foliaceus.

fusion with BP occurs if IgG deposits are also found by immunofluorescence.

Chronic bullous dermatosis of childhood. This is a bullous skin disease with very similar feature to LABD but it is characteristically seen in a younger age group.

PSORIASIS

Psoriasis is a common, disfiguring, chronic skin disease, affecting some 2% of Caucasians. The onset is usually at puberty or menopause, and the characteristic skin lesion is a red plaque covered by silvery skin scales. The disease has a relapsing remitting course, and the typical sites affected are the elbows, knees, scalp and buttocks. A combination of genetic and environmental factors are at play. The onset or relapse of the disease may be provoked by a variety of stimuli including trauma, infection (particularly with β-haemolytic streptococci), drugs, UV radiation and possibly stress. There is an association with the HLA alleles *Cw6* and *DR7*, the former giving a relative risk of 5–10 times the background population. Identical twins have a concordance rate for the disease of approximately 65%. Some 10% of patients may also be affected by an arthritis.

Pathogenesis

The underlying process giving rise to the skin manifestations of the disease is an increase in the rate of skin turnover, in association with abnormal epidermal maturation. The epidermis usually turns over every 30–40 days, but this epithelial layer of the skin may turn over every 5 days. There is no unifying hypothesis as to the pathogenesis of psoriasis, but several immune abnormalities have been described, suggesting that at the very least the immune system makes a contribution. The pathology of the skin disease shows that early lesions are associated with peri-vessel dermal infiltrates of lymphocytes and mononuclear phagocytes. Neutrophils may appear within the epidermis to create micro-abscesses and can occasionally be seen leaving the vessels in the dermal peri-vascular unit. Epidermal hyperplasia is a characteristic feature and with the excessive keratinisation this gives rise to the micro- and macroscopic features of the skin. Even in uninvolved skin, cell cycling of keratinocytes may be abnormal. Any unifying hypothesis regarding the pathogenesis of psoriasis must combine the characteristic infiltrate, containing lymphocytes in the early lesions followed by neutrophils, with the apparent dysregulation of the keratinocyte life cycle.

Neutrophils in psoriasis. Neutrophils are a relatively late feature of psoriatic skin lesions. There is evidence that neutrophils are activated within the blood and skin of psoriatic patients, and mediators found within diseased skin (C5a, leukotriene B$_4$, IL-8) are likely to be responsible for this. Interestingly, application of chemotactic factors to uninvolved skin in psoriatic patients induces microabscesses but not the typical skin lesions, suggesting that they contribute to persistence of the disease but are not primary factors.

Lymphocytes in psoriasis. As we have seen, in normal skin the great majority of T cells reside in the dermis, and most of these are in the dermal peri-vascular units. The CD4:CD8 ratio amongst these cells is one, and over 80% of the resident cells are activated. In psoriasis, certain changes to these populations of T lymphocytes occur. A T lymphocyte infiltration is seen that is predominantly CD4$^+$, and the CD4:CD8 ratio in psoriatic skin exceeds that in the patient's blood. This implies a selective accumulation, and E-selectin appears to act as a skin-related vascular addressin that preferentially attracts T lymphocytes of the memory phenotype, although the T cell ligand is not yet known. But perhaps the strongest evidence that these activated CD4$^+$ T cells are involved in the pathogenesis of psoriasis comes from the identity of two of the most potent antipsoriatic drugs — cyclosporin A and tacrolimus — both being powerful immunosuppressive agents that act by inhibition of T cell activation.

Antigen specificity. If these findings are accepted as strong evidence that activated CD4$^+$ memory T lymphocytes initiate/perpetuate the disease, two questions arise. What are the antigens against which the T cells are sensitised and how does their response result in profound changes in keratinocyte function? Little is known of the antigen specificity of skin T cells in psoriasis, but blood T cells from psoriatic patients proliferate to β-haemolytic streptococcal antigens, one of the better defined disease triggers, and there is cross-reactivity between antigens from these bacteria and human skin components. Once activated, CD4$^+$ T cells could release a variety of cytokines that have been shown to act

Psoriatic skin

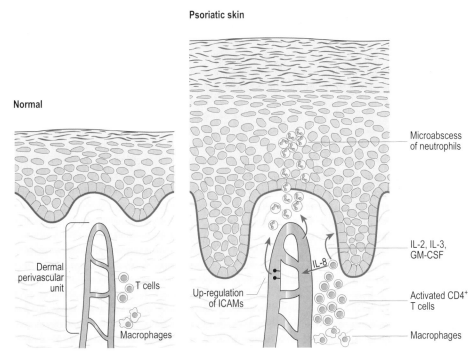

Fig. 17.8 **Possible immune mechanisms in the pathogenesis of psoriasis.**

on keratinocytes to induce stimulation in vitro (IL-2, IL-3, GM-CSF) (Fig. 17.8).

VITILIGO

Complete loss of skin pigment (depigmentation) in a patchy distribution is a common disorder, of which the best known cause is **vitiligo**. It is an acquired disorder, and the depigmentation results from destruction of melanocytes in the skin, which produce the pigment melanin. Affected patches appear totally white, whatever the racial origin, and hair affected typically grows white. Vitiligo is common, with an estimated incidence of up to 1%. Both sexes may be affected and, in a third of cases, there is a family history. The consensus view on the aetiology of vitiligo is that it is an autoimmune disease in which the immune system damages melanocytes irreparably. The evidence for this derives from:

- an association between vitiligo and the presence of other autoimmune disorders, notably thyroiditis, type 1 diabetes, pernicious anaemia and adrenal insufficiency; vitiligo is commonly found in patients with autoimmune polyglandular syndromes
- autoantibodies to pigmented human melanocytes are detectable in the circulation of a high proportion of patients (see below)
- CD4⁺ T cells bearing activation markers are seen in skin biopsies taken at the margins of new lesions
- the condition can be alleviated by topical use of glucocorticosteroids.

Vitiligo has a mixed prognosis. In some it may be very patchy and even resolve spontaneously. In others it is progressive; the social and psychological conse-quences, particularly in racially dark-skinned patients, can be devastating.

Recently, the nature of the molecular target of the antimelanocyte autoantibodies was identified. Working on the 'hunch' that the targets could be proteins involved in the synthesis or export of melanin, since this is the distinguishing feature of the target cells, a research group generated one of these molecules, tyrosinase, in a recombinant form. These workers were able to demonstrate antityrosinase autoantibodies in 77% of patients with vitiligo, but none of their controls. This finding may offer some direction for future attempts to stop the chronic autoimmune destruction of melanocytes.

Skin diseases

- In the blistering disorders, a variety of autoantibodies directed against components involved in cell adhesion, appear to have pathogenic roles.
- In several of the blistering disorders, an association with HLA genotypes in seen.
- Dermatitis herpetiformis is associated with pathology of the gastrointestinal tract (coeliac disease).
- In psoriasis, T lymphocyte recruitment and activation in the skin appears to be a key component in the dysregulation of keratinocyte function, which is central to the disease.
- In vitiligo anti-melanocyte autoantibodies indicate an autoimmune attack on melanocytes resulting in a loss of pigment. Tyrosinase, an enzyme involved in the synthesis and export of melanin, has been implicated as a target antigen.

The **blood–brain barrier** is an ill-defined obstacle, originally invoked to account for differences in penetration of proteins, salts and drugs into the CNS. It applies equally to immunological proteins, such as immunoglobulin, and may also be an effective barrier to cell-mediated responses. Therefore, the extent to which primary brain immune responses recruit immune effector cells from the periphery, and the extent to which inflammatory processes in the periphery affect primary brain immune responses are controversial. In no disease process is this controversy more hotly debated than in **multiple sclerosis**.

IMMUNE-MEDIATED DEMYELINATING SYNDROMES

MULTIPLE SCLEROSIS

Multiple sclerosis (MS) is a disease of unknown aetiology, characterised by numerous, circumscribed areas of demyelination within the brain and spinal cord. It is, therefore, one of the demyelinating diseases, a group of disorders in which loss of myelin occurs without axonal degeneration. The combination of intact axons and some capacity for myelin regeneration gives rise in approximately two thirds of patients to a repeated relapsing and remitting disease course, but with a general accumulation of disability over several years. In the remaining one third, the disease is slowly progressive. Considerable evidence has been amassed to suggest that MS is an autoimmune disease, arising on a distinct genetic background and influenced strongly by environmental factors.

MS is a common disorder, with a prevalence in the general population in Western Europe and the USA approaching 1 in 1000. The age of onset is usually between 10 and 60 years, with the median age between 25 and 30 years. It is more common amongst women, with estimates of the female:male ratio ranging between 2:1 and 7:1. The epidemiology of MS is fascinating. The incidence is unevenly distributed within the same country and appears to be related to latitude, with higher numbers affected in populations nearer the poles. Therefore, in the southern states of the North American continent the prevalence of MS is 0.1 per 1000, rising to 1.3 per 1000 in northern Canada. Some have argued that these differences could relate to ethnic and, therefore, genetic differences between populations. Careful studies in Australia, however, where northern and southern populations have a similar ethnic composition, show the same relationship between disease incidence and latitude, though in this case MS is more common in the southern areas. In the UK, the prevalence is at its highest in Scotland, where cases number up to 3 per 1000. The relationship between latitude and risk of MS argues for an environmental agent, possibly a virus prevalent in temperate regions, acting as an important trigger for the disease. Moreover, the

fact that the disease incidence peaks during the third decade argues for the main disease triggers operating during adolescence. Again, careful epidemiological studies have strengthened this concept. It appears, for example, that individuals migrating from a birthplace of relative high risk to one of low risk of MS, and vice versa, carry their level of disease susceptibility with them as long as they travel after the age of 15 years. In contrast, migration before the age of 15 incurs the level of susceptibility of the new environment.

What could the environmental factors be? Most would argue for a transmissible virus as one of the major triggers for the disease, although no single agent stands out. Common virus infections (e.g. measles, mumps, rubella) tend to affect MS patients at later ages than is typical; MS prevalence is higher in higher socioeconomic groups, who may be less likely to encounter

---

Lessons from an epidemiological study of the Faroe Islands

There have been several reports of epidemic outbreaks of MS, but none more convincing and intriguing than that in the Faroe Islands, a volcanic group in the north Atlantic Ocean and part of the state of Denmark. Between 1900 and the outbreak of the Second World War in 1939, there had been only two reported cases of MS amongst the 45 000 or so islanders. Both individuals affected had spent 3 or more years on mainland Denmark, where there is a high incidence of MS, some years prior to the onset of symptoms. However, between 1940 and 1979, 25 cases of MS were reported in islanders who were native born and had never lived anywhere else, and a further nine cases in islanders who had lived abroad for less than 2 years. What could have happened on the island during the war years to cause such a dramatic increase in incidence, which has now declined?

The answer appears to lie in the British Forces' occupation of the Faroe islands, which began on 13 April 1940 and ended 5 years later. At its peak, the British garrison had some 4000 soldiers in it, billeted on some 21 sites scattered throughout the islands. Of the 32 cases of MS occurring amongst the islanders over the next 40 years, only three occurred on sites where there were no troops, and only four occupation sites did not have a single case of MS on them.

This might argue for direct transmission of an agent from patient to patient. However, many studies have shown that the incidence of MS amongst spouses of affected patients is the same as in the background population, and the British Forces are unlikely to have contained large numbers of troops with significant neurological disease (i.e. potential carriers). What the Faroe Islanders' experience suggests is that the British Forces brought with them a transmissible agent not indigenous to the population but which is an important trigger in the train of events that leads to MS.

common viruses until secondary school or university; and MS may occur in mini-epidemics in sheltered island populations (see box: 'Lessons from an epidemiological study of the Faroe Islands'). Infectious agents could also be important in disease exacerbations. Clinical observations indicate that relapses frequently follow upper respiratory tract infections.

Genetic factors are also important in susceptibility to MS. Caucasians are much more vulnerable than African blacks, American Indians (mongolians) and some groups of mongoloid Asians, in whom the disease is extremely rare. Twin and HLA studies in MS have identified similar trends to those in type 1 diabetes (see p. 187), in that concordance for the disease is approximately 2.5% between dizygotic and 26% between monozygotic twins, who carry a relative risk for the disease of 3–400 times that of the background population. Interestingly, though, some 70% of unaffected monozygotic twins of MS patients will have CNS lesions typical of MS detectable by magnetic resonance imaging (see below), implying that subclinical demyelination could occur on a wider scale. Some 50–70% of patients with MS have the serologically defined *HLA-DR2* allele (present in 20–30% of the normal population), and in a recent study of Norwegian patients, 98% carried one of several *HLA-DQB1* genes that give rise to a common amino acid sequence at positions 23–31 amongst the β-pleated sheets on the floor of the antigen-binding groove of HLA-DQ. This argues strongly that the binding of an antigenic peptide at this site on the DQ molecule is critical to the development of the disease.

Pathology

The typical pathological lesion of MS is a perivenous inflammatory infiltrate in the peri-ventricular white matter, composed of $CD4^+$ and $CD8^+$ T lymphocytes, B lymphocytes, plasma cells and macrophages. Most frequently affected regions of the CNS are the cerebrum, brain stem, spinal cord and optic nerve. Predominant in the infiltrate is the T lymphocyte, with $CD4^+$ T lymphocytes in the majority in early lesions and $CD8^+$ T lymphocytes in the later stages. Myelin and oligodendrocytes are destroyed and, depending on the age of the lesion, there may be variable evidence of remyelination. There is localised oedema, and old lesions show evidence of gliosis (i.e. expansion of glial cells). Demyelination appears to be closely related to the presence of macrophages, and at the sites of these lesions macrophages are actively endocytosing myelin, often through interaction between surface Fc receptors and IgG attached to the sphingolipid. MHC class I molecule expression is present on most cells, and class II molecules are expressed on microglia, B cells, macrophages and astrocytes in the lesions and on the surrounding endothelium. Interferon-γ is present in the CSF in MS patients and may be of importance in enhancing class II MHC expression. The ensuing inflammatory process appears to result in local break-

down of the blood–brain protein barrier, since complement proteins and immunoglobulins are found extensively in active lesions.

The picture is painted of a cell-mediated immune process, probably orchestrated by $CD4^+$ T lymphocytes (Fig. 18.2). The target is the oligodendrocyte or its important product myelin. Macrophages may be the final effectors of damage or may just be clearing the debris. The process could be initiated from within the CNS, but evidence of the breakdown of the blood–brain barrier also suggests that exacerbations could be secondary to peripheral immune events.

Pathogenesis and immunological features

Apart from the immunological features in the CNS lesions, there are immune abnormalities in the cerebrospinal fluid (CSF), which bathes the CNS, and in the peripheral blood. The questions that need to be addressed in order to understand the pathogenesis of MS are what sensitises and triggers the T lymphocytes to become involved, the extent of the role of other immune effectors and which element delivers the *coup de grâce* to the oligodendrocyte. In addition, there needs to be some understanding of what factors are involved in the generation of exacerbations of the disease. This would seem to be an important determining factor in the clinical outcome, and the twin studies alluded to above suggest that asymptomatic MS lesions may be a common phenomenon.

In terms of the factors involved in the initiation of CNS lesions, T lymphocyte responses in the peripheral blood and CSF have been studied extensively using two main approaches: assays detecting proliferation of lymphocytes to putative autoantigens, and cloning from reactive cells to study TCR usage, antigenic epitopes and the HLA restriction elements. These approaches tend to examine $CD4^+$ T lymphocyte responses predominantly. One of the major trends in these studies has been to follow up findings initially made in the animal model of MS known as experimental allergic encephalomyelitis (EAE; see p. 122 and box: 'The experimental allergic encephalomyelitis model of MS').

Evidence that there are $CD4^+$ T lymphocytes in the peripheral blood and in the CSF that react with myelin basic protein (MBP) and proteolipid protein (PLP), the two main components of myelin, have been obtained through proliferation assays and T lymphocyte cloning studies. Although there is a slightly higher level of T lymphocyte proliferation to MBP in MS patients compared with controls, the frequency of responding cells has been shown to be similar in both groups; approximately 1 in 10^6 lymphocytes respond by proliferation when incubated with MBP. There are two main T lymphocyte epitopes in the centre of the MBP molecule, between amino acids 84 and 102, and 143 and 168. HLA-DR2 molecules appear to be capable of presenting both of these and other MBP peptides. In contrast with the EAE model, there is limited evidence that TCR variable chain usage is restricted in T lymphocyte

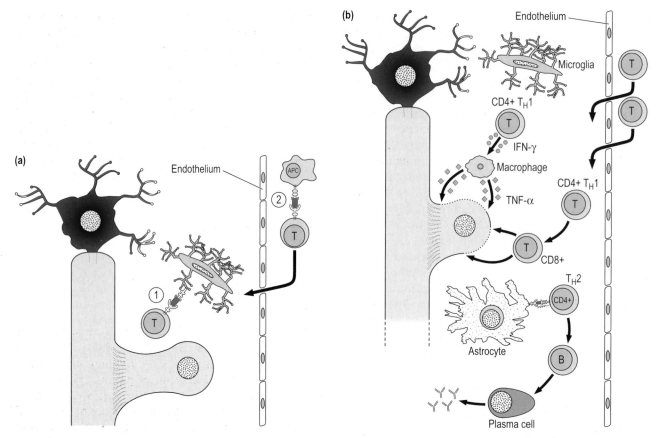

Fig. 18.2 **Demyelination in MS.**
(a) Mechanism of induction of demyelination. An antigen is presented to T lymphocytes. The peptide is possibly derived from a primary CNS autoantigen or from an infecting agent, but has epitopes cross-reactive with myelin components. The activation of these autoreactive T lymphocytes may take place within the CNS (1), or is an external event (2) followed by migration through the brain endothelium. (b) Mechanisms of perpetuation of demyelinating plaques. Autoantigen-sensitised CD4⁺ T_H1 cells arriving from the peripheral blood stimulate CD8⁺ cytotoxic T lymphocytes or macrophages, resulting in damage to oligodendrocytes and myelin by direct cytotoxicity or through cytokines such as TNF-α. A range of myelin-derived peptides are presented by microglia and macrophages. Astrocytes, with their phagocytic properties and the capacity to express class II MHC molecules, may also become involved in antigen processing and presentation. Clones of B lymphocytes within the CNS may become activated as bystanders, producing the oligoclonal immunglobulin bands seen in the CSF.

The experimental allergic encephalomyelitis model of MS

Experimental allergic encephalomyelitis (EAE) is induced by intravenous injection of constituents of brain, either from the same or another species. The inducing antigens may be crude brain homogenate, myelin sheath, myelin basic protein (MBP), myelin proteolipid protein (PLP) or shorter peptides from these myelin proteins. Within 2–3 weeks, the animals become lethargic, paralysed and lose sphincter control. In some immunising regimens in some strains, the disease has a relapsing remitting course, making it a particularly appropriate model for MS. The CNS pathological lesion in the animals is almost identical to that in MS. T lymphocytes, which proliferate when cultured with MBP or PLP, arise in the peripheral blood during the development of EAE and are capable of transferring the disease to unaffected animals. In one mouse strain, restriction of the T lymphocyte receptor usage of these cells, to the V_β8.1 chain, has been reported. Equally, the epitopes on the MBP and PLP

molecules that are recognised are highly restricted. The disease is inducible in certain strains of mice, rats and guinea-pigs, with one of the determining factors in susceptibility being the MHC type. Therefore, EAE has the features of an autoimmune disease with well-defined autoantigens presented by a restricted range of MHC molecules to activated clones of T lymphocytes with a restricted T lymphocyte receptor repertoire. Manipulation of any of these features can lead to permanent recovery from the demyelination; for example, targeting the V_β8.1-positive T lymphocytes with a specific monoclonal antibody or giving peptides that occupy and block the MHC-binding site. The question of great importance is whether the immunological features of this model, induced by injection of auto-antigen in the periphery, fit with those of the spontaneous human disease. Hence the search in MS for T lymphocyte reactivity, restriction of antigenic epitopes, T lymphocyte receptor usage and HLA restriction.

responses in MS. For example, even when clones reacting with a particular MBP epitope (e.g. amino acids 84–102) are generated from patients with MS, several different V_β genes may be used. If MBP-reactive T lymphocyte clones are present at the same frequency in patients and controls, do not have absolute requirements for particular HLA molecule presentation or antigenic epitopes, and do not use a distinctive set of variable TCR genes, can we still assume that the T lymphocyte response is critical to the development of the disease?

It seems probable that we can. One possibility to account for the existence of MBP-reactive T lymphocytes in healthy individuals without evidence of demyelination is that these T lymphocytes need to become activated in order to become pathogenic. Activation of the T lymphocytes not only enables clonal expansion and recruitment of other lymphocytes and macrophages, but is also followed by the expression of adhesion molecules which will be important in the ability of circulating MBP-reactive T lymphocytes in the periphery to gain access to the CNS. Using a new assay that detects antigen-reactive *activated* T lymphocytes, it has been shown that the circulating MBP-reactive T lymphocytes in MS patients are activated; those in healthy controls are not. The requirement for autoreactive T lymphocytes to become activated in order to become involved in an autoimmune disease process is likely to be a general rule applicable to other autoimmune disorders, such as type 1 diabetes.

Can all of these strands of evidence be brought into a single, tangible theory of the pathogenesis of MS? The epidemiology and genetics argues for a virus; the immunology and animal data indicate sensitisation against myelin components as being a critical feature. Bringing these together is evidence to support the possibility that a virus, acting through the mechanism of molecular mimicry, could induce an autoimmune response in the CNS, since several close homologies exist between short viral peptide sequences (e.g. measles, rubella and varicella) and myelin. Despite the attraction of this theory, viruses have not been demonstrable in the CSF or in MS lesions, and injection of homogenates of affected brain into primates does not induce disease. Myelin and oligodendrocyte damage is induced by TNF-α in vitro, lending support to the argument that a T_H1 lymphocyte response, with macrophage activation, is an important component of the pathogenesis of MS. As for the exacerbations, these appear to follow 'viral illnesses' in up to 80% of cases. The resulting brief inflammatory process could give rise to cytokine release with enhanced activation of autoreactive T lymphocytes and damage to the brain endothelium, allowing sensitised T lymphocytes access to their targets.

Clinical features

The initial clinical picture in patients presenting with MS is variable. Pyramidal tract features such as weak-

ness and hyper-reflexia are common, and ataxia caused by cerebellar involvement may also be seen. When the brain stem is affected, there may be cranial nerve involvement. Blurred vision is also a frequent presenting symptom, indicating optic neuritis. Optic neuritis may also occur as a single entity, without evidence of dissemination of the demyelination, but it is estimated that 50–80% of such patients will ultimately develop MS. In younger patients, the relapsing remitting course is more typical. In patients presenting in late middle age, however, it may be possible to elicit a longer history of neurological disturbance.

The diagnosis of MS, at one time made on essentially clinical grounds, can now be supported by several investigations:

1. measurement of IgG levels in CSF
2. CSF electrophoresis for oligoclonal bands
3. visual evoked potentials
4. magnetic resonance imaging.

Examination of the CSF reveals an increased number of cells, predominantly lymphocytes, though this is not diagnostic. IgG levels in the CSF are modestly raised in MS. This could be the result of plasma cell secretion within the CNS, or in the periphery. To differentiate these two, the CSF IgG:albumin ratio can be compared with that in serum, since albumin is not synthesised in the CNS. A rise in the IgG:albumin ratio in CSF is a reasonably specific but not very sensitive test for MS. In contrast, CSF electrophoresis reveals **oligoclonal bands** in some 80–90% of MS patients (Fig. 18.3). Oligoclonal bands are not diagnostic of MS, since they may be seen transiently in other CNS inflammatory conditions (e.g. post-infectious encephalomyelitis), but

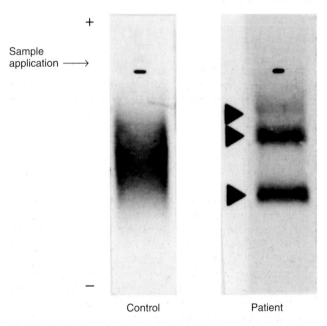

Fig. 18.3 **Electrophoresis of cerebrospinal fluid from a healthy control and a patient with multiple sclerosis.**
In the control, immunoglobulins are diffusely stained, indicating polyclonality. In the patient, at least 3 discrete oligoclonal bands can be seen, indicating synthesis of immunoglobulins within the CNS by a small number of B cell clones. (Courtesy of Dr J. P. Frankel).

persistence of the bands is a typical feature of this re-lapsing/remitting demyelinating disease. Despite intensive research, it is still not clear against what the IgG in the bands is directed. Antimyelin antibodies form a small proportion (5%) and some 75% of MS patients have raised CSF titres of anti-measles antibody. The slowing of transmission of **visual evoked potentials** demonstrates the impairment of nerve function typically associated with demyelination. A relatively new, but well-established examination for MS is the **magnetic resonance image** (MRI), which demonstrates plaques of demyelination, usually in several sites (Fig 18.4).

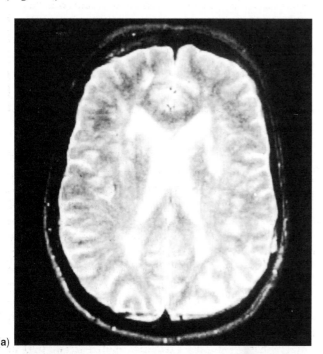

(a)

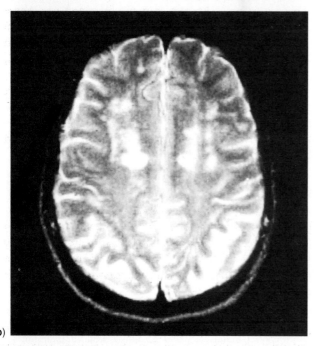

(b)

Fig. 18.4 **Magnetic resonance images of the brain of a patient with MS, showing the typical peri-ventricular plaques of demyelination.**
The plaques appear as white regions. (Courtesy of Dr E. J. Evanson)

Treatment

There is no specific therapy for MS and no entirely satisfactory non-specific therapy. The relapsing and remitting nature of the symptoms and signs has meant that clinical trials have often been difficult to perform and interpret. MS is a disease in which the requirements for randomisation, placebo and blindness of both patients and physicians to the treatment could not be greater. Intravenous corticosteroids may reduce the severity of acute exacerbations and speed their resolution, without having any effect on the course of the disease. In recent years, therapy with interferon β_1b (a synthetic analogue of IFN-β) has shown considerable promise in clinical trials. A reduction in the frequency of exacerbations of some 30% seems to be achieved, and the treatment is well tolerated. There does not appear to be any effect on the presence of brain lesions detected by MRI, and cost may be a proscriptive factor (some $10 000 per patient per year), although the therapy could be restricted and may become cheaper as it is used more widely.

Over the next few years, it is likely that immune-based therapies, shown to be effective in the EAE animal model of MS, will undergo clinical trials, as a recent report on the effectiveness of inducing oral tolerance to MBP suggests (see box: 'Induction of oral tolerance in the treatment of MS').

ACUTE DISSEMINATED ENCEPHALOMYELITIS

Acute disseminated encephalomyelitis (ADEM) is a rare disorder associated with extensive, central, perivenous demyelination occurring during or closely following an infection or vaccination.

Pathology

In fatal cases (up to 25%) post-mortem analyses reveal a swollen and congested brain and spinal cord. There is an intense peri-vascular inflammatory cell infiltrate, and at these sites there is extensive demyelination. There is some evidence that neutrophils predominate in early lesions and that macrophages and lymphocytes are dominant thereafter, with a majority of the lymphocytes being CD8+.

Pathogenesis and immunological features

Little is known about the nature of the immune response in ADEM. Typically the illness follows infection with viruses (e.g. rubella, measles), or vaccination against infectious agents (e.g. rabies), and, therefore, it is assumed that cross-reactivity occurs against myelin components. In many cases, ADEM resembles the EAE syndrome induced in animals (see the box on p. 246) in which the neurological disease is frequently monophasic rather than relapsing and remitting.

Clinical features

Patients present with a rapid (a few days) onset of fever, headache, declining level of consciousness and

Induction of oral tolerance in the treatment of MS

One approach to immune-based therapy in the autoimmune diseases is attempting to induce tolerance to autoantigens by administering them orally. The fact that antigens given by the oral route tend to be ignored by the immune system is presumed to be a natural mechanism to prevent continuous reactivity to food antigens from plants and animals. If this process leading to tolerance can be harnessed for autoantigens, a relatively painless therapy can be envisaged. Encouraged by the beneficial effects of administering autoantigens orally in animal models (e.g. MBP in EAE, insulin in diabetes, collagen in arthritis and retinal S-antigen in uveitis), a group in Boston recently organised a double-blind pilot trial of oral tolerisation in 30 patients with MS, randomised to receive 300 mg bovine myelin daily (which contains both MBP and PLP) or placebo, over a 1 year period. 12 of the placebo versus six of the myelin-treated group had at least one major disease exacerbation. These results give some encouragement for the future use of this therapy and there appeared to be no evidence of toxicity or side effects.

The mechanism of oral induction of tolerance to autoantigens is not clear. In the MS study, the frequency of MBP-reactive T lymphocytes in the myelin-treated group (between 0.1 and 1 per million cells) decreased significantly, but it remained static in the placebo-treated group. This reduction could lead to a fall in T lymphocyte infiltration and inflammation within the CNS. One other possible mechanism is that suppressive cytokines are secreted in response to antigens administered via the oral route. There is some evidence from animal models, for example, that TGF-β release plays a part in suppressing autoreactive T lymphocyte responses.

---

occasional focal signs such as convulsions, optic neuritis, cranial nerve palsies and transverse myelitis. CSF analysis reveals no organisms but a moderate lymphocytosis. Recovery is the rule, and the frequency and severity of sequelae (weakness, mental retardation in children) relate to the severity of the disease at presentation. One of the key questions that remains unanswered is whether patients with ADEM have a higher risk of proceeding to MS.

Demyelinating syndromes

- Multiple sclerosis is a demyelinating disease that results from a subtle interplay of genetic (e.g. *HLA-DR2*) and environmental factors (e.g. a virus).
- The pathological lesion is one of plaques of CNS demyelination, infiltrated by T lymphocytes and with evidence of macrophages actively phagocytosing the myelin sheath.
- The presence of activated T lymphocytes in the peripheral blood and CNS that recognise components of myelin suggests that these cells initiate and/or perpetuate the CNS lesions.
- A rare syndrome of monophasic demyelination, ADEM, is probably immune mediated but resolves without evolving into a chronic autoimmune disease.

THE GUILLAIN–BARRÉ SYNDROME

The Guillain–Barré syndrome (GBS) is an inflammatory peripheral polyneuropathy named after the two French Army neurologists who linked clinical and CSF findings in the early part of this century. It is preceded by a viral-like illness in some 60–80% of patients and has an acute onset, beginning with paraesthesiae affecting the toes and finger tips, and evolving into a global, symmetrical, motor neuropathy with weakness of the legs and subsequently of the muscles of the arms, face and pharynx. Frequently there is also some deep muscle pain, but in general, sensory nerve loss is rare. The severity varies from mild weakness to quadriplegia and the need for supported mechanical ventilation for several months. The cause is unknown, but the consensus view is that there is immune system involvement in the destruction of myelin and nerve axons.

GBS has an annual incidence of 0.5–2/100 000 of the population. Although it may affect any age, there are two peaks of incidence, at 16–25 years and 45–60 years of age, and a slight male preponderance. No convincing genetic associations have been identified, and the disease has an essentially sporadic nature.

Despite advances in the treatment of GBS, most notably in the area of cardiorespiratory support, there is still a significant mortality, and refinement of immune-based interventions introduced in recent years should have some impact on this.

Pathology

A mononuclear cell infiltration, comprising lymphocytes and macrophages, is well established within days of the onset of symptoms. Such lesions are extremely unusual in the CNS, and signs of CNS involvement are rare. There is patchy myelin destruction and in some cases axonal destruction.

Pathogenesis and immunological features

Potential candidate antigens in this immune response are only beginning to be characterised, and the mechanism of damage remains unclear.

Evidence of immune mechanisms in the pathogenesis of GBS are:

- mononuclear cell infiltration of affected peripheral nerves
- antibodies to myelin components
- peripheral T lymphocyte activation
- two animal models in which T lymphocytes and antibody, respectively, may transfer disease
- the clinical efficacy of plasma exchange and intravenous immunoglobulin (p. 312).

The targets and prevalence of antimyelin antibodies in GBS are currently the focus of much research effort. The major pathogenic element to the disease is damage to the myelin sheath around peripheral nerves, which is generated by Schwann cells. Myelin, or the Schwann cells themselves, could be the targets of the immune attack. There are several candidate target antigens.

Animal models of Guillain–Barré syndrome

There are two main animal models of GBS, which offer quite different perspectives on the disease. In one, rats and mice immunised with the P_2 myelin protein develop a flaccid quadriplegia, from which there is recovery after 1–2 weeks. The animal disease can be transferred into virgin syngeneic recipients by T lymphocytes; the critical epitope on the P_2 molecule capable of inducing the neuropathy is between amino acids 53 and 78. There has been some controversy as to how the P_2-activated T lymphocytes mediate nerve damage and which cells in the peripheral nervous system present antigen, with some groups suggesting that the Schwann cell is important in APC function. This has been elegantly resolved in a series of experiments using the 'P_2' animal model established in Lewis rats. T lymphocytes from this strain are unable to transfer the disease to another rat strain, DA, because of class II MHC incompatibility. However, if the recipient DA rats are irradiated to disable bone marrow function and then reconstituted with bone marrow from the F1 generation animals of a Lewis × DA cross, the disease is tranferrable using Lewis-derived T lymphocytes. This implies that bone marrow-derived APCs bearing Lewis rat class II MHC molecules emanate from the transplanted bone marrow to present antigen to the pathogenic T lymphocytes, and it confirms that cells of the monocyte/macrophage lineage are necessary for the induction of the nerve damage.

The second main animal model of GBS is induced in rabbits by injection of galactocerebroside, with resulting quadriplegia. Serum from the affected rabbits is able to transfer the disease into rats.

These animal models have directed research into the pathogenesis of GBS towards these two antigens, in much the same way that MBP- and PLP-induced EAE has in MS. It would appear, however, that immune reactivity to P_2 and galactocerebroside is more difficult to pinpoint in GBS.

Two of these, the **P_2 protein** component of myelin and **galactocerebroside** are implicated because of a clear role in animal models of inflammatory polyneuropathy (see box: 'Animal models of Guillain–Barré syndrome'). Evidence of T lymphocyte reactivity to any of these in humans is poor, with only one report of proliferative responses to P_2, and antibodies to P_2 and galactocerebroside have not been detectable in GBS. Other potential autoantigens include gangliosides, which are important components of lipid membranes particularly in the nervous system. Antibodies to the **ganglioside LM_1**, the major ganglioside in peripheral nerve myelin, are present in approximately 50% of patients with GBS, and antibodies to **sulphatide**, the major acidic glycosphingolipid in myelin, in 65%.

Several events appear to be capable of triggering GBS:

- viral-like illness in 60–70%
- immunisation in 5%
- pregnancy
- surgical procedure
- lymphoma.

The main viruses involved are cytomegalovirus and Epstein–Barr virus. One well-documented outbreak of GBS in 1976 following immunisation with an influenza vaccine has suggested that sporadic cases could follow immunisation, a recent history of which is found in 5% of patients. In pregnancy, GBS may occur in the third trimester, and the fact that the unborn fetus is not affected suggests that antibody-mediated myelin damage is not a feature of this form. A recent study has indicated that 38% of GBS patients have circulating antibody to the intestinal pathogen *Campylobacter jejuni*, and a cross-reactivity between the target of these antibodies and peripheral nerve myelin components, such as gangliosides, has been postulated but requires confirmation.

The controversy over the pathogenesis of GBS is clearly being fuelled by new findings. A recent study has found elevated levels of intact membrane attack complexes (C5b6789) of the terminal complement pathway, adding support to the role of antibody to myelin in nerve damage. Levels of the C5b6789 complex reached a peak on the 4th day after admission to hospital and declined thereafter, to become undetectable by 1 month. A mechanism of antibody- and complement-mediated nerve damage (Fig. 18.5) would also explain why intravenous immunoglobulin is effective in the disease since it is known to 'mop up' complement components and reduce their availability to pathogenic antibodies.

Clinical features

The diagnosis of GBS is essentially clinical. None of the autoantibodies described has yet acquired clinical usefulness. Protein levels in the CSF are raised, characteristically without the presence of cells; rarely there may be oligoclonal bands that are transient. The autonomic nervous system may be affected, leading to bradycardia and the need for endocardial pacing. In a

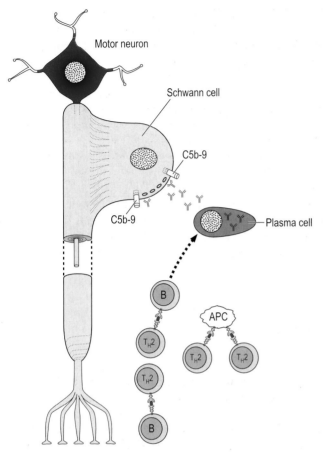

Fig. 18.5 A putative mechanism of immune pathogenesis in Guillain–Barré syndrome.
T$_H$2 lymphocytes are activated in response to antigens presented by APCs within the peripheral nerve. The nature of this antigen, and whether it is an autoantigen or a component of a microorganism mimicking one, is not known. The B lymphocytes activated as a result recognise myelin components (e.g. ganglioside LM$_1$, sulphatide) and recruit complement, with resulting nerve damage.

Table 18.1 **Autoantibody targets in immune-mediated neuropathies**

Disorder	Target antigen	Prevalence
Guillain–Barré syndrome	Peripheral nerve myelin components (e.g. ganglioside LM$_1$, sulphatide)	Up to 100%
Amyotrophic lateral sclerosis	Ganglioside GM$_1$	20%
Paraprotein-associated polyneuropathy	Myelin-associated glycoprotein (MAG)	Up to 50%
Paraneoplastic subacute sensory neuropathy	Hu	Unknown
Paraneoplastic cerebellar degeneration	Purkinje cells	Unknown

of MND, termed **amyotrophic lateral sclerosis** (ALS), initially tends to affect the cervical spinal cord alone and, therefore, has no cranial nerve signs but does show a combination of lower motor neuron signs in the upper limbs and upper motor neuron deficit in the upper and lower limbs. In ALS, antibodies to the ganglioside GM$_1$ have been detected.

In another group of patients, demyelinating polyneuropathy is associated with the presence of a paraprotein, without paresis of the other immunoglobulin classes (a condition termed **monoclonal gammopathy of undetermined significance** MGUS; see p. 298). In 50% of patients with neuropathy associated with MGUS, the IgM paraproteins are directed against a neuronal target, **myelin-associated glycoprotein** (anti-MAG) and the serum from these patients is able to transfer nerve damage passively to animals.

Two other disorders worthy of mention are associated with carcinomas. One is **paraneoplastic sensory neuropathy**, associated with small cell cancer of the lung. Patients with this complication have antibodies to an antigen termed **Hu**, which has a molecular mass of 35–40 kDa and is thought to be a protein involved in neurogenesis and neuronal maintenance. The other is paraneoplastic cerebellar degeneration, associated with antibodies to the Purkinje cells in the cerebellum.

typical case, the full syndrome takes some 4 weeks to develop, followed by a plateau of symptoms and neurological deficit lasting up to 1 month, and then recovery, which takes a median of some 9 months. In 30% of patients, the syndrome is sufficiently severe that elective ventilation is undertaken. Mortality in some series is up to 8% and while some 70–80% of patients show an almost complete recovery, 20–30% of surviving patients have a significant neurological deficit.

OTHER IMMUNE-MEDIATED INFLAMMATORY POLYNEUROPATHIES

Several other neuropathies, much less common than the Guillain–Barré syndrome, have features that suggest an immune component in the development of nerve damage (Table 18.1). Autoantibodies have been searched for in **motor neuron disease** (MND), a progressive degenerative disease of unknown aetiology affecting upper and lower motor neurons. One variant

Guillain–Barré syndrome and other immune-mediated neuropathies

- Guillain–Barré syndrome is often preceded by a viral-like illness; the cause is unknown but myelin and nerve axons are destroyed.
- GBS may require cardiorespiratory support and carries a significant mortality risk.
- Other neuropathies may have immune components involved in nerve damage and different target antigens have been proposed.

MYASTHENIC SYNDROMES

Myasthenia is defined as a fatiguable weakness of striated muscle. It is the result of a defect of transmission of impulses from nerve to muscle at the neuromuscular junction (NMJ). The normal anatomy and physiology of the NMJ is shown in Figure 18.6. There are two clearly defined autoimmune disorders in which synaptic transmission at the NMJ is interfered with by an antibody-dependent mechanism. In **myasthenia gravis** (MG), an autoantibody is generated against the **acetylcholine receptor** (AChR), on the post-synaptic membrane. In the **Lambert–Eaton myasthenic syndrome** (LEMS), an autoantibody interferes with the pre-synaptic process of acetylcholine release by binding to voltage-gated calcium channels (VGCC). Of great interest in the pathogenesis of these disorders are the roles of the thymus and of neoplasia: MG is associated with thymic hyperplasia and occasionally thymic neoplasia, whilst LEMS typically occurs in association with a small cell carcinoma of the lung.

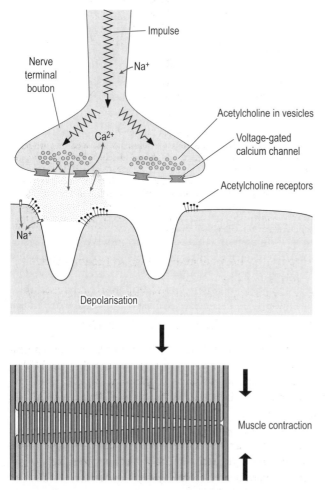

Fig. 18.6 **The ultrastructure of the neuromuscular junction.** The depolarising action potential arriving in the nerve terminal causes voltage-gated calcium channels to open, with movement of acetylcholine-containing vesicles to the pre-synaptic membrane and release of the neurotransmitter into the synaptic cleft. Binding of acetylcholine to its receptor on the crests of the post-synaptic clefts causes opening of Na^+ channels and depolarisation of the muscle fibre, with subsequent contraction.

MYASTHENIA GRAVIS

The characteristic symptom of MG is muscle weakness arising with repeated usage. Any striated muscle may be affected, but those served by the cranial nerves, and especially the eye muscles, are affected in over 50% of patients. Patients often present after stressful events — infection or anaesthesia — with weakness that worsens as the day progresses, or after repeated usage of particular muscles. The characteristic laboratory finding is of a circulating antibody to the AChR, detectable in nearly 90% of patients. The prevalence of MG appears consistent throughout the world, at around 5–10 cases per 100 000 of the population.

Although there is an overall sexual bias in favour of women by 2 to 1 and the disease may occur at any age, distinctive clinical subgroups emerge when large numbers of patients are pooled for analysis. In 'classical' MG, which accounts for 55% of patients and occurs between adolescence and the 20s, females predominate. In Caucasians, this group also has an excess of the serologically defined HLA alleles *B8 DR3*, and histological analysis of the thymus typically reveals hyperplasia. In another subgroup (20% of patients), MG onset occurs equally in males and females over the age of 40 years. In these patients, there is an association with the serologically defined HLA alleles *B7 DR2*, and the thymus is atrophic on histological analysis. Yet a third group of patients (10%) have a thymoma; the sexes are equally affected and there is no genetic linkage. Finally, in some 10–15% of patients, antibodies to the AChR are not detectable, so-called 'seronegative' MG.

There is a strong association of MG with other autoimmune disorders, notably type 1 diabetes, autoimmune thyroiditis and rheumatoid arthritis.

Pathology

Typically, there is a small collection of mononuclear inflammatory cells (lymphocytes, macrophages) near the NMJ, with occasional evidence of degeneration of the muscle fibres. Staining for IgG and complement components (C3, C5b6789 complexes) at the NMJ is positive. Electron microscopy reveals a widening of the post-synaptic cleft. The thymus is usually examined for enlargement radiologically using computed tomography; thymectomy for thymic enlargement reveals hyperplasia or a thymoma, which may be malignant or benign. Hyperplasia is often associated with the existence of lymphoid germinal centres within the thymus.

Pathogenesis and immunological features

The existence of a thymoma and therapy with D-penicillamine are the only factors known to provoke MG. For example, 30–40% of patients with a thymoma develop an autoimmune disease, one third having MG. In addition, approximately 1% of patients with rheumatoid arthritis treated with D-penicillamine develop a myasthenic syndrome, with anti-AChR antibodies that

Myasthenia gravis in a bone marrow-transplant recipient: a rare complication

Some convincing evidence for the hypothesis that MG arises from an immune response involving autoreactive B lymphocytes comes from a case report in 1983. A young girl with aplastic anaemia received bone marrow from her HLA-identical brother (*A3 B40 DR4/A2 B7 DR2*). Apart from the development of graft-versus-host disease, the transplant was a success. Some 2 years later, however, she developed ptosis and diplopia. The clinical diagnosis of MG was supported by a Tensilon test and the presence of anti-AChR antibodies. The existence of repeated serum samples dating from before the transplant allowed the clinicians in charge to establish that the anti-AChR antibodies had first appeared within 3 months of her receiving the bone marrow. Serum samples from the girl's brother and parents were negative for the autoantibodies. The first important question to answer was whether the clones of B lymphocytes producing the anti-AChR antibody were from the girl or her brother. Molecular techniques were not as advanced in the early 1980s as they are now, but the investigators were able to establish that all of the peripheral blood lymphocytes and bone marrow cells in her circulation carried a Y chromosome, which must have derived from her brother. The second question was why had the brother not developed the disease? It is conceivable that the presence of the autoreactive B cell clones alone is not sufficient to generate MG. MG in this age group is more common in females, as are several autoimmune diseases, and it may be that the manifestation of MG in members of this family required the presence of the 'female milieu'. Alternatively, it is possible that the autoreactive B lymphocytes in the brother were held in check by immunoregulatory T lymphocytes. These could have been inadequately represented in the bone marrow transplanted to his sister or were particularly sensitive to the methotrexate and steroids given to treat the graft-versus-host disease.

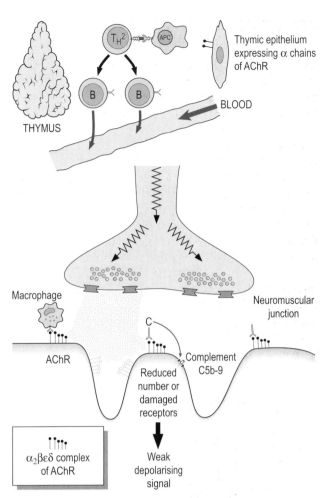

Fig. 18.7 **Pathogenesis of myasthenia gravis.**
Acetylcholine receptors (AChR) are damaged, reduced in number or blockaded by circulating anti-AChR antibodies. T_H2 lymphocytes are sensitised, possibly in the thymus, to the α subunit of the AChR. B lymphocytes become activated, leading to the generation of high-affinity, complement-fixing IgG autoantibodies to the AChR. These block binding of ACh, or damage the receptors and the motor end-plate by complement-mediated lysis or recruitment of Fc-receptor-bearing macrophages.

- complement-mediated damage to the end-plate with AChR loss
- decreased synthesis and increased degradation of AChRs
- antagonist action by receptor blockade.

The presence of IgG and complement C5b6789 (membrane attack complex) deposition at affected NMJs, with heaviest deposition at the NMJs with the least remaining AChRs, strongly supports the hypothesis of complement-mediated damage. Second, injection of MG sera into mice increases the daily turnover rate of AChRs by approximately three-fold, with catabolism outstripping synthesis. Finally, serum from some patients is capable of blocking depolarisation of cultured muscle cell lines in vitro.

There are several lines of evidence that support the hypothesis that autoantibodies to the AChR are involved in the pathogenesis of myasthenia gravis:

- 90% of patients have anti-AChR antibodies, which are undetectable in healthy controls

disappear along with the symptoms when the therapy is stopped. The events that lead to all other 'idiopathic' cases of MG remain to be defined.

The idiopathic cases of MG are united for the most part by the presence of anti-AChR antibodies and reduced numbers of AChRs at the motor end-plates. The questions to be addressed regarding the immunopathogenesis of MG are whether these two factors are causally related, and what incites the production of the autoantibody. The AchR has four subunits forming a complex ($\alpha_2\beta\epsilon\delta$). The α chain, which contains the binding site for ACh and the snake neurotoxin α-bungarotoxin (a venom that causes paralysis), is the target of the autoantibodies in MG. There are three mechanisms by which the presence of circulating anti-AChR antibodies results in loss of receptor (Fig. 18.7):

- one in eight babies born to mothers with MG have a transient myasthenic syndrome (neonatal MG) which lasts 2 to 3 weeks
- injection of MG sera into mice causes a myasthenic syndrome
- IgG and complement are seen at the NMJ in MG.

The explanation for the production of anti-AChR antibody by patients with MG remains elusive. No convincing cross-reactions between the receptor and microorganisms have been proposed to support a theory of molecular mimicry at the B cell level, and interest has concentrated more recently on the role of T helper cells in giving rise to these high affinity IgG autoantibodies. An intriguing association in this respect is the link between thymomata, thymic hyperplasia and MG. Recent analysis of thymoma material from patients with MG using monoclonal antibodies to the AChR has identified a protein with sequences highly homologous to the AChR α subunit. In the case of MG associated with a thymoma, then, it is possible to hypothesise that intrathymic T cells become sensitised to the AChR α subunit indirectly, having encountered a highly homologous protein within the thymic environment, possibly as part of an anti-tumour response. Encountering novel antigens within the thymus is likely to involve specialised APCs and could lead to a particularly vigorous T cell response; indeed, there is evidence that T cells extracted from a thymoma show stronger proliferative responses than peripheral blood T cells when stimulated with AChR α subunit in vitro.

The histological appearance of hyperplastic thymus, found in the majority of patients with 'classical' MG, is of a gland largely taken over with germinal centres and surrounding T cell areas. When these glands are removed, dispersed and the cell suspensions cultured in vitro, there is spontaneous synthesis of anti-AChR antibodies, suggesting that this is the main site of antibody production in vivo. This evidence has led many to suggest that pathogenic events in the hyperplastic thymus in MG are probably similar to those in thymomatous MG. In support of this, the AChR α subunit-like protein described in thymomata may also be seen in normal glands; there is also a muscle-like myoid cell present in the thymus in very small numbers that expresses complete AChR molecules.

Studies in which clones of T cells have been generated from peripheral blood and the thymus of patients with MG have revealed that the main T cell responses are directed against the α subunit of the AChR. However, as yet no part of the molecule dominates the immune response, and no class II MHC molecule has emerged as being critical in antigen presentation. In addition, T cell clones with a similar specificity have been generated from healthy controls.

The pathogenesis of so-called 'seronegative' MG, in which anti-AChR antibodies are not found, is also unclear. However, there is evidence to support the existence of a serum factor that gives rise to the syndrome. For example, patients with seronegative MG may benefit from plasmapheresis; mice injected with serum from these patients develop myasthenic features; and a baby born to a mother with the condition has developed neonatal MG. However, the identity of the serum factor responsible remains to be established.

Clinical features

The diagnosis of MG is made on clinical grounds, along with autoantibody testing, single fibre electromyography and the Tensilon test. A suggestive history is supported by an examination, which may reveal fatiguability and weakness, particularly of muscles supplied by the cranial nerves (e.g. difficulty in holding a vertical gaze). Tendon reflexes are present. Anti-AChR autoantibodies, found in 85–90% of patients, are detected using a sensitive immunoassay in which purified human AChRs are labelled with radioactivity using [^{125}I]-labelled α-bungarotoxin, which complexes with the AChR. In the Tensilon test, 5–10 mg edrophonium, a cholinesterase inhibitor, is given intravenously. It has the effect of making more ACh available at the NMJ and this can overcome the lack of functional AChRs, reversing the myasthenic symptoms temporarily for several minutes. Autoantibodies to striated muscle are detected in over 90% of patients with thymoma and a small proportion of other patients.

Treatment

The treatment of MG is based around the use of pyridostigmine, a long-acting cholinesterase inhibitor. Corticosteroids and azathioprine are occasionally added in an attempt to reduce anti-AChR levels with apparent benefit, though prospective trials have not been performed. Plasmapheresis may be used to remove autoantibodies to the AChR during acute MG exacerbations or prior to surgery. Evidence of a thymoma should be sought with regular follow-up, and since local tumour spread may be life threatening, thymectomy is recommended even though improvement in the myasthenic

---

Myasthenia gravis

- The presence of high-affinity, IgG autoantibodies to the acetylcholine receptor leads to myasthenia gravis, a syndrome of fatiguable weakness associated with loss of these receptors at the neuromuscular junction.
- The disease is multifactorial and has different subtypes; the most common form of the disease has many features typical of other autoimmune diseases (young, female predominance, HLA association).
- There is an intriguing link with events in the thymus: some patients have thymic neoplasia, others thymic hyperplasia; a protein homologous to the acetylcholine receptor, present in the gland, may be the focus of the initial immune response.

symptoms is unusual. Thymectomy is beneficial if performed early in other cases, and in 30–50% of young patients with hyperplastic thymuses containing many germinal centres, it may induce a long period of remission. More recently, clinical improvement has been reported with intravenous gammaglobulin, which is thought to work either by soaking up activated complement components or by blockading Fc receptors on macrophages surrounding the motor end-plates.

LAMBERT–EATON SYNDROME

The Lambert–Eaton myasthenic syndrome (LEMS) is typified by proximal muscle weakness, increased muscle strength during isometric contraction (post-tetanic potentiation), loss of tendon reflexes and autonomic dysfunction. The onset is usually acute, and in roughly half the patients there is an associated malignancy. In over 80% of patients, the tumour is a small cell carcinoma of the lung (SCLC), with myasthenic symptoms preceding the detection of the cancer by up to 5 years. The LEMS is approximately 10 times less frequent than MG, although it may go undiagnosed in some patients with SCLC, and probably affects 3% of patients with this type of neoplasm.

The diagnosis of LEMS is made on electrophysiological tests, which include post-exercise recruitment, repetitive nerve stimulation and single fibre electromyography. Antibodies to the voltage-gated calcium channels (VGCC) are detected using a radioimmunoassay similar in principle to that used in the diagnosis of MG; here, VGCCs are solubilised and radioactively labelled using a different toxin, [^{125}I]-labelled-ω-conotoxin. Anti-VGCC antibodies are present in approximately 65% of patients.

Pathology

The abnormality at the NMJ is best revealed by electron microscopy, which shows a reduction in the so-called 'active zones' on the presynaptic membrane that contain the VGCCs.

Pathogenesis and immunological features

The electrophysiological abnormalities seen in electromyography reflect a reduction in the pre-synaptic release of acetylcholine quanta. That this could be associated with autoantibodies was first suggested by the successful use of plasmapheresis, which gave clinical and electrophysiological improvement. Classical passive transfer experiments of a patient's IgG into mice then reproduced the syndrome, as well as the electrophysiological abnormalities. The reduction in VGCCs does not appear to be complement dependent, since the same changes were seen in mice genetically deficient in complement component C5 and, therefore, unable to construct the membrane attack complex, C5b6789. It appears that divalent antibody (as opposed to Fab fragments) is essential to recreate the lesion of LEMS in passive transfer models, indicating that the abnormality

is not caused by blockade but may arise from cross-linking of VGCCs, with subsequent internalisation.

The remaining question is what initiates the production of anti-VGCC antibodies, most notably in patients with SCLC. Evidence that VGCC-like molecules may be represented within the tumour comes from the fact that cultures of SCLC cells support voltage-gated calcium flux, which is inhibited by serum from LEMS patients. In addition, LEMS improves markedly when SCLC are removed surgically. These findings suggest that, like MG associated with a thymoma, LEMS associated with SCLC may arise as a result of an immune response to antigens expressed within the tumour.

Clinical features

Symptoms of fatiguability are similar to those in MG, but patients may get autonomic symptoms, with dry mouth, impotence and sphincter dysfunction.

Treatment with 3,4-diaminopyridine improves acetylcholine release and improves symptoms, as does any appropriate antitumour therapy. In LEMS not associated with cancer, prednisolone and azathioprine may give neurological improvement.

> **Lambert–Eaton syndrome**
> - The Lambert–Eaton myasthenic syndrome is associated with antibodies to presynaptic structures, the voltage-gated calcium channels, which have a critical role in the release of the neurotransmitter acetylcholine.
> - Some 50% of patients with this disorder have a tumour, small cell carcinoma of the lung, which has neuroendocrine origins.
> - Calcium channels homologous to those seen on the pre-synaptic membrane may be expressed within the small cell carcinoma and could represent the autoantigenic targets involved in the initiation of this autoimmune disorder.

STIFF MAN SYNDROME

Stiff man syndrome (SMS) has already been encountered in the discussion of autoantigens in type 1 diabetes (see p. 185). The recognition that SMS patients have serum antibodies to glutamic acid decarboxylase (GAD) and autoantibodies to pancreatic islets by indirect immunofluorescence led to the identification of GAD as an important islet autoantigen in type 1 diabetes, as well as marking SMS as an autoimmune disease. SMS is characterised by symptoms of tightness and stiffness, with slowly progressive axial and abdominal wall rigidity.

Pathology

Post-mortem studies in patients with SMS are rare and have not produced any clear pattern of pathological abnormalities.

Pathogenesis and immunological features

The most striking immunological feature is the presence of autoantibodies to GAD in a high proportion (>60%) of SMS patients. Other autoantibodies (anti-thyroid microsomal, thyroglobulin, gastric parietal cell antibodies) are frequently found, making SMS one of the rarer components of polyendocrine disorders. Anti-GAD antibodies in SMS patients differ from those found in patients with type 1 diabetes. The titres tend to be higher in SMS patients, whose autoantibodies also tend to bind so-called 'linear' epitopes of the GAD molecule, whilst those of diabetic patients bind only to conformational epitopes. The relationship between anti-GAD antibodies and SMS remains to be established, although therapeutic manoeuvres that impede autoantibodies (e.g. plasmapheresis) have been reported to be successful.

Stiffness occurring in association with breast carcinoma has also been reported as a paraneoplastic complication, and these patients do not have anti-GAD antibodies, but their sera do contain autoantibodies to a brain protein of 128 kDa, as yet unidentified.

Clinical features

As a polyendocrine disorder, SMS is frequently associated with type 1 diabetes (60%) as well as thyroid autoimmune disease, pernicious anaemia and vitiligo.

Initial treatment is usually with diazepam or baclofen, but steroids, with or without plasmapheresis, have been used successfully, as has intravenous immunoglobulin in anecdotal reports.

IMMUNE-MEDIATED EYE DISEASE

The eye is prone to involvement in immune-mediated disease, either secondarily as a result of systemic illness or as a primary event. Some special features of the eye are of importance in considering its involvement in disease. Microorganisms, allergens and other forms of antigens may enter the eye through the mucous membranes of the conjunctiva, or through the blood. Some structures (the conjunctiva, retina and uveal tract) are well vascularised, whilst others are normally avascular (cornea and sclera) and may only become vascular during inflammatory responses, with important consequences for visual acuity. Immune protection in the eye includes secreted proteins in tears, such as lysozyme and IgA, as well as the physical properties of the fluid itself. Diseases of the eye will be considered here according to the different anatomical locations affected (Fig. 18.8). Immune responses affecting the eye secondarily will be mentioned briefly, with full accounts of the underlying pathological processes (e.g. connective tissue disease) in the relevant chapters.

SKIN AND MUCOUS MEMBRANES

Like other mucosal and skin surfaces, the eye may be

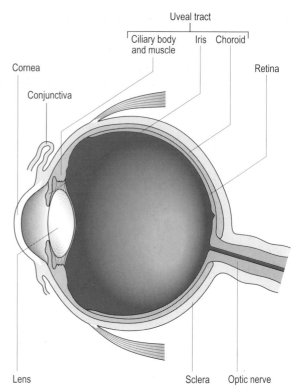

Fig. 18.8 **Anatomy of the eye.**

affected by IgE-mediated allergic reactions (Ch. 10). Contact sensitivity (type IV hypersensitivity; p. 144) can arise in response to topical ocular medications and cleaning and preservation fluids used for contact lenses. Cicatricial pemphigoid, the term used to describe involvement of mucosal membranes in bullous pemphigoid (p. 237), can affect the conjunctiva as well as the oral cavity and is a difficult ophthalmic problem to treat. There may be extensive scarring of the conjunctiva and the formation of adhesions between its two surfaces, leading to distortion of the eye lids and lashes. In addition, the cornea may become secondarily vascularised, and blockage of lacrimal ducts leads to a dry-eye syndrome.

CORNEA

Inflammation of the cornea, the avascular structure forming the anterior wall of the anterior chamber, is termed **keratitis**. Infective keratitis caused by herpes simplex infection may become recurrent, in a process that is believed to involve the generation of cellular immune responses to normal corneal components. **Keratoconjunctivitis sicca** is an inflammatory process involving the cornea and conjunctiva associated with lack of lacrimal secretions. The lacrimal glands are infiltrated with lymphocytes and plasma cells and become atrophic. The condition of dry eyes gives symptoms of grittiness, pain and dryness worsening as the day goes on and may be diagnosed formally using the **Schirmer test**, in which a thin strip of filter paper (0.5 × 3.5 cm) is inserted under the eyelid for 5 minutes. A positive test is one in which less than 10 mm of the paper has been moistened by tears. The triad of keratoconjunctivitis sicca plus a similar condition affecting the salivary glands resulting in a dry mouth and a connective tissue disease such as rheumatoid arthritis is **Sjögren's syndrome** (p. 178).

SCLERA AND EPISCLERA

The sclera is the tough, fibrous outer coat of the eye that has a white appearance and abuts the bony socket. It is nourished from a highly vascular coating, the episclera. **Episcleritis** results in pain, redness, photophobia and tenderness and is usually a benign, self-limiting condition of unknown aetiology. **Scleritis** is less common and is most frequently secondary to a chronic inflammatory process elsewhere in the body. Symptoms are similar to those of episcleritis, but usually more severe. A number of conditions give rise to this potentially blinding condition:

- Connective tissue diseases
  — ankylosing spondylitis
  — rheumatoid arthritis
  — Wegener's granulomatosis
  — polyarteritis nodosa
  — systemic lupus erythematosus.
- Type IV hypersensitivity states
  — tuberculosis
  — sarcoidosis
  — leprosy.

The underlying pathogenic processes leading to scleritis are likely to be the same as those of the primary condition (e.g. circulating immune complexes, vasculitis). In rheumatoid arthritis, the sclera may become thinned and ultimately perforate, a complication termed **scleromalacia perforans**.

UVEAL TRACT AND RETINA

Uveitis refers to inflammation of the uveal tract, a structure that includes the iris (coloured, circular membrane in front of the lens), ciliary body (ciliary processes and muscle suspending the lens) and choroid (vascular structure between the retina and sclera). Uveitis is generally divided into anterior (iritis and iridocyclitis) and posterior (choroiditis and choroidoretinitis). Uveitis is a relatively common condition, and in half the patients it arises either as a result of infection or secondary to a chronic, systemic illness, frequently a connective tissue disease. There is an unknown aetiology for 50% of cases, but there is considerable evidence to suggest that this 'idiopathic' form of uveitis is an autoimmune disease. Causes of immune-mediated uveitis include:

- Chronic inflammatory diseases
  — ankylosing spondylitis
  — autoimmune hepatitis
  — inflammatory bowel disease
  — juvenile rheumatoid arthritis
  — multiple sclerosis.
- Type IV hypersensitivity states
  — tuberculosis
  — sarcoidosis.
- Primary autoimmune (idiopathic) disease.

Uveitis usually presents with pain, photophobia and blurring of vision. There are several serious sequelae of the inflammatory process associated with this disorder, ranging from glaucoma precipitated by the formation of adhesions between the iris and lens, through cataract formation, to blindness caused by retinal detachment.

Idiopathic (autoimmune) uveitis typically affects the posterior segment of the uveal tract. On histological examination, there may be granulomatous lesions, containing macrophages, epithelioid cells and CD4$^+$ and CD8$^+$ T lymphocytes. Like other autoimmune diseases, this finding suggests a chronicity to the disease at presentation and makes it difficult to decipher the events and (auto)antigens that have incited the inflammation. Some of the best evidence for an autoimmune basis for uveitis, therefore, has come from an animal model, experimental autoimmune uveitis (EAU). Similar to EAE, the model of multiple sclerosis, EAU follows 9–10 days after systemic injection of animals with retinal photoreceptor-related antigens, the best known being retinal S-antigen. In the early phase, CD4$^+$ T cells accumulate around blood vessels in the retina and choroid, while macrophages infiltrate the same site. An abundance of local macrophages probably leads to efficient endocytosis and presentation of autoantigens within the posterior uveal tract. This phase is followed by a CD8$^+$ T cell-dominated infiltration. As in EAE, there is evidence of restricted T cell receptor V$_\beta$ chain usage, predominantly to V$_\beta$8 and V$_\beta$2. In addition, feeding animals retinal S-antigen orally provides protection from subsequent systemic injection of the same autoantigen.

Current conventional therapy for acute autoimmune uveitis involves the use of immunosuppressants such as corticosteroids and, more recently, cyclosporin A. Doses of these two drugs for chronic treatment may be reduced if azathioprine is added. Topical mydriatics are important to prevent adhesion of the iris.

Sympathetic ophthalmia is a potentially devastating condition following some weeks or months after an injury or perforation of one eye. A granulomatous, CD4$^+$ T cell-mediated inflammatory process is established in the uninjured eye (hence 'sympathetic'), leading to pan-uveitis, with the potential for loss of vision in both eyes. The condition is believed to result from the release of photoreceptor antigens (such as retinal S-antigen) and subsequent activation of sensitised CD4$^+$ T cells. CD4$^+$ T cells expressing the IL-2 receptor are seen in the infiltrate in the early phases of the disease. This implies that the state of tolerance to photorecep-

Left eye

Right eye

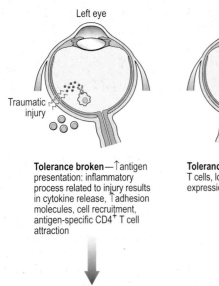

Traumatic injury

Tolerance broken—↑antigen presentation: inflammatory process related to injury results in cytokine release, ↑adhesion molecules, cell recruitment, antigen-specific CD4⁺ T cell attraction

Tolerance—no responding T cells, low level of autoantigen expression

Healing

Tolerance broken in normal eye because of the arrival of activated autoantigen-specific T cells

Fig. 18.9 **Possible sequence of events leading to sympathetic ophthalmia.**
T cell tolerance to retinal photoreceptor proteins is maintained by lack of presentation of the autoantigens. Once released through trauma, autoantigen presentation leads to recruitment and activation of CD4⁺ T cells. The mechanism by which the non-traumatised eye becomes sympathetically involved is not clear. Possibly low levels of retinal photoreceptor autoantigens are normally presented and tolerance is broken by the presence in the circulation of sensitised, activated T cells.

tor autoantigens is normally maintained by their being 'hidden' from the immune system, or present in only very small quantities. Release of large amounts of the autoantigens, associated with a small, trauma-induced local inflammatory infiltration, cytokine release and up-regulation of endothelial adhesion molecules, is sufficient to lead to autoantigen-specific T cell activation (Fig. 18.9). Interestingly, the arrival of these T cells in the non-traumatised eye, where autoantigens are present at 'normal' levels, is then in turn sufficient to break local tolerance and lead to ocular damage. Treatment is prophylactic in the first instance: sympathetic ophthalmia is very rare if the traumatised eye is removed within 10 days of injury. Once established, sympathetic ophthalmia should be treated vigorously with corticosteroids and/or cyclosporin A. Removal of the traumatised eye now is unwise: it may eventually prove to be the better of two damaged eyes.

A similar condition, termed **lens-induced uveitis** may follow lens surgery. Leakage of 'hidden' lens proteins (remember the lens is avascular and, therefore, has no immune surveillance) leads to the establishment of an immune response, usually involving the formation of autoantibodies. Typically, it is the eye with the damaged lens that is affected, and sympathetic inflammation is rare.

Immune-mediated eye disease

- The skin and mucosa of the eye are frequently affected by hypersensitivity or autoimmune diseases such as perennial allergy and pemphigoid.
- Other disorders affect the eye secondarily to a systemic autoimmune disease, particularly the connective tissue diseases and vasculitic diseases.
- Uveitis may arise spontaneously as an autoimmune disease, or in response to trauma and release of 'hidden' autoantigens.

The consequences of a failure in the immune system should now be apparent: an increased risk of infection, autoimmune disease, hypersensitivity or even cancer. A malfunction that results directly in the development of such disorders is the clinical state of immunodeficiency. For the most part, immunodeficiencies lead to increased susceptibility to infection, while autoimmunity, hypersensitivity and malignancy are commonly associated features. Immunodeficiency may arise either as a primary event, through congenital or genetic abnormality, or secondary to another condition or therapy. Secondary immunodeficiency is by far the more common, particularly in association with the widespread use of steroids, cytotoxic agents and immunosuppression for organ and bone marrow transplantation. A primary immunodeficiency, however, such as congenital absence of the thymus (the DiGeorge anomaly), may only be encountered every 100 000 births, so that a teaching hospital would only see a case every 25 years.

What, then, is the justification for the detailed accounts in this chapter of several rare primary immunodeficiencies? The explanation is that they provide our best possible insights into the roles of different components of the human immune system. In addition, they offer the opportunity to define a framework for the investigation of a clinically suspected immunodeficiency. The importance of such an algorithm is graphically illustrated by the appearance in the early 1980s of a new disease: the acquired immunodeficiency syndrome.

CLASSIFICATION

The nature of the diseases that arise in an immunodeficient individual depends upon which part of the immune system is affected. For example, pyogenic infections affecting mucosal sites such as the upper and lower respiratory tracts are typical of selective IgA deficiency. Any classification which is to be useful in guiding the clinician to a diagnosis must take account of this. For this reason, the conventional subdivision of immunodeficiency into primary and secondary may be of little value. It is preferable to classify immunodeficiency states according to the component of the immune system that is impaired, to include T lymphocytes, B lymphocytes, or both, neutrophils and complement. As a result of the co-operation between different components of the immune system, and the fact that some defects may cripple more than one element, some immunodeficiencies are difficult to compartmentalise (Table 19.1).

CLINICAL FEATURES

Immunodeficiencies may arise at any age, but the infections associated with them have several typical features:

- they are often chronic or recurrent
- they may resolve only partially with conventional therapy
- the organisms involved may be unusual.

Organisms typically described as 'opportunistic' are often involved. These are pathogens of low virulence

Table 19.1 **Classification of immunodeficiencies and the main diseases in each category**

Imune component	Disease
T lymphocyte deficiency	Third and fourth pharyngeal arch syndrome (DiGeorge anomaly) Acquired immunodeficiency syndrome Chronic mucocutaneous candidiasis
B lymphocyte deficiency	X-linked agammaglobulinaemia (Bruton's syndrome) Selective IgA deficiency IgG subclass deficiency Common variable immunodeficiency Transient hypogammaglobulinaemia of infancy

Combined T and B cell defects	Severe combined immunodeficiency
	   Adenosine deaminase deficiency
	   Purine nucleoside phosphorylase deficiency
	   Defective IL-2 production
	   MHC expression defects
	   Congenital TCR deficiency
	   X-linked hyper IgM syndrome
	Wiskott–Aldrich syndrome
	Ataxia telangiectasia

Neutrophil defects	Chronic granulomatous disease Leukocyte adhesion deficiency
Deficiency of complement components	Classical pathway Alternative pathway Common pathway Regulatory proteins

that are easily held in check by an intact immune system but that take their moment to invade when the host's guard is lowered.

Patterns of infection may be typical of certain immune deficiencies (Table 19.2). B lymphocyte and antibody defects, for example, result in infections with pyogenic organisms. T lymphocyte deficiency is associated with infection with fungi, protozoa and intracellular microorganisms, such as viruses and myco-bacteria, whilst deep skin infections, abscesses and

osteomyelitis are seen in patients with phagocyte defects. Other features relate more specifically to particular syndromes. Congenital or genetic deficiencies of antibody production are typically not revealed for several months after birth, for example, since the half-life of IgG is 28 days and maternal antibody remains at protective levels for only 5–6 months.

A family history, possibly of unexplained infant death, may be helpful in indicating a heritable disorder that has affected other siblings, whilst the sex of affected children gives a clue to the mode of inheritance. Consanguinity is a predisposing factor to any disorder with an autosomal recessive inheritance pattern. Finally, autoimmunity is inextricably linked to immuno-deficiency, and autoimmune disease is occasionally the mode of presentation.

Graft-versus-host disease (GVHD; p. 151) is a frequent complication of both primary and secondary T cell immunodeficiency. For GVHD to arise, the prerequisites are impaired T cell function in the recipient and the transfer of immunocompetent T lymphocytes from an HLA non-identical donor. In patients with T cell immunodeficiency, GVHD usually arises from therapeutic interventions such as transfusion of red blood cells or platelets, or transplantation of bone marrow. Transfusions destined for patients with suspected T cell deficiency should first be irradiated to inactivate donor T lymphocytes. GVHD has also been described in association with solid organ transplants during which the recipient is immunosuppressed to avoid graft rejection.

ASSESSING IMMUNE FUNCTION

In order to diagnose immunodeficiency, the immune

Table 19.2 **Patterns of infectious organisms encountered in immunodeficiency**

Infective agent	B cell deficiency	T cell deficiency	Phagocyte deficiency	Complement classical pathway deficiency	Complement membrane attack pathway deficiency
Bacteria	Haemophilus influenzae, Streptococcus pneumoniae, Staphylococcus aureus		Staphylococcus aureus, Staphylococcus epidermidis, Pseudomonas aeruginosa, Serratia marcescens, Escherichia coli	Haemophilus influenzae, Streptococcus pneumoniae, Staphylococcus aureus	Neisseria meningitidis, Neisseria gonorrhoeae
Viruses	Echoviruses	Cytomegalovirus; herpes zoster			
Flagellate parasites	Giardia lamblia				
Intracellular microorganisms		Mycobacterium tuberculosis, M. avium intracellulare			
Fungi		Candida albicans	Candida albicans, Aspergillus flavus		
Protozoa		Pneumocystis carinii, Toxoplasma gondii			

Table 19.3 **Useful screening tests for the assessment of immune function in the investigation of immunodeficiency**

Tests	T lymphocytes	B lymphocytes	Phagocytes	Complement
Enumeration	CD3$^+$ lymphocytes CD4$^+$, CD8$^+$ subsets	CD20$^+$ lymphocytes Ig$^+$ cells Immunoglobulin levels IgG subclass levels	Neutrophil count	
Assessment of in vitro functioning	PHA stimulation Antigen-specific stimulation IL-2 production		NBT test	CH$_{50}$
Assessment of in vivo functioning	Delayed hypersensitivity reaction to purified protein derivative (PPD) of *M. tuberculosis*	Specific antibody levels: isohaemagglutinins; anti-*E. coli*; antitetanus, antidiphtheria toxins (with booster injections if necessary)		

NBT, nitroblue tetrazolium

system must be examined: an obvious point, you may think. Yet our access to the sites of active immunity — lymph nodes, spleen, infective foci — is severely limited and almost all tests must be performed on blood samples (Table 19.3). Proteins such as IgG may diffuse to maintain equilibrium between the blood and the tissues; white cells may be actively sequestered out of the circulation and other proteins, such as those of the complement system, may be synthesised locally at inflammatory sites. For these reasons, some laboratory tests provide only an indirect assessment of immune function and require careful interpretation.

T LYMPHOCYTES

Counting the numbers of circulating cells is a useful initial test. T lymphocytes and their subsets are identified with monoclonal antibodies directed against relevant CD markers: CD3, CD4, CD8, as the main functional subsets. The percentages of T lymphocytes or subsets can be measured using flow cytometry (p. 83) and converted to a cell concentration (cells/μl) using a full blood count and white cell differential and these are the parameters of most use in the diagnosis and monitoring of lymphocyte immunodeficiency. Further differentiation to measure the ratio CD4:CD8 is of little diagnostic value as this is subject to considerable variation in health and has a wide normal range.

Tests of T lymphocyte function, however, tend to be difficult to standardise and are rarely antigen specific. The best known is stimulation of T lymphocytes with **mitogens** (compounds capable of inducing mitosis) followed by detection of their proliferative response. Lectins such as **phytohaemagglutinin** (PHA) are potent mitogens, capable of stimulating all T lymphocytes through a mechanism independent of TCR recognition and, therefore, not antigen specific. Other methods of assessing the proliferative capacity of T cells are stimulation with the T cell growth factor IL-2, or using allogeneic cells as a stimulus in **mixed lymphocyte reactions** (MLR). The MLR relies upon the fact that foreign MHC molecules are potent stimuli of many TCRs. More information may be gained by measuring the production of cytokines, notably IL-2, in response

to a mitogenic stimulus. In general, impaired proliferation to mitogens is only detectable in relatively severe T lymphocyte deficiencies. If possible, mitogens should be replaced in such assays by antigens most have been exposed to, such as the mycobacterium-derived purified protein derivative (PPD) or *Candida albicans*.

Other T cell functions may also be assessed in vitro. The ability of T lymphocytes to provide help to B lymphocytes during culture together can be assessed by measuring immunoglobulin production in the supernatant. For this an extra stimulus, from specific antigen or more usually from the T and B lymphocyte stimulator **pokeweed mitogen** (PWM) is required. Alternatively, the ability to inhibit antibody production by B lymphocytes can be used to examine suppressor activity in a population of T lymphocytes.

Assessment of the integrity of T lymphocyte functions in vivo is performed using intradermal injection of an antigen and measurement of the degree of induration and erythema after 48–72 hours caused by a **delayed hypersensitivity** reaction (p. 144). This is exemplified by the Heaf test, used to assess immunity to *Mycobacterium tuberculosis* in schoolchildren.

B LYMPHOCYTES

Measurement of the levels of circulating IgG, IgA and IgM and the number of circulating B lymphocytes are the most apt screening tests for B cell dysfunction. Immunoglobulin levels are best measured directly by nephelometry or radial immunodiffusion (see box: 'Detection of serum levels of immunoglobulin, complement and other immune mediators'; Fig. 19.1), since protein electrophoresis is insensitive and not quantitative. In the investigation of immunodeficiency in childhood, it is important to note the age dependence of immunoglobulin levels, which tend to increase with age until the late teenage. B lymphocytes are counted by flow cytometry using monoclonal antibodies to CD19, CD20 or surface immunoglobulin (sIg).

As for T lymphocytes, there are few antigen-specific tests of B lymphocyte function. Levels of specific antibody can be measured to assess the ability to mount directed immune responses. The most widely used targets are the blood group antigens of the ABO system, vaccines such as tetanus and diphtheria, and common pathogens such as *Escherichia coli*. IgM class anti-A and/or anti-B antibodies (the **isohaemagglutinins**) should be detectable in all individuals of blood groups A, B and O (about 97% of the population of the UK). Antitetanus or antidiphtheria antibodies are found in recently immunised individuals. Booster injections may be required, therefore, bearing in mind that live vaccines should never be given to individuals with suspected primary immunodeficiency.

PHAGOCYTES

The number of circulating neutrophils is usually available from the full blood count and should be interpreted in the light of any concurrent illness that would normally induce a neutrophilia. Tests of neutrophil functions centre upon phagocytosis, killing of microorganisms and chemotaxis. When neutrophil dysfunction is suspected, the **nitroblue tetrazolium** (NBT) test serves as a robust screening technique to assess neutrophil killing. NBT is a yellow dye that is added to a culture of neutrophils (pre-activated with endotoxin)

✎ Detection of serum levels of immunoglobulin, complement and other immune mediators

In the clinical immunology laboratory, measurement of proteins such as the immunoglobulins and complement components is typically carried out using two assays based on the use of specific polyclonal antisera: these are raised in animals using the analyte to be measured (e.g. anti-IgG, anti-C3, etc) as the antigen. In one assay, radial immunodiffusion (RID), the specific antiserum is added to an agarose gel just before it is poured (Fig. 19.1a). Wells are then cut, and the test sample is added to one well, and standards of known concentration to others. As the analyte (e.g. IgG) diffuses out into the gel, it is complexed to the antiserum present, forming a white precipitate. The distance the

analyte diffuses before all has been precipitated will depend upon its concentration. Therefore, at the end-point of the assay, the concentration of the analyte is proportional to the diameter of the precipitation ring.

A more automated and sensitive assay is based upon nephelometry: the measurement of light scattering immune complexes (Fig. 19.1b). Here, the specific antiserum is added to the test serum containing the protein of interest and incubated in a cuvette to allow analyte/antibody complexes to form. A laser light source is passed through, and the light scatter detected depends upon the density of complexes, which depends in turn upon the concentration of the analyte.

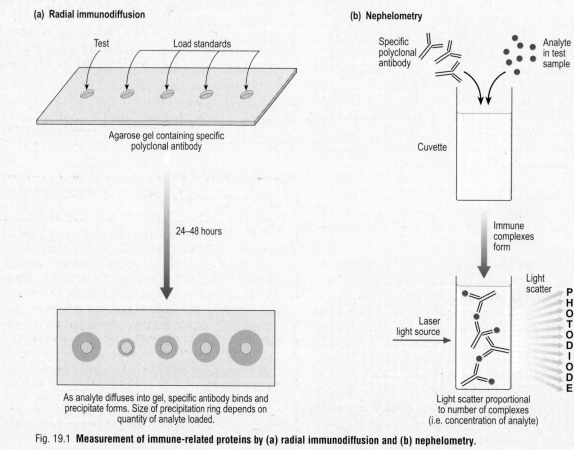

Fig. 19.1 **Measurement of immune-related proteins by (a) radial immunodiffusion and (b) nephelometry.**

along with an appropriate target, usually fungi of the *Candida* species. Healthy, activated neutrophils engulf and kill the *Candida*, employing toxic metabolites generated by the respiratory burst (p. 29). As a direct result of this metabolic burst, NBT is converted to a blue/black precipitate, formazan, which can be viewed by light microscopy within the neutrophil cytoplasm. Phagocytosis can be assessed in a straightforward way by counting the number of neutrophils successfully engulfing *Candida*. Chemotaxis is more difficult to study, and the best known technique employs a Boyden chamber. Neutrophils are attracted from the upper part of the chamber towards the lower part, which contains a potent chemoattractant (for example casein or f-Met-Leu-Phe) (see p. 22). Between the levels of the chamber is a cellulose membrane with small (3 μm) pores. The chemotactic factor diffuses through the membrane towards the cells, creating a gradient along which neutrophils will move. After 1 hour, the distance moved by the cells within the membrane is assessed microscopically following conventional staining of the filter.

A deficiency of neutrophil adherence has been described in which a subunit common to the leukocyte function-associated antigen-1 (LFA-1) and CR-3 complement receptor is absent. The diagnosis can be made, therefore, using specific monoclonal antibodies and flow cytometry as described above.

COMPLEMENT

Complement is a series of approximately 40 serum and membrane-bound proteins, and there are numerous, well-described deficiency syndromes. Levels of individual complement components can be measured directly by techniques such as radial immunodiffusion, but a better approach is to screen the functioning of the whole cascade, from attachment of C1qrs to antibody through to insertion of the membrane attack complex. In the **complement haemolysis assay**, antiserum raised against sheep red blood cells is incubated with patient's serum as a source of complement. The CH_{50} unit relates to the complement required to haemolyse 50% of the targets and is an arbitrary measurement of the lytic ability of the complement within the serum. A complete deficiency of a component between C1 and

C9 will be revealed as a CH_{50} of zero. Once a defect in the classical pathway is defined, individual complement components can be measured directly.

Deficiency of regulatory proteins in the cascade may lead to uncontrolled complement activation, resulting in disease. When such a condition is suspected, individual proteins should be measured directly.

T LYMPHOCYTE DEFICIENCIES

THIRD AND FOURTH PHARYNGEAL ARCH SYNDROME/DiGEORGE ANOMALY

Pathogenesis

In this congenital abnormality, there is failure of development during the 12th week of gestation of the third and fourth pharyngeal arches, which normally give rise to the parathyroid glands and the thymus. Diagnostic criteria hinge upon the demonstrable absence, or failure of descent, of the thymus and upon neonatal hypocalcaemia with low levels of parathormone (see box: 'The DiGeorge anomaly: an experiment of nature'). Associated features that aid diagnosis are aortic arch abnormalities, characteristic facies (micrognathia, 'fish-mouth', low set ears and hypertelorism) and T lymphocyte abnormalities. The features are somewhat variable, however, which has led to the use of the term **partial DiGeorge anomaly** for those children in whom the abnormalities are less severe and who may be managed more conservatively. The anomaly usually arises spontaneously in association with chromosomal abnormalities or a history of exposure to teratogens (e.g. alcohol), though some cases may be inherited in Mendelian fashion.

Clinical features

The frequency of the DiGeorge anomaly is somewhere between 1 and 5 per 100 000 of the population. It is

---

Assessing immune function

- Primary immunodeficiency is rare but instructive.
- Secondary immunodeficiency is relatively common and is often associated with the use of steroids, cytotoxic drugs and immunosuppression.
- The clinical features of immunodeficiency conform to patterns which should indicate appropriate laboratory tests and aid diagnosis.
- Laboratory tests screen for activity in the different components of the immune system.

The DiGeorge anomaly: an experiment of nature

By a coincidence, Angelo DiGeorge, a paediatrician in Philadelphia, attended a scientific meeting in 1965 in which the results of seminal studies on the effect of bursectomy and thymectomy on the immune system in chickens were being presented. Bursectomised chickens were unable to produce immunoglobulin, whilst thymectomy rendered the birds incapable of rejecting grafts but immunoglobulin levels remained normal. Through his interest in hypoparathyroidism, DiGeorge had seen four children with associated thymic agenesis. He was able to relate his own observations on this experiment of nature in which, as in the thymectomised chicken, immunoglobulin levels were indeed normal in the absence of a thymus gland.

usual for the anomaly to present in the newborn period as a result of hypocalcaemic tetany or cardiac defects rather than with episodes of infection, which may take several months to appear. Viral, protozoal, fungal and bacterial infections are typically found and infants fail to thrive.

Immunological features

The three typical findings, which may be of diagnostic help, are reduced T lymphocyte number (the CD4 count is usually less than 400/μl; normal range > 600/μl), reduced proliferative response to PHA and an increase in B cell number. Immunoglobulin levels may be normal despite severely impaired specific antibody responses (see box: 'Immunological reconstitution in DiGeorge anomaly').

Management

Calcium supplements and vitamin D, correction of cardiac abnormalities and prophylactic treatment with sulphonamides to avoid *Pneumocystis carinii* pneumonia will be required once the diagnosis is made. There have been three different therapies used in an attempt to reverse the immunodeficiency and each can claim some success. Early therapy centred upon thymic transplants using fetal tissue. Subsequently, cultured, mature thymus tissue has been used and, more recently, bone marrow transplant from HLA identical siblings has been successful. Thymus transplant carries a reasonable prognosis, with continued survival in more than 50% of patients, the longest period of follow-up being more than 15 years.

CHRONIC MUCOCUTANEOUS CANDIDIASIS

Pathogenesis

This is a condition characterised by candidal infections of the skin and mucous membranes. The disorder is associated to a variable extent with endocrine organ failure, affecting the parathyroid and adrenal glands predominantly. The aetiology of the disorder is not known, but it has a familial tendency.

Clinical and immunological features

The disease presents in the first two decades, either as candidal infections or endocrinopathy.

Lymphocyte numbers and PHA responses are normal, but a consistent finding is variable impairment of in vitro T cell responses and delayed hypersensitivity to *Candida albicans*. Interestingly, infection with other fungi is rare, and T cell responses to other fungi remain intact. Autoantibodies reflecting organ-specific autoimmunity may be detected, leading to the suggestion by some that at the heart of this disorder is an autoimmune disease.

Treatment

Apart from aggressive treatment of candidal infections with a variety of antifungal agents (clotrimazole, ketoconazole, miconazole and amphotericin B), Addison's disease (adrenocortical insufficiency) is the major concern, since it is a potentially life-threatening complication. The prognosis is considered to be poor, with many patients dying within the first three decades of life.

T lymphocyte deficiencies

- Isolated T cell deficiency, as in the DiGeorge anomaly, is rare but has devastating consequences.
- The molecular basis for severe T cell deficiences is becoming better defined, and relates to the function of cytokines, their receptors, and antigen recognition molecules.
- Bone marrow transplantation from an HLA identical donor can reconstitute T cell immunity.

B LYMPHOCYTE DEFICIENCIES

Deficiencies in B lymphocyte function can result from lesions occurring at multiple sites in the pathway of production of mature active B cells (Fig. 19.2). Lesions can result in one of the B lymphocyte deficiency diseases discussed here or in one of the combined B and T cell defects discussed below.

X-LINKED AGAMMAGLOBULINAEMIA/BRUTON'S SYNDROME

Pathogenesis

Since the first description of this disorder in 1952, several other X-linked primary immunodeficiencies have been described:

- agammaglobulinaemia (Bruton's syndrome)

 Immunological reconstitution in DiGeorge anomaly

The question arises as to how T cell immunity may be reconstituted from a bone marrow transplant in patients with the DiGeorge anomaly. Two explanations offer themselves. The first is that the marrow is a source of mature, post-thymic memory T cells capable of division, which reconstitute the immune system of the affected children. Second, it has been proposed that the patients in whom this therapy is successful have only a partial anomaly, with some residual thymus, which has failed to descend to the mediastinum. In this case, T cell precursors from the transplanted marrow would undergo thymic maturation. The question then arises as to why children with such residual thymus tissue should be immunodeficient at all, for which we do not have an answer.

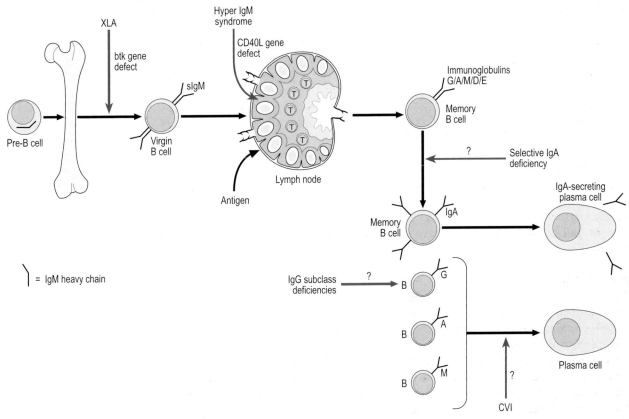

Fig. 19.2 Scheme of the major lesion sites leading to B cell immunodeficiency.
XLA, X-linked agammaglobulinaemia; CVI, common variable immunodeficiency.

- severe combined immunodeficiency syndrome caused by IL-2 receptor γ chain deficiency
- hyper IgM syndrome
- Wiscott–Aldrich syndrome
- chronic granulomatous disease.

In X-linked agammaglobulinaemia (XLA), affected males have IgG levels less than 2.0 g/l and all five classes of immunoglobulins are affected, with total levels of less than 2.5 g/l. Pre-B cells staining positive for cytoplasmic μ chains are present in normal numbers in the bone marrow, although these IgM heavy chain molecules lack the variable region segment. There are no subsequent members of the B cell lineage, however, and B lymphocytes are absent from the peripheral blood and lymph nodes. Until recently, the disease was thought to be a result of a defect in B cell growth stimulation; in 1993 the gene defective in the disease, encoding a novel tyrosine kinase, was identified.

Clinical features

Children present after the age of 5–6 months, when the protective benefits of placentally transferred maternal IgG have worn off (Fig. 19.3). Recurrent infections of the upper and lower respiratory tract with pyogenic organisms are typical, whilst enteritis and malabsorption is frequently associated with the presence of *Giardia lamblia* in the gut. Morbidity and mortality are related mainly to chronic lung disease and potentially fatal CNS infections with echoviruses.

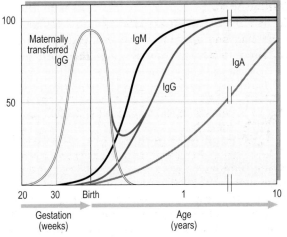

Fig. 19.3 Serum immunoglobulin levels in the fetus during the last trimester and in the newborn period.
Transfer of maternal IgG rises sharply during the last 8 weeks of pregnancy and then declines after birth, with a half-life of 28 days. Immunoglobulins produced by the baby are at low levels at birth but increase rapidly thereafter, with IgM being the first class produced. There is a trough in IgG levels occurring within 6 months after birth (physiological hypogammaglobulinaemia). Interference with the transfer of maternal IgG (e.g. through prematurity) prolongs the trough. Antibody deficiencies become symptomatic at the age of 5–6 months after maternal antibody has declined below protective levels.

Immunological features

Immunoglobulin levels are low and specific antibody is undetectable. B lymphocytes and plasma cells are not found, and lymph nodes are depleted of B cell areas. T lymphocyte function is normal. The X chromosome gene defective in XLA has been identified as a member of a non-receptor tyrosine kinase family, now named Bruton's tyrosine kinase, or Btk. It is presumed that it has a critical role in early signalling for B cell differentiation.

Treatment

Infections should be treated appropriately until cleared, but prophylactic antibiotics may be counterproductive. Chest physiotherapy is important in established lung disease. Intravenous administration of gammaglobulins (IVIG) has transformed the management of this disease. Previously, intramuscular immunoglobulin was given, but this treatment suffered several disadvantages: the injections were often painful, adequate quantities of immunoglobulin could not always be achieved by this route and adverse reactions, including anaphylactoid episodes probably resulting from IgG or IgA aggregates, occurred in 10–20% of patients. Refinement of the processes used to purify immunoglobulin has removed these drawbacks and additional steps such as heat treatment and donor screening have further reduced early problems of viral transmission. Home treatment with IVIG after proper training in hospital is becoming more widely used, and subcutaneous administration of immunoglobulin by a pump is also used, particularly in patients with a previous history of adverse reactions to intramuscular or intravenous administration. The aim of therapy is that the trough IgG concentration, taken just before the next infusion, remains within the normal range (i.e. > 5–6 g/l). Administration of IVIG appears to improve lung function, and use of preparations with high antiviral titres may retard the progression of echovirus infections.

Many patients now survive into the third decade, but by this age chronic lung disease and lymphomas are life-threatening complications, so that the prognosis remains poor.

SELECTIVE IgA DEFICIENCY

Pathogenesis

Serum IgA levels of < 0.05 g/l, with normal levels of IgG and IgM, is termed selective IgA deficiency, which is found in approximately 1/700 northern Europeans, making it the most common primary immunodeficiency. B lymphocytes bearing surface IgA are present in the circulation, but IgA-producing plasma cells are markedly reduced in number or absent. The immunoglobulin α heavy chain genes are normal and no abnormalities in the heavy chain switch region have been demonstrated. The pathogenesis of IgA deficiency remains unknown, but there is evidence to support the proposal that an immunoregulatory defect leads to arrested B lymphocyte differentiation (Figs 19.2 and 19.4).

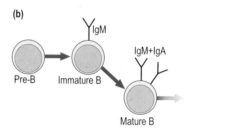

Fig. 19.4 **Selective IgA deficiency.**
Maturation of B lymphocytes to give IgA memory cells and IgA-secreting plasma cells. (**a**) In normal individuals, mature B lymphocytes with surface IgM and IgA become activated and differentiate into memory B cells with surface IgA. (**b**) In IgA deficiency, development is arrested at the surface IgA$^+$, IgM$^+$ stage.

Clinical features

IgA deficiency may be asymptomatic or may be associated with recurrent infections with pyogenic organisms affecting mucosal sites, predominantly in the upper respiratory tract. Symptoms may begin at any age, and

The pathogenesis of IgA deficiency

IgA-bearing B lymphocytes in IgA deficiency appear to be arrested at the surface IgA$^+$, IgM$^+$ stage (Fig. 19.3). This implies either a defect in the maturational signals they receive or in their ability to respond. T lymphocytes from IgA-deficient individuals can support normal differentiation of IgA B cells from healthy individuals in vitro, suggesting that T cell function is normal. However, bone marrow transplanted from an IgA-deficient individual into a histocompatible non-IgA-deficient sibling transfers the deficiency, implying that the defect resides at an early stage of stem cell development within the marrow.

Another intriguing aspect of IgA deficiency is the variable penetrance of the clinical manifestations. It has been proposed that the immune system compensates for absent IgA by increased production of specific antibodies in other isotypes, thus maintaining protection. If IgA-deficient patients were unable to produce specific antibacterial antibodies in another isotype, there might be increased susceptibility to infection. Support for this explanation comes from the identification of IgG2 and IgG4 subclass deficiencies in some symptomatic IgA-deficient patients. IgG2 is particularly important in production of antibodies to polysaccharide antigens such as those found on bacterial capsules.

associated disorders include allergy and autoimmune disease:

- rheumatoid arthritis
- systemic lupus erythematosus
- Sjögren's syndrome
- haemolytic anaemia
- type 1 (insulin-dependent) diabetes
- autoimmune hepatitis
- Addison's disease (adrenocortical insufficiency)
- myasthenia gravis
- coeliac disease.

Immunological features

Both IgA1 and IgA2 subclasses are reduced or absent, as is secretory IgA. B and T lymphocyte numbers are normal and they have intact in vitro responses to mitogen and antigens. Circulating autoantibodies, largely of the organ-specific type, are a common finding, though the relationship between these and the increased incidence of autoimmune disease is not known. There is a strong association between IgA deficiency and certain HLA alleles (see box: 'HLA genes and IgA deficiency').

Treatment

Of great clinical importance is the tendency to produce anti-IgA antibodies of the IgG and IgE class. Infusion of exogenous IgA, as would occur in blood transfusion, can result in anaphylaxis. All IgA-deficient patients should be screened for anti-IgA antibodies, and, if necessary, transfused with washed red cells, blood from an IgA-deficient donor or with their own blood which has been stored. Infections should be treated aggressively as they arise. In theory, immunoglobulin-replacement therapy is of little value in IgA deficiency: preparations contain little IgA, will not benefit secretory IgA levels and what little IgA there is may be sufficient to provoke adverse reactions in sensitised individuals. The rare exceptions to this rule may be patients with an associated IgG subclass deficiency in whom the therapy gives demonstrable benefit. The prognosis is reasonably good as long as the diagnosis is made before life-threatening complications such as chronic lung disease have become established.

IgG SUBCLASS DEFICIENCY

Pathogenesis

Antibody responses to certain bacterial antigens may belong to a particular IgG subclass because of its unique effector functions. The inability to respond by production of this isotype could, therefore, result in immunodeficiency. The field of IgG subclass deficiency is somewhat controversial, however, and though subclass deficiency syndromes have been described, many are of questionable clinical significance. Perhaps the exception is selective absence of IgG2 associated with increased susceptibility to infection with organisms such as *Streptococcus pneumoniae* and *Haemophilus influenzae* type b. The physiological basis for such a deficiency is the fact that antibody responses to polysaccharide antigens in bacterial capsules are normally of the IgG2 isotype.

More recent studies have concentrated upon measuring antibody responses to specific pathogens. It appears that the ability to make a particular isotype response may be of more relevance than the total level of that subclass.

Clinical and immunological features

IgG2 subclass deficiency most commonly presents with recurrent upper and lower respiratory tract infections.

Levels of IgM and IgA are normal (unless there is associated IgA deficiency) and total IgG levels may be unaffected by a deficiency of one or other subclass. Subclass levels should be interpreted in the light of the appropriate normal ranges, which take age and ethnic origin into consideration. Antibody responses to a range of potential pathogens (tetanus and diphtheria toxoids and pneumococcal and *H. influenzae* type b capsular polysaccharides) should also be measured.

Treatment

Antibiotic therapy is the first line of treatment. Repeated *Haemophilus* infections may benefit from immunisation with the *H. influenzae* type b polyribose phosphate vaccine. IVIG may be used when there is a demonstrable subclass or specific antibody defect and conventional treatment fails. Commercial immunoglobulins vary in their subclass compositions and their antibacterial titres, so the preparation best suited to

---

HLA genes and IgA deficiency

Based on the assumption that a defect in immunoregulation may underlie IgA deficiency, many studies on the MHC have been carried out. In addition to finding associations with individual alleles, however, they have demonstrated increased frequencies of particular combinations of MHC genes inherited en bloc: so called **supratypes**. A typical supratype in IgA deficiency contains *HLA-B8*, deleted complement *C4A* and 21-hydroxylase genes and *HLA-DR3*. The question arises as to whether within this stretch of chromosome 6 there is the true IgA deficiency-susceptibility gene or whether gene deletions, such as those of the complement proteins, could influence antibody production. Recent evidence suggests that the latter may be the case: individuals deficient in classical pathway complement components have impaired production of IgG4 and to a lesser extent of IgG2, but not of IgG1 and IgG3.

Interestingly, sequence studies on the HLA-DQβ chain in IgA deficiency have shown a similar picture to that in insulin-dependent diabetes, namely that when position 57 is occupied by a neutral amino acid, susceptibility to the disease is conferred; when it is occupied by a charged amino acid, such as aspartate, there is protection.

replacing the deficiency should be chosen. The prognosis of symptomatic IgG subclass deficiency remains to be established.

COMMON VARIABLE IMMUNODEFICIENCY

Pathogenesis

Hypogammaglobulinaemia in association with cellular immune defects is termed common variable immunodeficiency (CVI), and is the second most common primary immunodeficiency after IgA deficiency. The defects are heterogeneous in nature, implying that there are several syndromes that produce overlapping types of immunodeficiency. The dominant feature of CVI is usually antibody deficiency and, for this reason, it is considered here rather than in the section on combined T and B cell defects. However, T cell defects do occur and, when severe, give a clinical picture in which T cell deficiency is dominant (see Table 19.2). Another reason for considering CVI in this section is that it shares several features in common with IgA deficiency, combined IgA and IgG2 subclass deficiency and IgG subclass deficiency, suggesting that these might be different components of a spectrum of immunoglobulin deficiencies. In addition, the HLA associations in IgA deficiency and CVI are very similar and there is an increased incidence of IgA deficiency in first-degree relatives of patients with CVI. Several abnormalities that could account for CVI and that possibly represent different immunopathogenetic subgroups have been described:

- reduced numbers of B lymphocytes or T lymphocytes
- T lymphocytes that fail to promote B cell differentiation
- B lymphocytes that fail to secrete antibody
- circulating autoantibodies to B cells.

Clinical features

The incidence of CVI is between 6 and 12 per 10^6 of the population. There appear to be two peaks of disease onset, in the first decade and between the ages of 15 and 30 years. Recurrent upper and lower respiratory tract infections with organisms typical of antibody deficiency, chronic bronchiectatic lung disease, and malabsorption and diarrhoea secondary to giardiasis are the presenting features. Malignancy in patients with CVI has a high incidence, as do autoimmune diseases, particularly pernicious anaemia and autoimmune cytopenia. Rarely, patients present with features of T cell immunodeficiency.

Immunological features

Total immunoglobulin levels are less than 3 g/l and the concentration of IgG is less than 2.5 g/l. Specific antibody production is impaired, but circulating B cell numbers are usually normal. Typically, T lymphocyte numbers are also normal but reduced levels are present in those patients with more severe cellular defects.

Management

Appropriate antibiotic therapy, including metronidazole for giardiasis, should be readily available. Replacement therapy with IVIG should also be employed if the severity of the immunodeficiency warrants it. In the absence of complications such as chronic lung disease and haematological malignancy, the prognosis is good. Impairment of T cell mediated immunity carries a worse prognosis.

TRANSIENT HYPOGAMMAGLOBULINAEMIA OF INFANCY

Pathogenesis

Abnormally low levels of IgG occurring after maternal IgG has disappeared and persisting for up to 2 years is known as transient hypogammaglobulinaemia of infancy. The aetiology of this condition, which in some texts is confusingly labelled 'physiological hypogammaglobulinaemia' is not known, although a temporary defect in T cell help has been proposed.

Transfer of maternal IgG begins at around the 16th week of gestation but is maximal during the 3rd trimester (Fig. 19.3). Maternal IgG has a half-life of 4 weeks and the majority has been catabolised by 5–6 months, before the infant's own IgG synthesis is fully under way. The resulting trough, which is found in all healthy babies, is a period of **physiological hypogammaglobulinaemia**. It may be of importance clinically when it is prolonged, as in transient hypogammaglobulinaemia, or when maternal transfer is incomplete, as in prematurity.

Clinical and immunological features

In transient hypogammaglobulinaemia of infancy, recurrent, severe respiratory tract infections after 5–6 months of age produce a clinical picture similar to X-linked agammaglobulinaemia.

IgG levels remain in the trough that follows the decline in levels of maternal antibody (Fig. 19.3) in infants with transient hypogammaglobulinaemia. However, IgA and IgM levels begin to rise as expected and circulating B lymphocyte numbers are normal, making this easily differentiated from X-linked agammaglobulinaemia.

Treatment

Infections should be treated as appropriate. Replacement IVIG therapy may be needed in prolonged transient hypogammaglobulinaemia. An obvious question is whether premature babies with prolonged physiological hypogammaglobulinaemia on neonatal intensive care units should be given prophylactic IVIG. The results of current randomised trials are awaited. Clinical trials carried out up to now are inconclusive, two showing significant benefit and two not. Two studies carried out using IVIG to 'rescue' septic neonates have provided encouraging results.

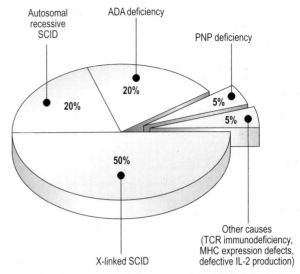

B lymphocyte deficiencies

- Agammaglobulinaemia with low IgG and no B lymphocytes is treated with intravenous gammaglobulins (IVIG) to reduce infections.
- IgA deficiency is the most common primary immunodeficiency. It has variable clinical manifestations and functional immunodeficiency in this condition may relate to associated IgG subclass deficiency.
- Anti-IgA antibodies in the circulation of IgA-deficient patients can give rise to potentially lethal anaphylactoid reactions.
- Intravenous immunoglobulin-replacement therapy is effective in replacing IgG class deficiencies and may be carried out at home.
- Common variable immunodeficiency (CVI), IgA deficiency and IgG subclass deficiencies appear related and may have a common pathogenesis.

Fig. 19.5 **Distribution of the different types of SCID and their incidences.** ADA, adenosine deaminase; PNP, purine nucleoside phosphorylase.

COMBINED T AND B LYMPHOCYTE DEFICIENCIES

SEVERE COMBINED IMMUNODEFICIENCY

Severe combined immunodeficiencies (SCID) are a heterogeneous group of rare, genetically determined disorders resulting from impaired T and B cell immunity (Table 19.4; Fig. 19.5). The condition is diagnosed in 1–5 live births per 500 000, though its severe nature suggests that it may often be a cause of undiagnosed infant death. The combined T and B cell deficiency gives rise to the early onset of susceptibility to infection by virtually all types of microorganism. Approximately 50% of SCID results from an X-linked, lymphopenic disorder with low T but normal B cell numbers. The genetic basis for this, a defect in the IL-2 receptor γ chain, has been defined recently (see below).

In autosomal recessive SCID, both T and B cell numbers are reduced, presumably as a result of failure of stem cell differentiation.

Other forms of SCID for which the basis is clearly defined are:

- defects of the purine salvage pathway enzymes: adenosine deaminase (ADA) and purine nucleoside phosphorylase (PNP)
- defective production of IL-2
- absence of surface expression of class I MHC and class II MHC molecules
- a defect in the TCR–CD3 complex.
- an inherited deficiency of the TAP transporter, resulting in absent class I MHC molecule expression
- a defect in ZAP-70, a TCR-associated tyrosine kinase involved in signalling and activation.

Table 19.4 **Severe combined immunodeficiency and related forms of combined immunodeficiency**

Designation	Cell numbers	Inheritance
X-linked SCID	T lymphocytes ↓ B lymphocytes normal	X-linked
Autosomal recessive SCID	T lymphocytes ↓ B lymphocytes ↓	Autosomal recessive
Adenosine deaminase deficiency	Progressive T lymphocytes ↓ Progressive B lymphocytes ↓	Autosomal recessive
Purine nucleoside phosphorylase deficiency	Progressive T lymphocytes ↓ B lymphocytes normal	Autosomal recessive
TCR immunodeficiency	CD2+ T lymphocytes normal B lymphocytes normal	Autosomal recessive
MHC class II deficiency	T lymphocytes normal B lymphocytes normal	Autosomal recessive
Defective IL-2 production	T lymphocytes normal B lymphocytes normal	Not known

↓, reduced levels

SCID caused by failures of antigen presentation or recognition

A rare cause of SCID, **TCR immunodeficiency**, has recently been described in which T cell function is impaired because of the absence of a key component of the CD3 complex. This transduces activation signals following interaction between the TCR heterodimer (α/β or γ/δ) and antigen and is composed of five polypeptides (p. 84). In TCR immunodeficiency, there is an impaired association of the CD3 ζ chain with other components of the CD3 complex, resulting in inhibition of complex assembly and transport to the cell surface. As a result, levels of the TCR–CD3 complex on the T lymphocyte surface are 10-fold lower than in healthy individuals. A clinically milder version, in which TCR–CD3 complex expression is less affected, has been described. Antigen-specific PHA responses are impaired in the severe form of TCR immunodeficiency and, to a lesser extent, in the mild version, whilst responses to T cell stimulation with the mitogen phorbol myristate acetate, anti-CD2 monoclonal antibody and IL-2, all of which provide TCR-independent stimulatory signals, remain intact.

Absence of surface expression of MHC class I molecules with normal class II expression (the '**bare lymphocyte syndrome**') has been described in association with combined immunodeficiency, but also in healthy individuals. In **MHC class II deficiency**, however, combined T and B cell immunodeficiency is a consistent finding.

The IL-2 receptor γ chain was the last component of the receptor to be identified. Once its gene was known to be located on the X chromosome, an immediate examination of IL-2 receptor γ chain genes in patients with X-linked SCID was prompted, revealing that each had a mutation at this site. However, one puzzle remained. Why was the defect in X-linked SCID so severe, in comparison, say, with children with IL-2 deficiency (Table 19.4), in whom T lymphocyte numbers are normal? It was reasoned that the IL-2 receptor γ chain might have other functions; one obvious possibility was that it acts as a receptor for other cytokines. This was soon shown to be the case, with receptors for IL-4, IL-7, IL-9 and IL-15 requiring the γ chain for normal function. This explains the profound T cell abnormalities seen in γ chain deficiency.

In **ADA deficiency**, the enzyme substrates adenosine and deoxyadenosine and the metabolite deoxyadenosine triphosphate preferentially accumulate in lymphoid cells and interfere with their development. The syndrome is diagnosed by measuring ADA activity, and screening studies have revealed partial ADA deficiency that is not associated with immunodeficiency. **PNP deficiency** is somewhat rarer, with some 30–40 patients identified worldwide. Impairment of B cell function is variable: in some cases there is even a normal response to childhood immunisations.

Clinical features

In SCID of whatever form, persistent infections usually develop by the age of 3 months. Candidal infections of the mouth and skin, protracted diarrhoea and failure to thrive are typical presenting features; if the underlying condition is left untreated, *Pneumocystis carinii* pneumonia is one of the most frequent causes of death.

Immunological features

The results of B and T lymphocyte phenotype analysis in peripheral blood are variable. As a general principle, when sufficient lymphocytes are available for analysis, T and B lymphocyte functions are severely impaired when assessed in vitro by mitogenic or antigenic stimulation. Occasionally, the presence of healthy maternal lymphocytes in the child's circulation may interfere with functional tests. Such cells can also give maternofetal GVHD in some 10% of affected children.

Treatment

The most successful treatment for all forms of SCID has been bone marrow transplantation from a healthy HLA-identical donor, such as a sibling. Figures obtained in a recent European study indicate that in HLA-identical transplants performed since 1983, 97% of children were alive and had successful T and B lymphocyte engraftment after a median follow-up of 41 months. Only 40% of affected children will have a related, matched donor, however, and haploidentical donors, usually a parent, are the next best option. In this case, the donated marrow is purged of T lymphocytes using monoclonal antibodies to avoid GVHD. In addition, there is evidence that treatment of the recipient with cytotoxic agents such as cyclophosphamide and busulphan (a **conditioning regimen**) enhances the chances of successful engraftment, particularly of donor B lymphocytes. With haploidentical donors, the best results were obtained using both T lymphocyte purging and a conditioning regimen, giving 86% sustained engraftment after a median of 47 months' follow-up.

Other therapies have been used in certain forms of SCID. Red blood cell transfusions were used as a source of enzymes to correct accumulation of toxic substances in ADA and PNP deficiency, and bovine ADA bound to polyethylene glycol ('antifreeze') is effective therapy in ADA deficiency.

X-LINKED HYPER IgM SYNDROME
Pathogenesis

An X-linked immune deficiency, characterised by an inability to produce mature immunoglobulin isoforms (IgG, IgA), but with an over-production of IgM, has been recognised for some years and termed the hyper IgM syndrome. Interestingly, although the predominant immunological manifestation suggests a B cell deficiency, patients are also prone to infection with organisms such as *Pneumocystis carinii*, more typical of

Gene therapy in SCID

The insertion of the genetic sequence encoding a deficient protein into carrier cells and thence into a recipient is a milestone of modern medicine. Preliminary studies to establish the safety of the technique were carried out in 1990 in patients suffering from advanced cancer. They were being given a treatment in which tumour infiltrating lymphocytes (TIL) are removed and activated with cytokines to increase their tumoricidal activity. TILs from some patients also had the gene for neomycin resistance inserted as a marker to enable clinicians to follow the distribution of the cells following reinfusion. The demonstration that the addition of a gene to the lymphocytes caused no side effects suggested that gene therapy is safe and encouraged the development of new therapies.

The first trial of gene therapy for any condition was carried out in two patients with ADA deficiency. Peripheral T cells were removed, activated with anti-CD3 and IL-2 to produce T cell expansion, and the gene for ADA introduced. Approximately 10^{10} cells were reinfused. In a 4-year-old girl, T cell ADA activity increased from 1 to 35% of normal, T cell numbers increased, titres of isohaemagglutinins appeared and normal delayed hypersensitivity and in vitro proliferative responses developed. Repeated cycles of T cell infusion are required, however, to maintain the effect. Future research will need to address the question of how to achieve prolonged benefits, possibly by insertion of genes into stem cells. Gene therapy could also be applied to TCR immunodeficiency and other causes of SCID in which the genetic basis is known and the gene sequence is available.

T cell immunodeficiency. In 1993, the basis for the disorder was identified as a defect in the gene encoding the ligand for CD40 (CD40L; it does not yet have its own CD designation). Interaction between CD40 on virgin B cells that have been activated by antigen and the CD40L on T cells in the germinal centre is a key process in the generation of class-switched, affinity-matured B cells (Figs 19.2 and 19.6).

Clinical and immunological features

Children usually present with recurrent pyogenic infections, although other complications, such as neutropenia and haemolytic or aplastic anaemia, may also be seen.

Levels of IgG, IgA and IgE are low or undetectable, whilst IgM is typically normal or raised (up to 10.0 g/l: normal upper limit in adults 2.0 g/l). There are no germinal centres in the lymph nodes.

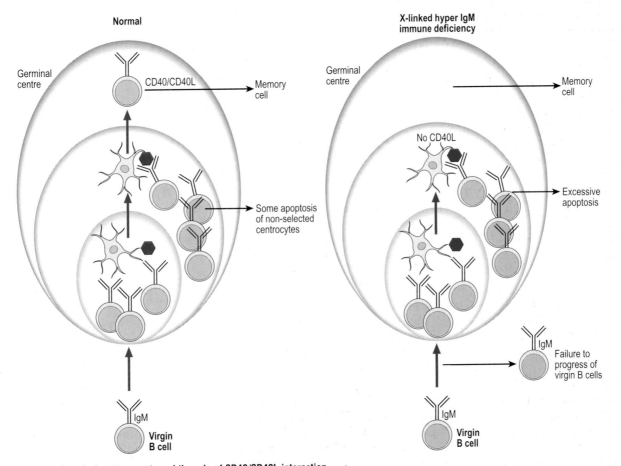

Fig. 19.6 Germinal centre events and the role of CD40/CD40L interaction.
In the absence of this interaction, B cells are destined to apoptosis or to remain as IgM-producing virgin B cells.

Treatment

At present, children with hyper IgM syndrome are managed with IVIG in much the same way as patients with X-linked agammaglobulinaemia. However, the additional risk of opportunistic infections owing to T cell immune deficiency makes this only a partial treatment. Hyper IgM syndrome is another of the immune deficiencies for which gene therapy may be indicated in the future.

WISKOTT–ALDRICH SYNDROME

Pathogenesis

This rare X-linked immunodeficiency is characterised by eczema, thrombocytopenia with abnormally small platelets, and recurrent pyogenic and opportunistic infections caused by a combination of T and B cell immune deficiency. In 1994, the genetic basis for the disorder was localised to an X chromosome gene encoding a novel protein, termed WASP (Wiskott–Aldrich syndrome protein) since as yet no function can be assigned to it.

Clinical and immunological features

Male infants usually present early in life with infections and bleeding. Eczema is a feature by the age of 1 year and there is an increased risk of lymphoreticular malignancy.

Levels of IgA and IgE are increased, IgM is decreased and IgG is normal. Isohaemagglutinins are reduced and responses to polysaccharide antigens are impaired. The number of circulating B and T lymphocytes are initially normal, but there is progressive T and B lymphopenia.

Treatment

Supportive therapy includes antibiotics and IVIG, but curative measures centre upon the use of HLA-identical bone marrow transplant preceded by a conditioning regimen of irradiation or busulphan to remove any remaining T cell function. The progressive nature of the immunodeficiency in Wiskott–Aldrich syndrome implies that without successful 'cures', such as bone marrow transplantation, the prognosis is poor.

ATAXIA TELANGIECTASIA

Pathogenesis

A failure of repair of chromosomal damage is thought to underlie this disease, which has an autosomal inheritance. Ataxia is apparent when affected infants begin to walk, and after 5 years, telangiectases develop on exposed parts of the body. Abnormalities of gene rearrangements have been invoked to account for characteristic immunoglobulin deficiencies, and recent studies on T lymphocytes suggest that the same mechanism may affect TCR usage.

Clinical and immunological features

Pyogenic infections of the respiratory tract and viral and fungal infections reflect the degree of reduction in T cell number and function.

IgM levels are increased; this is in keeping with the hypothesis that a failure occurs in the gene rearrangements that accompany isotype switching. Thus IgA levels are reduced in 80% of patients and a deficiency of IgG2 and IgG4 is common. The ratio of T cells using the $\gamma\delta$ to those using the $\alpha\beta$ TCR is between two and five times higher in patients with ataxia telangiectasia compared with healthy individuals, tending to support the hypothesis that gene rearrangements are abnormal.

Treatment

Treatment centres upon adequate therapy to treat infections. IVIG appears to reduce infective episodes, but information on thymus and bone marrow transplantation is not yet available. Death occurs in the second and third decades as a result of infection or malignancy, usually lymphoreticular.

Combined B and T lymphocyte defects

- SCID of T and B lymphocyte functions is rare but usually fatal unless treated.
- Bone marrow replacement is an effective and successful therapy in SCID.
- Gene replacement therapy has been used for the first time to treat the human disease adenosine deaminase deficiency.

NEUTROPHIL DEFECTS

CHRONIC GRANULOMATOUS DISEASE

Pathogenesis

Chronic granulomatous disease is an immunodeficiency that results from a defect in neutrophil killing. Two thirds of cases are X-linked and the remainder have an autosomal recessive inheritance. The functional defect, in generating the respiratory burst to produce superoxide, hydrogen peroxide, oxidised halogens and hydroxyl radicals for bacterial killing, is common to all types of chronic granulomatous disease. There are several genetic bases for the same functional defect, however. The respiratory burst requires a series of electron transfers using NADPH, a flavoprotein, a quinone and a unique cytochrome b_{558} (Fig. 19.7). Cytochrome b_{558} is a heterodimer composed of 91 kDa and 22 kDa chains. In the X-linked form of chronic granulomatous disease, the 91 kDa chain is deficient and the cytochrome is undetectable. In the majority of autosomal recessive chronic granulomatous disease a 47 kDa phosphoprotein, which is probably part of the electron transport chain, is deficient. Two rare autosomal recessive conditions exist, one in which the 22 kDa chain is absent, and one in which another oxidative protein in the chain, of 67 kDa, is missing.

Clinical and immunological features

The disease has an incidence of approximately 1 in 10^6. By the age of 2 years, children with chronic granulomatous disease will have begun to experience infections; these typically affect the deep tissues (lymphadenitis, osteomyelitis and skin abscesses) as well as causing pneumonia and periodontitis.

Neutrophil numbers are either normal or increased in response to intercurrent infection. The qualitative NBT test reveals a complete deficiency of neutrophils capable of undergoing a respiratory burst.

Treatment

Aggressive treatment of infections, with surgical drainage of deep abscesses, enhances survival. Antibiotic and antifungal therapy should be prolonged for 5–6 weeks. With this management, survival into the second and third decades can be achieved (see box: 'IFN-γ treatment in chronic granulomatous disease').

IFN-γ treatment in chronic granulomatous disease

This therapy has recently been attempted in a controlled trial of 128 patients, on the basis of results obtained in vitro that showed that IFN-γ added to patients' neutrophils partially corrected the defect in superoxide production. The therapy increased the time between serious infections (i.e. those requiring hospitalisation) and decreased the number of such episodes by half, irrespective of the type of chronic granulomatous disease. There remains some controversy as to whether the treatment augments superoxide production in vivo. In the majority of cases, it probably does not, and its efficacy may be a result of enhancing oxygen-independent antimicrobial pathways, or through the action of other arms of the immune system, such as T and B cell function.

LEUKOCYTE ADHESION DEFICIENCY

Pathogenesis

Leukocyte adhesion deficiency (LAD) results from defects in the family of immune cell surface glycoproteins, termed the integrins (see p. 25). The β_2 integrin family have a common β chain, CD18, which combines with different α chains (CD11a, CD11b and CD11c) to form heterodimers including the complement receptor 3 (CD11b/CD18, receptor for the opsonin iC3b) and LFA-1 (CD11a/CD18), which is important in lymphocyte, monocyte and phagocyte adherence. Leukocyte adhesion deficiency-1, or LAD1, results from absence of CD18 so that the receptors are non-functional, leading to decreased adherence, phagocytosis and chemotaxis by neutrophils, and impaired T cell-mediated cytotoxicity.

A second form of LAD, LAD2, has been described. In this rare autosomal recessive condition, infants are unable to synthesise fucose from GDP mannose and cannot form the Lewis X ligand for some of the selectin molecules.

Clinical and immunological features

LAD1 has autosomal recessive inheritance and may present almost immediately after birth, with delayed umbilical cord separation. Recurrent infections similar to those in chronic granulomatous disease appear during the first decade of life. The clinical picture is similar in LAD2, but the children also have mental retardation.

In LAD1, monoclonal antibodies directed against CR-3 and LFA-1 demonstrate their absence on neutrophils, monocytes and lymphocytes. In LAD2, the sialyl Lewis X molecule is not detectable.

Treament

Patients require aggressive treatment with antimicrobial and antifungal agents.

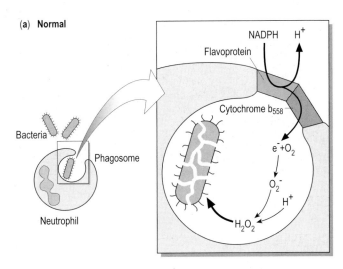

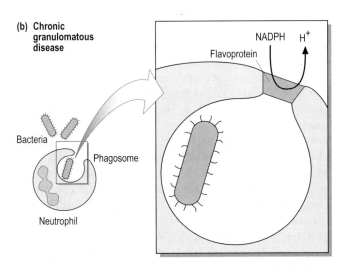

Fig. 19.7 Neutrophil killing.
Mechanisms involved in the development of toxic oxygen metabolites (O_2^-, H_2O_2) to mediate death of microorganisms within the phagosome of a neutrophil in a normal individual (**a**) and in a patient with chronic granulomatous disease (**b**). These patients lack cytochrome b_{558} and are unable to generate a respiratory burst.

> **Neutrophil defects**
>
> - Primary defects of neutrophil function arise rarely but have severe clinical consequences.
> - The NBT test is diagnostic of a defect in the neutrophil respiratory burst, found in chronic granulomatous disease.
> - IFN-γ therapy in chronic granulomatous disease reduces the incidence of serious infections.

DEFICIENCY OF COMPLEMENT COMPONENTS

The consequences of deficiency of complement proteins, whether pro-inflammatory or regulatory components, can be predicted from knowledge of their functions (Table 19.5). Broadly speaking, the main physiological roles of complement are in enhancing neutrophil-mediated lysis of bacteria and in solubilising and removing immune complexes. Failures in these will lead to impaired non-specific immunity with an increase in bacterial infections, and a tendency to immune complex diseases such as SLE. Whilst it is easy to accept that complement deficiency predisposes to infection with pyogenic bacteria, it is somewhat unexpected to find that neisserial infections are often encountered in patients with complement defects, particularly defects of the membrane attack complex. Therefore, complement deficiency reveals a function of the cascade that might not otherwise have been uncovered, to mediate lysis of *Neisseria* directly.

The inheritance pattern of factor D deficiency is not yet known, but most other deficiencies are inherited in

Table 19.5 **Deficiencies of the complement cascade and associated syndromes**

Deficiency	Number of cases/prevalence	Associated features
Classical pathway		
C1q, C1r/C1s	>50	SLE-like syndrome; pyogenic infections
C4	17	SLE-like syndrome
C2	>100	SLE-like syndrome; vasculitis
C3	16	Pyogenic infections
Alternative pathway		
Factor D	1	Neisserial infection
Properdin	>50	Neisserial infection
Membrane attack pathway		
C5, 6, 7, 8	>130	Neisserial infection, SLE
C9	Common in Japan (1/1000)	None/neisserial infection
Regulatory proteins		
Factors H, I	27	Pyogenic infections, SLE
C1 inhibitor	Prevalence of 1/150 000	Hereditary angioedema

an autosomal recessive pattern with two notable exceptions: properdin deficiency is X-linked and C1 inhibitor deficiency has an autosomal dominant inheritance. Deficiencies may also result from increased consumption: loss of C2 and C4 resulting from uncontrolled classical pathway activation in C1 inhibitor deficiency can result in immune complex disease.

Classical pathway

Classical pathway defects are often associated with an increased risk of infection and immune complex disease, because of their critical role in the solubilisation of antigen–antibody complexes. Defects of C1r and C1s occur together, probably as a consequence of their close genetic linkage on chromosome 12. Complete C4 deficiency requires the inheritance of non-functional ('null') alleles at all four *C4A* and *C4B* loci. More than two thirds of patients with C4 deficiency will have an autoimmune disease, and it has the highest incidence proportionally of SLE amongst the complement deficiencies. C2 is the most common homozygous complement deficiency in northern Europeans, with a prevalence of between 10 and 30 per 100 000 of the population.

Alternative pathway

Defects in alternative pathway components are mainly associated with increased susceptibility to infection, notably with *Neisseria*, reflecting the role of this part of the cascade in immediate and innate responses to microorganisms.

Common pathway

The component C3 lies at the convergence of the classical and alternative pathways, has a major role in opsonisation and must be activated before the membrane attack pathway can proceed. Given its pivotal role, therefore, it is not surprising that no homozygous C3-deficient patient has been reported who is disease free. Approximately one fifth of C3-deficient patients will have a disorder that is usually attributed to damage mediated by circulating immune complexes: SLE, vasculitis or glomerulonephritis.

Absence of any one of the components between C5 and C8 in the membrane attack complex results in a significantly increased risk of infection with *Neisseria meningitidis* and *N. gonorrhoeae*; SLE is a rare complication. Meningococcal infections are often repeated and may involve unusual serotypes. Homozygous deficiency of C9 is common in Japan (1/1000 individuals) and in early studies was not associated with increased meningococcal disease. Careful studies taking into account the lower incidence of meningococcal infection in Japan have shown that C9 deficiency does confer a risk of disease but at a lower level than for other membrane attack components.

Complement regulatory proteins

Amongst the complement regulatory proteins, deficiency of factors H and I are rare. Unrestrained activation leads to an acquired state of C3 deficiency, giving an increased risk of pyogenic infections. Deficiency of **C1 inhibitor** (also termed C1 esterase deficiency) was first described in 1881. This enzyme is involved in regulation of several plasma enzyme systems (e.g. the kinin system) and its continued consumption means that the resulting 50% of normal production, as occurs in heterozygotes for the C1 inhibitor gene deletion, barely copes with the demand. Under minimal stress, therefore, uncontrolled activation of complement and the kinins may occur. The clinical picture is then one of progressive oedema of the deep tissues affecting the face, trunk, viscera and the airway, hence the name **hereditary angioedema** (HAE). Laryngeal oedema may be fatal unless the acute attack fades or is treated. The increase in fluid loss into the tissues may be a result of bradykinin release or C2 kinin derived from complement. Uncontrolled classical pathway activation leads to reductions in C2 and C4, but controls at the C3 level are intact and other pathways are not affected. Treatment of acute attacks previously relied upon fresh frozen plasma as a source of C1 inhibitor, but purified preparations are now available. Plasmin inhibitors (tranexamic acid, ε-aminocaproic acid) may control C1 inhibitor consumption and can be used prophylactically to cover surgical procedures. Prophylactic therapy centres upon drugs belonging to a class called **impeded androgens** or **anabolic steroids**, of which the most commonly used is danazol, which increases C1 inhibitor levels by an unknown mechanism.

Some 85% of patients with HAE have symptoms resulting from an absence of C1 inhibitor (type 1 HAE) and in the remainder the protein is present but non-functional (type 2 HAE). An acquired version of the syndrome (AAE) is described in association with B cell lymphoproliferative disorders (type 1 AAE) or an autoantibody to C1 inhibitor (Table 19.6).

Deficiency of complement components

- Complement defects are associated with an increased risk of infections with pyogenic organisms and immune complex-mediated diseases such as SLE (classical pathway), neisserial infections (alternative pathway) or a combination of neisserial infections and lupus (membrane attack pathway).
- C1 inhibitor deficiency is relatively common and can result in life-threatening laryngeal oedema.

SECONDARY IMMUNODEFICIENCY

As stated in the introduction, secondary causes of immune deficiency, particularly of neutrophil and antibody function, are relatively common. These may arise secondary to treatment, neoplasia or viral infection. Steroids are widely used as immunosuppressants in autoimmune and other inflammatory conditions and have a range of deleterious effects on most parts of the immune system. Cyclosporin A is used in transplantation to control graft rejection and has direct inhibitory effects on T cell function. Infections with *Candida albicans*, *Pneumocystis carinii*, herpes zoster and cytomegalovirus are relatively common sequelae, therefore. Cytotoxic drugs and radiotherapy are used to treat

---

Immunological therapies in secondary immunodeficiency

Recent therapeutic advances in the management of secondary immunodeficiencies promise to reverse some of the damage inflicted upon the immune system by drugs and tumours. Double-blind trials of IVIG therapy in B cell chronic lymphatic leukaemia have shown a reduction in the incidence of infections in the treated group. However, an attempt to apply the rules of economics to this therapy suggest that conventional antibiotic treatment may be more cost effective, so that it is not clear whether IVIG will be generally adopted. The results of trials in multiple myeloma are awaited.

A therapy gaining wider acceptance is the use of recombinant human colony-stimulating factors such as G-CSF in treatment-induced neutropenia. G-CSF induces a prompt and selective increase in blood neutrophils, which is of use in hastening marrow recovery after chemotherapy or bone marrow transplant. This reduces the period of neutropenia when patients are at high risk of infection and require hospitalisation, though a question mark remains over whether CSFs could actually worsen the course of some myeloid malignancies.

Table 19.6 **Function and presence of C1 inhibitor and classical pathway components in hereditary and acquired angioedema**

	C1 inhibitor function	C1 inhibitor antigen	C1q	C2	C4
Hereditary angioedema					
Type 1	↓	↓	N	↓	↓
Type 2	↓	N or ↑	N	↓	↓
Acquired angioedema					
Type 1	↓	N or ↓	↓	↓	↓
Type 2	↓	N or ↓	↓	↓	↓

N, normal; ↓, reduced levels; ↑, raised levels
Low levels of C2 and C4 are helpful in the diagnosis, particularly if measured during an attack. To distinguish hereditary and acquired angioedema, measurement of C1q may be useful.

leukaemia and lymphoma, either directly or as part of the marrow ablation required before bone marrow transplantation. Prolonged states of lymphopenia and neutropenia may follow, during which patients are acutely susceptible to infection. Finally, lymphoproliferative disorders, particularly those affecting the B cell compartment, such as B cell chronic lymphatic leukaemia (CLL) and multiple myeloma, can result in functional antibody deficiency.

Secondary immunodeficiency

- Secondary immunodeficiency is common and results mainly from chemotherapy and neoplasia.
- New therapies with colony-stimulating factors and intravenous immunoglobulin are improving its management.

Human immunodeficiency virus and AIDS

In June 1981, the Centers for Disease Control (CDC: American equivalent of the Public Health Laboratory Service in the UK) reported an unexplained cluster of five cases of *Pneumocystis carinii* pneumonia in Los Angeles, all in homosexual men. Until then, this infection was typically seen in immunocompromised individuals, most frequently in immunosuppressed transplant recipients and patients with haematological malignancies undergoing cytotoxic therapy. The report resonated throughout America, where physicians began to recognise that for up to 2 years they had been witnessing unusual disorders in young men: CNS infection with the protozoal parasite *Toxoplasma gondii*, severe herpes skin infections, widespread infection with *Candida albicans*, as well as manifestations unrelated to infections, such as extreme weight loss, fevers, lymphadenopathy and the appearance of a tumour, Kaposi's sarcoma, previously associated with elderly men. The disease was labelled the acquired immunodeficiency syndrome (AIDS) and was destined to engender not only a mini-revolution in social behaviour but also an unprecedented level of international scientific controversy.

A novel retrovirus, now named the human immunodeficiency virus type 1 (HIV-1), was isolated from a patient at risk of the disease in 1983 and subsequently from patients with AIDS in 1984. 2 years later another retrovirus (HIV-2) associated with a clinical immunodeficiency syndrome resembling AIDS was isolated from patients in West Africa. Much of the controversy alluded to has surrounded the question of whether HIV *causes* AIDS, although a causal link between the two is certainly a view held by the vast majority of scientists in the field. The dominant immunopathogenic feature of the syndrome is an absolute deficiency of circulating CD4+ helper/inducer T lymphocytes.

In America, the death toll from AIDS is now in excess of 100 000. Estimates of the scale of the problem vary, but there may be 50–100 thousand HIV carriers in the UK, and 8–10 million worldwide.

HIV may be considered as an infectious disease like any other, in that transmisission is largely related to behaviour: changes in sexual and social behaviour, therefore, offer the best hope of controlling the disease. Where this is not possible, a safe and effective vaccine will be required and may ultimately offer the opportunity of eradicating the virus.

EPIDEMIOLOGY

MODES AND RISK OF TRANSMISSION OF HIV

HIV has been isolated from virtually all body fluids, including blood, semen, vaginal secretions, tears, urine, saliva and breast-milk. The most common form of transmission is through sexual contact, the next most frequent in developed nations being the parenteral route because of needle-sharing drug abusers. Blood or blood-product transfusion remains a risk where antibody testing of donors is not performed. Other recognised transmissions are maternal–fetal and mother–baby during breast-feeding. There are approximately five cases worldwide of HIV seroconversion (development of antibodies to HIV as evidence of infection) following skin or mucous membrane exposure to contaminated blood, although the risk of such transmission is considered negligible if standard precautions in the handling of bodily fluids are taken. There are no reported cases of transmission via kissing or food, drink or casual contact, from infected doctors to their patients, or from mosquito bites.

The danger of acquiring HIV infection is difficult to quantify and the best estimates are given in Table 20.1. The likelihood of transmission from an infected mother to the child during pregnancy is high, with an even higher risk if the baby is then breast-fed. Intriguingly, transmission to the first-born of a pair of twins is more common than to the second-born, possibly because the first twin makes the most difficult and traumatic passage through the birth canal, increasing the chance of contact with virus carried by the mother.

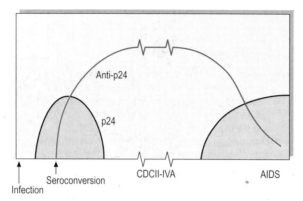

Fig. 20.4 Diagnostic markers of HIV infection.
p24 antigen appears soon after infection and declines following
seroconversion and production of anti-p24 antibody. This pattern is
reversed in the later stages of the disease.

enzymes are contained within a core surrounded by
capsid proteins (Fig. 20.3). This in turn is enveloped
by a lipid membrane which is anchored internally to
viral matrix proteins and crossed by integral envelope
glycoproteins that protrude into the external milieu.
The constituents of the virus are denoted by a p (for
protein) or gp (for glycoprotein) followed by their
molecular weight. Antibody responses to capsid, matrix
and envelope proteins are detectable in the serum of
infected patients. For the most part, responses such
as these, mainly to p24 and gp120, are sufficient
for diagnosis. In the early stages of infection, before
seroconversion, free p24 in the blood may be used
diagnostically. Most cases of infection with HIV will
follow the pattern shown in Figure 20.4, in which the
antigen, in this case p24, and anti-p24 antibody run
a reciprocal course. In a minority of cases antibody is
not detectable, and evidence of HIV infection is only
obtained by amplification of HIV DNA using the
sensitive polymerase chain reaction, which can detect
a single copy of the genome.

The HIV genome may be divided into three regions:
one encoding the capsid and matrix proteins (*gag*), one
the reverse transcriptase, a protease and an integrase
(*pol*) and one the envelope proteins (*env*). Various other
genes, including *tat*, *rev* and *nef* have been identified as
having regulatory effects on viral assembly, and drugs
that modulate these functions are actively being sought.

THE IMMUNOPATHOGENESIS OF HIV INFECTION

There is little consensus as to how HIV causes AIDS
and, indeed, there remains a vocal minority which says
that it does not. Undoubtedly the main component of
the immunodeficiency is the CD4⁺ T lymphopenia,
and various mechanisms for the pathogenesis of this
have been invoked; all have in vitro data in their support and some are outlined here. Additional components are effects on macrophage and B cell function.

CD4 is the HIV receptor

As soon as HIV had been isolated, the recognition that
marked depletion of CD4⁺ T lymphocytes was the hall-

The origins of HIV

The apparent abruptness of the appearance
of a new disease and aetiological agent have led to
intense speculation on the origins of HIV. It is unlikely that the virus suddenly materialised in the late
1970s. Clues to the origin of the virus come from its
similarity in structure to simian immunodeficiency
virus (SIV), first isolated from captive macaques
with an immunodeficiency syndrome resembling
AIDS. Antibody responses to HIV-1, HIV-2 and
SIV show cross-reactivity and there are sequence
similarities between them. SIV has been isolated
from wild African green monkeys, who are, surprisingly, disease free. HIV-2 and SIV share the greatest
proportion of sequence homologies, suggesting that
they have a common ancestor which itself shares
origins with HIV-1. The host in which the progenitor
of HIV developed, and the means of transfer to
humans remain open to speculation.

mark of AIDS led to the identification of CD4 as the
viral receptor (Fig. 20.5a). HIV has a tropism for cells
bearing CD4, the accessory molecule that stabilises
interactions with class II MHC in antigen recognition
(p. 82). Whilst there may be other mechanisms that
allow HIV entry into a cell, by far the most important
factor is the possession of surface CD4.

The envelope protein gp120 binds CD4 with a high
affinity constant (K_d 10^{-9} M). A change in conformation of the envelope proteins ensues and fusion and
viral entry is mediated by gp41 (Figs 20.5b and 20.6).
Recent evidence indicates that fusion requires the presence on the target cell of additional receptors. One had
been identified as fusin, and another as a B chemokine
receptor, CC CKR5. Intriguingly, it has recently been
reported that chemokines (a family of small molecular
weight peptides with diverse inflammatory effects) are
capable of inhibiting HIV replication in vitro, presumably by blockade of their cell surface receptors, inhibiting HIV fusion and entry. Once inside the CD4⁺
cell, the virus is uncoated and viral RNA transcribed to
DNA using the enzyme reverse transcriptase. Double-
stranded DNA is then circularised and inserted into the
host cell genome. What follows, latency or viral replication, is dependent upon the state of activation of the
cell (Fig. 20.5c,d and box). When virus is assembled
and leaves the cell, it does so by budding, incorporating
host cell membrane into its coat (Fig. 20.5e).

Cells derived from the monocyte/macrophage lineage have low surface levels of CD4, and are capable of
sustaining HIV infection. These include:

- alveolar macrophages
- microglial cells
- Langerhans cells in the skin
- myelo-monocytic bone marrow precursors
- thymocyte precursor cells
- dendritic cells.

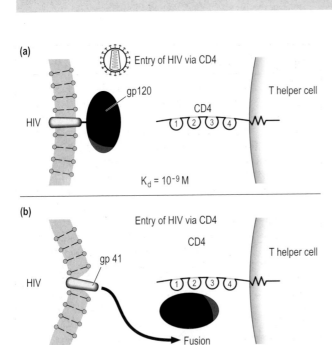

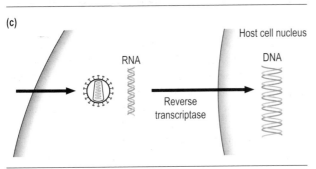

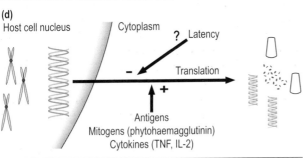

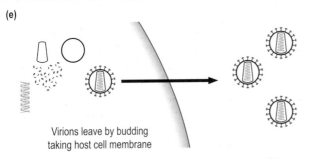

Fig. 20.5 **HIV infection of a cell, from binding to the CD4 molecule to viral budding.**

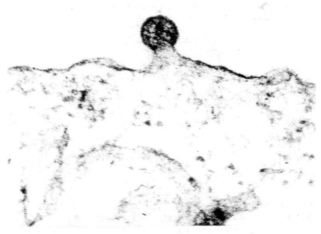

Fig. 20.6 **Electron micrograph of HIV fusing with cell membrane of a CD4+ T lymphocyte.**
(Reproduced with permission from Stein et al 1987 Cell 49: 659–668.)

Latency and hypermutation contribute to the pathogenesis of HIV infection

There are several important features about HIV that have a bearing on the nature of the infection, particularly its latency, as well as having implications for vaccine development. The first is that the genetic information of the virus is permanently incorporated into the genome of the infected cell. Second, the regulatory genes that govern viral replication and assembly are under the influence of activities within the host cell and there is evidence that activation of infected cells, by mitogen, antigen or cytokines such as TNF, up-regulates viral replication. This suggests there may be some benefit in avoidance of inter-current illnesses in HIV-infected patients. Third, the virus has a hypermutability, largely the result of the error-prone nature of the reverse transcriptase that catalyses DNA synthesis from viral RNA. This gives the possibility of mutant strains arising within an infected individual that are resistant either to immune attack or to drugs. One example is the appearance of syncytium-inducing (SI) strains (see Fig. 20.8b below), which may be more cytopathic. Evidence of AZT-resistant strains has already been acquired and these are likely to be under strong positive selection pressures. One theory adopts this principle to explain the latency of HIV infection as a period in which wave after wave of new escape-mutants of HIV are dealt with effectively but by a slowly dwindling immune system, until there is no more protection against the virus, and symptomatic immunodeficiency ensues.

Interestingly, HIV is not cytopathic to these cell types, and their role in the pathogenesis of the infection is believed to be as a reservoir of infection. They do not remain functionally intact, however, and impaired macrophage chemotaxis and cytotoxic ability may contribute to infections at mucosal sites in the lung and gut.

Is HIV directly cytopathic?

The answer to the question is yes — maybe. In vitro, there is little doubt that HIV infection of CD4+ T lymphocyte cell lines can lead to cell death, and two mechanisms have been invoked. In the first, large numbers of viral particles budding simultaneously from

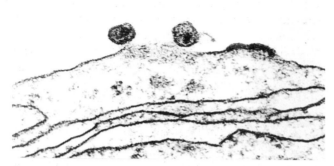

Fig. 20.7 **Electron micrograph of HIV virions budding from the cytoplasm of a CD4⁺ T lymphocyte.**
(Reproduced with permission from Stein et al 1987 Cell 49: 659–668.)

the cell can fuse with CD4 on the same cell's surface, destroying membrane integrity in an 'auto-fusion' (Figs 20.7 and 20.8a). This mechanism is dependent upon a high concentration of surface CD4, as seen on T lymphocytes but not on macrophages and dendritic cells, which could explain why they form an effective reservoir without being lysed. The second mechanism centres upon the observation in vitro that infected cells fuse to form large, multinucleate giant cell syncytia that have a markedly reduced half-life compared with intact cells (Figs 20.8b and 20.9).

In the past, there were several reasons for doubting that these mechanisms explain the loss of CD4⁺ T lymphocytes in HIV infection. First, the frequency of cells in the circulation that were infected appeared to be too low for syncytia to form. However, early estimates of 1/10 000 cells infected have been revised in the light of studies with more sensitive techniques, particularly the polymerase chain reaction. In early infection 1/100 cells may contain virus and this rises to 10% in patients with ARC and AIDS. Despite this, the lack of demonstrable syncytia in the circulation, lymph nodes or other sites militates against this theory. However, the possibility that large-scale viral budding kills CD4⁺ T lymphocytes remains an attractive hypothesis.

Cytotoxic responses to HIV-infected cells

CD8⁺ T cells isolated from asymptomatic HIV-infected individuals are capable of destroying target cells expressing autologous class I MHC molecules presenting antigenic sequences of the p24 gag peptide and also env- and pol-derived peptides (Fig. 20.8c). Since cytotoxic T cells are an important line of host defence against intracellular viruses, it is reasonable to suppose that they are important in protection against HIV infection. The double-edge of this protective sword is apparent when one considers that the infected cells are CD4⁺ T helper/inducer lymphocytes, depletion of which leads to clinical immunodeficiency.

Other cytotoxic responses have also been demonstrated in vitro. Serum from HIV infected patients lyses target cells in an antibody-dependent cell cytotoxicity (ADCC) reaction (p. 109). The specificity of the antibodies is not known, but it has been speculated that

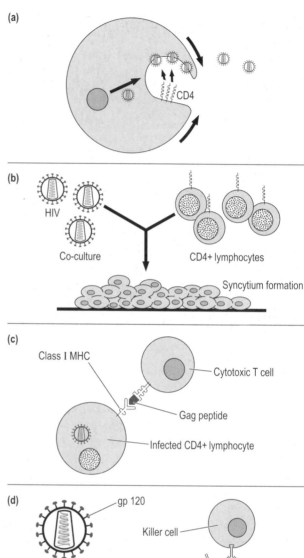

Fig. 20.8 **Mechanisms of CD4⁺ T cell dealth.**
(**a**) Large-scale viral budding leads to 'auto-fusion'. (**b**) Cell death caused by fusion of cells to form giant cell syncytia. (**c**) Cytotoxic T cells can destroy target cells expressing class I MHC molecules presenting viral peptides (gag). (**d**) Antibody-dependent cell toxicity.

free gp120 binding to CD4 on the cell surface could render T helper cells as targets for ADCC reactions in patients with anti-gp120 antibodies (Fig. 20.8d), which is a sizeable majority.

Apoptosis: programmed cell death

Programmed cell death (PCD; also known as apoptosis) is a physiological process, which we have already encountered during clonal deletion in the thymus (see p. 93). There is some evidence to support the hypothesis that PCD is initiated by HIV in T lymphocytes in infected patients. First, one of the early characteristics

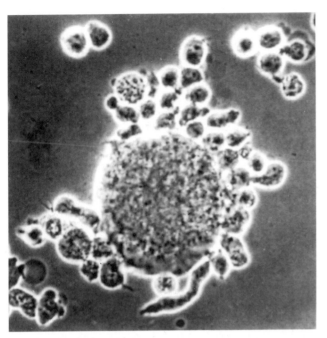

Fig. 20.9 **CD4+ lymphocytes cultured with HIV forming a large syncytium by repeated cell–cell fusions.**
(Reproduced with permission from Stein et al Cell 49: 659–668.)

and T_H2) was beginning to germinate, and it was subsequently proposed that the immune dysfunction in HIV infection could be accounted for by an imbalance between T_H1 and T_H2 cells. Therefore, T_H1 activity (cell proliferation through production of IL-2) was being overpowered by the actions of T_H2 cells (immunoglobulin production), bearing in mind that these subsets are mutually antagonistic. In recent years, there has been much activity in laboratories throughout the world to substantiate the theory that profound immunodeficiency and AIDS develop after HIV infection as a result of T_H1/T_H2 imbalance. In one analysis, T cell clones derived from a patient just before HIV seroconversion were predominantly T_H1, producing IL-2, but 3 years later were mainly IL-4-secreting T_H2 cells. Following the theory to its logical conclusion, one might expect that HIV-infected patients who remain well some years after seroconversion ('long-term survivors') might have T_H1 responses intact; indeed, there is evidence to support this. The search is on for therapies that may selectively enhance T_H1, and dampen T_H2 responses, although one obvious candidate, IL-2, has been tried and appears not to work.

of CD4 lymphocytes in HIV infection is their reduced responsiveness to recall antigens, associated with reduced IL-2 secretion. This is also an early feature of T lymphocyte PCD. Second, there is the progressive depletion of CD4 lymphocytes, an obvious consequence if PCD is widespread. Finally, CD4 and CD8 lymphocytes from patients with HIV infection show early signs of PCD after in vitro culture, and this is hastened by cell activation. The mechanism through which the virus acts is unknown, but it may involve interaction between surface CD4 molecules and soluble gp120 or endogenous anti-CD4 antibodies.

B lymphocytes in HIV infection

Hypergammaglobulinaemia, with elevated levels of IgG and IgA, is an early feature of HIV infection. This finding is something of a paradox, since one might predict that a lack of T cell help would result in poor B cell function. In fact, patients with HIV infection acquire a functional antibody deficiency, since IgG and IgA hyperproduction is poorly directed and results in polyspecific antibodies. Response to immunisation tends to be poor, and the functional antibody deficiency may lead to infection with pyogenic organisms such as *Streptococcus pneumoniae*. The mechanism of the hypergammaglobulinaemia is not known but may relate to high circulating levels of IL-6.

The balance of T_H1/T_H2 in HIV infection

Two early observations in laboratory studies on HIV infection were that T cell proliferation in response to mitogens and the ability to produce IL-2 tend to decline and that immunoglobulin levels rise. In the early 1990s, the concept of functional CD4 subsets (T_H1

HIV immunopathogenesis

- HIV is an RNA retrovirus, relying upon a reverse transcriptase to translate its genome into DNA: this and other essential enzymes are potential drug targets.
- Latency and a tendency to mutate are features of the virus that add to its pathogenicity.
- The predominant effect of HIV infection is depletion of CD4+ T lymphocytes, but B cell and macrophage immunity is also compromised.
- The precise mechanism by which HIV mediates destruction of CD4+ T lymphocytes is unknown.

TREATMENTS OF THE FUTURE

NOVEL DRUG APPROACHES

The complex nature of the life cycle of HIV offers several opportunities for modulation by drugs. Interference with reverse transcriptase activity by AZT may be improved upon with dideoxycytidine (ddC) and dideoxyinosine (ddI), related thymidine analogues that work via the same mechanism but may have less side effects.

Other targets of drug research are the integrase enzyme necessary for insertion of viral DNA into the host cell genome, the protease that is required for extracellular processing of *gag*- and *pol*-encoded structural proteins, and the regulatory proteins such as nef, tat and rev, which control viral replication. These new protease inhibitors have already become available.

VACCINES

There are various issues overshadowing the quest for an effective, inexpensive and safe vaccine to protect against HIV infection:

- sterile versus protective immunity
- virus hides within cells
- viral genome inserted in host cell
- cell-to-cell passage
- reservoirs of infection
- nature of protection unknown
- virus is hypermutable
- no good animal models of HIV infection.

First, there is the question of what type of immunity is required. The optimal vaccine is that most closely resembling the natural infection, and live attenuated viruses generally give the best protection. However, since HIV copies its genome into the host cell, it is unlikely that a live vaccine will be acceptable. Many vaccines work on the principle of providing 'protective immunity', in which infection is allowed but disease is controlled. Again, this may be difficult in a disease in which the viral genome is inserted into host cells and in which it appears that ultimately infection always leads to disease. Protective immunity will also require very high vaccination levels in the population, since infected, protected individuals will remain able to pass on the virus, at least theoretically. Another option is to prevent infection completely, so-called 'sterile immunity'. This requires a constant, high level of protection, which may be difficult to maintain.

Another problem that is faced is the fact that viral transmission may not take place through the passage of free virions, but through infected cells. In this case, the virus is hidden from the high-titre antibodies that might otherwise protect. Should infection occur, the virus hides intracellularly, has an integrated genome, cell reservoirs of infection and may pass from cell to cell through direct contact without becoming exposed to the immune system. One of the most difficult aspects is the unknown nature of protection — it appears that all cases of HIV infection will ultimately result in immunodeficiency despite adequate antibody and cytotoxic T cell responses in the early stages. Hypermutability is undoubtedly a problem in vaccine design, which must cover all strains of infective virus.

Despite these caveats, many vaccines have been developed and tried, mainly in chimpanzees. There is evidence from these studies and others on mother–child transmission, in which high levels of maternal anti-gp120 antibodies transferred across the placenta protect the fetus from infection, that sterilising immunity may be achievable. Subunit vaccines, comprising components such as the gp120 envelope glycoprotein, have been tried extensively. Phase 1 trials, using volunteers to establish dosages and safety, have shown vaccines composed of gp120 to cause no ill effects and to produce antibodies that are neutralising in vitro. An attractive option is to administer combinations of gp120 peptides with slightly different sequences in the immunogenic regions and thus attempt to induce immunity to several strains.

Treatments of the future

- Drugs that inhibit reverse transcriptase are effective in reducing the progression of HIV infection, and better formulations as well as therapies aimed at other viral components are in hand.
- Several features of the virus, such as its hypermutability and its location within cells, present grave problems in vaccine design.
- For vaccines, aiming towards sterile immunity may be the most logical choice for protection, but the most difficult to achieve.

CHAPTER 21

Immunological manifestations of haematological disease

Malignant neoplastic expansions of red and white blood cells give rise to diseases such as leukaemia, lymphoma and myeloma. The diagnosis and management of the neoplastic diseases of blood are largely the realm of the haematologist, and these aspects are not covered in any depth in this chapter. The effects of such diseases on the functioning of immune cells are several. First, marrow replacement by malignant cells and suppression of normal haemopoiesis may result in reduced or defective generation of healthy immune effectors, such as neutrophils, leading to **secondary immunodeficiency**. Second, a malignant neoplastic expansion of cells of the B lymphocyte lineage can lead to disease as a result of an inability to regulate normal antibody production (i.e. **secondary antibody deficiency**). Finally, **autoimmune disorders** may arise, either as a consequence of the nature of antibody produced by a neoplastic clone or as a result of defective immune regulation. These are secondary, immune manifestations of malignant haematological cancers.

Autoimmune diseases affecting white and red blood cells result in shortening of cell survival and cytopenias (reduction in cell numbers) if production cannot compensate. These conditions may arise as primary disorders, or as complications of haematological malignancies, autoimmune disease, infections or drug therapy.

AUTOIMMUNE DISEASES OF THE BLOOD

AUTOIMMUNE HAEMOLYTIC ANAEMIA

Autoimmune haemolytic anaemia (AHA) is a relatively uncommon disease, which, in its mildest form, may manifest as a compensated normochromic normocytic anaemia but may rarely present acutely as a life-threatening haemolytic disease. It may arise as a primary condition, or secondary to a range of other malignant, autoimmune or inflammatory diseases (Fig. 21.1). The cause of the haemolysis is the presence of circulating autoantibodies to red blood cell surface antigens, which reduces the survival of red blood cells. The bone marrow compensates for the reduced survival by increasing cell production. It is the combination of reduced survival, increased production and increased metabolism of haem that makes up the clinical and laboratory manifestations of haemolytic anaemia.

One of the features of these disorders is the distinctive physicochemical nature of some of the autoantibodies. The majority (80–90%) of anti-red blood cell autoantibodies (Fig. 21.2) react optimally with their targets at physiological temperatures (i.e. 37°C) and

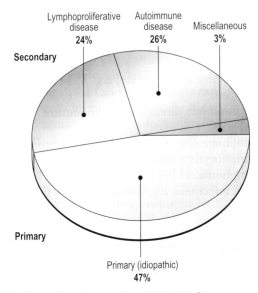

Fig. 21.1 **Causes of autoimmune haemolytic anaemia.**

DRUG-INDUCED HAEMOLYSIS

Drug-induced haemolysis may arise as an immune-mediated process with certain therapeutic agents. At least three well defined mechanisms have been described (Fig. 21.6). The most common results in a haemolytic syndrome indistinguishable from warm AHA, in which IgG autoantibodies to Rh antigens are formed. This form of drug-induced haemolysis has been most frequently associated with α-methyldopa, a drug formerly used in hypertension but now rarely prescribed. Some 20% of patients on treatment developed a positive direct Coombs' test, and 1% have clinically relevant haemolysis. The precise mechanism by which anti-Rh autoantibodies develop secondary to such drug therapy is unclear. The most plausible theory is that the drug

binds to red blood cell surface antigens, rendering them immunogenic in the process. This may operate through a T cell bypass mechanism (see Ch. 9) in which the drug provides a new T cell epitope on the red blood cell surface antigen, to bypass the existing control of potentially autoreactive anti-rhesus B lymphocytes.

In the second and third mechanisms, it has been postulated that the drugs act as haptens: in other words they need to bind to a macromolecule in order to become immunogenic. In one process (typically associated with penicillin and the cephalosporins), the drug requires attachment to a protein molecule on the erythrocyte surface before antibodies are generated. These then bind drug–cell complexes and the cells are open to immune damage. In the final proposed mechanism, used to account for haemolysis associated with quinine-

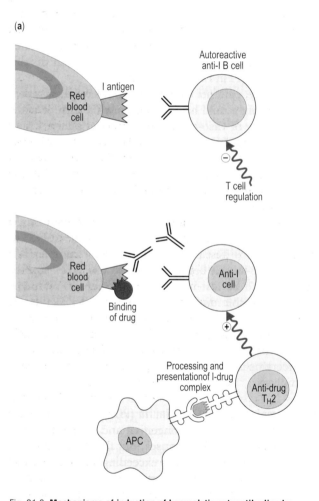

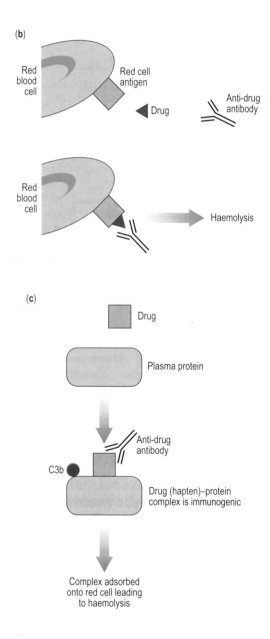

Fig. 21.6 **Mechanisms of induction of haemolytic autoantibodies by drugs.**
(a) In healthy individuals, anti-I antibodies are not produced because autoreactive B cells are controlled by regulatory T cells. Binding of drug to the I antigen may lead to processing and presentation of the complex, which behaves as a novel antigen. A T_H2 lymphocyte reactive with epitopes on the I–drug antigen promotes autoantibody production, bypassing the T-cell control. (b) The drug, behaving like a hapten, is not antigenic until bound to a macromolecule, in this case a red blood cell surface protein. The drug now induces antibody production, indirectly targeting the red blood cell. (c) The haptenic drug complexes with a plasma protein to induce antidrug antibodies. The immune complex formed is adsorbed onto the red blood cell, which is now prone to phagocytosis in the spleen.

What is the explanation for drug-induced haemolysis?

Although the three explanations given in the text are popular accounts for drug-induced direct Coombs' test-positive haemolysis, there are several flaws in the argument. First, two of the mechanisms rely upon drug binding to the red blood cell surface, yet this is very difficult to demonstrate convincingly. Second, two of the mechanisms rely upon the drug becoming a hapten after binding to the red blood cell surface or plasma-derived proteins. However, according to the classical theory (see p. 290) a hapten becomes the target of the antibody. Therefore, it should be possible to adsorb out antidrug antibodies from a patient's serum using the free drug; again, this has not been demonstrable.

A new explanation, which unites all of the theories as well as their flaws, is as follows. The drug, or its metabolite, bind to the red blood cell surface and creates a complex termed a 'neoantigen'. For example, an epitope on the neoantigen might be composed of part of the drug and part of a red blood cell protein. Antibodies to the neoantigen lead to haemolysis. Since it is a neoantigen, pure drug alone will not absorb out the antibodies. In addition, the generation of an immune response to the neoantigen on the red blood cell allows the production of true 'auto' antibodies, through T cell bypass. These auto-antibodies could target the Rh system, a group of red blood cell surface antigens frequently involved in Coombs' test-positive drug-induced haemolysis. Understandably, the 'neoantigen' theory is difficult to prove, but it remains an attractive compromise.

based drugs, the hapten (drug) binds to a soluble plasma protein to become immunogenic. The immune complex subsequently formed is absorbed onto the red blood cell surface through recruitment of classical complement components, and haemolysis results.

AUTOIMMUNE THROMBOCYTOPENIA

Destruction of platelets by immune mechanisms is a much more common clinical problem than autoimmune haemolysis. Again, the syndrome may be primary (**idiopathic thrombocytopenic purpura**, ITP) or occur as an **autoimmune thrombocytopenia** secondary to a range of disorders:

- Virus infection: occurs frequently in childhood with common viruses, usually follows acute infection by 3 weeks; HIV.
- Autoimmune disease: SLE; rheumatoid arthritis; autoimmune hepatitis.
- Lymphoproliferative disorders: chronic lymphocytic leukaemia; non-Hodgkin's lymphoma.
- Drugs: similar mechanisms to haemolytic syndromes are presumed.

Purpura in ITP refers to the purple skin rash that typically appears in any form of thrombocytopenia, resulting from subcutaneous haemorrhages. Other clinical presentations include bruising and, in severe disease, active mucosal bleeding (bleeding gums or nose, melaena, bleeding per rectum, haematuria, fundal haemorrhage). Any secondary disease or associated cytopenia may also be apparent.

The laboratory diagnosis is made on the platelet count (usually $< 80 \times 10^9/l$). Bone marrow response to thrombocytopenia, in the form of increased production, may be detected on a bone marrow aspiration as elevated numbers of megakaryocytes or in the blood as an increase in the mean platelet volume, since immature platelets are large. Various assays for the detection of platelet-bound and circulating antiplatelet autoantibodies may be performed, all based on the principle of the Coombs' test. Typically bound or circulating autoantibody of the IgG class is detected ($> 90\%$) but IgM and IgA autoantibodies may also be detected in up to half the patients.

The pathogenesis of autoimmune platelet destruction revolves around the presence of surface-bound autoantibody. IgG autoantibodies probably lead to platelet loss in the spleen, in a process analogous to that of warm AHA. IgM antiplatelet autoantibodies are presumed to operate through the recruitment of complement. Autoantibodies may interfere with the role of platelets in haemostasis, leading to platelet dysfunction.

In secondary autoimmune thrombocytopenia, the management of the primary disease should be addressed. In autoimmune thrombocytopenia, through whatever cause, the platelet count can be increased in 80% of patients by the administration of corticosteroids. Intravenous immunoglobulin (IVIG) may be used, either to enhance the response rate to steroids or as a means of elevating the platelet count immediately prior to surgery (e.g. splenectomy). IVIG is thought to operate through blockade of splenic Fc receptors, halting the phagocytic destruction of platelets. As such, it has also been used in haemolytic anaemia. However, it provides a transient respite in the disease, is relatively expensive to administer and offers no long-term cure in either condition. When reduced levels of platelets lead to evidence of mucosal blood loss, there is a real risk of intracranial haemorrhage. This life-threatening complication should be treated with platelet infusions and high-dose corticosteroids combined with IVIG. Another recent proposal is the use of extracorporeal immunoglobulin-binding columns, which specifically remove IgG antibodies.

AUTOIMMUNE NEUTROPENIA

Primary autoimmune neutropenia (AIN) is a rare disease typically affecting infants. The low neutrophil concentrations in the blood and tissues gives rise to infectious diseases typical of this type of immune defi-

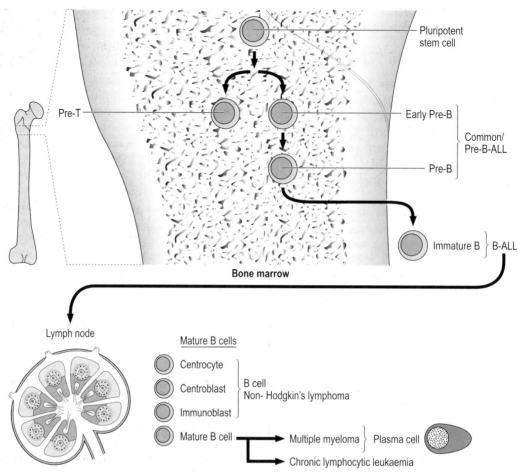

Fig. 21.8 **Origins of malignant B cell tumours in relation to the normal development of the cell.**

3. In 88% of chronic lymphocytic leukaemia it is the mature B lymphocyte that is affected, and mature B cells are also probably the origin of the so-called 'hairy' leukaemia cell.
4. Lymphomas of the non-Hodgkin's type are of B cell origin in approximately 90% of patients. These arise from B cells resident in the lymph nodes and are differentiated according to their morphology and degree of maturation (from immature to mature: lymphocytic, centrocytic, centroblastic and immunoblastic).
5. Neoplastic expansions of mature antibody-secreting plasma cells give rise to multiple myeloma, Waldenström's macroglobulinaemia, monoclonal gammopathy of unknown significance, and heavy chain disease. Tumours affecting plasma cells are often also referred to as **plasma cell dyscrasias**.

These disorders have different incidences, natural histories, therapies and prognoses. Apart from B-ALL, however, these neoplasms may be associated, to a greater or lesser extent, with complications related to immunoglobulin produced by the abnormal clone:

- hyperviscosity syndromes
- secondary antibody deficiency
- autoimmune phenomena.

Disease can, therefore, arise secondary to the excessive production of an immunoglobulin (e.g. a hyperviscosity syndrome); reduced production of protective immunoglobulins (e.g. secondary antibody deficiency); as a result of the nature of the target of the antibody produced by the neoplastic clone (e.g. autoimmune cytopenias); or as a result of a disturbance of regulation of idiotype/anti-idiotype networks, allowing expansion of polyclonal autoantibodies directed against surface antigens on circulating blood cells and platelets. This section will concentrate upon these immune complications and the diseases which give rise to them. Detailed information regarding the diagnosis and management of the B cell leukaemias and lymphomas is available in textbooks of haematology.

MULTIPLE MYELOMA

Multiple myeloma is an abnormal proliferation of malignant plasma cells typically characterised by the excessive production of an immunoglobulin molecule of single heavy and light chain type (termed a **paraprotein**). It is the most prevalent and clinically important plasma cell neoplasm and accounts for 10% of all haematological malignancies. Approximately four per 100 000 of Western Europeans and North Americans

Growth factors in multiple myeloma

Although there is an association between the development of multiple myeloma and radiation, the effect is weak and only demonstrable in individuals exposed to high doses or for long periods. The trigger(s) for the disease in the vast majority of patients remains unknown. However, recent studies have increased our knowledge about some of the factors that influence malignant plasma cell growth and have offered the potential for new therapies.

Several strands of evidence have implicated IL-6 as a growth factor for healthy plasma cells. Mice transgenic for IL-6 have a massive polyclonal increase in plasma cells, many of which enter the circulation. There is also a human condition, cardiac myxoma, in which high levels of IL-6 are associated with a plasma cell expansion. When attempts are made to grow plasma cells from such patients in vitro, the resulting cultures are dependent upon the addition of supplements of IL-6. This led several groups to look at the role of IL-6 in the growth of malignant plasma cells. High levels of IL-6 are found in the circulation of approximately one third of patients with multiple myeloma. When the plasma cells from these patients are cultured in vitro, they only grow in the presence of stromal support cells (e.g. macrophage-like cells and fibroblasts from the bone marrow). It has been shown that, in these culture systems, IL-6 is secreted into the supernatant by the stromal cells: more importantly, antibodies to IL-6 added to the culture completely inhibit the growth of the plasma cell clone. These exciting findings suggest that IL-6, and possibly other cytokines that synergise with it (IL-3, IL-5 and GM-CSF), promote plasma cell growth in vitro; interfering with these factors in vivo is currently being explored as a new therapy for myeloma.

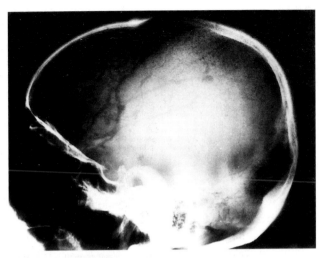

Fig. 21.9 X-ray demonstrating the typical 'punched out' appearance of lytic bone lesions in a patient with multiple myeloma.
(Courtesy of Dr E. J. Evanson)

Table 21.1 **Diagnosis of multiple myeloma and its remission**

Major criteria
I. Plasmacytoma (i.e. solid plasma cell tumour)
II. Plasma cells in bone marrow > 30%
III. Paraprotein level > 35 g/l (IgG); > 20 g/l (IgA), or Bence Jones proteinuria > 1 g in 24 hours

Minor criteria
a. 10–30% plasma cells in bone marrow
b. Paraprotein present but less than in III above
c. Lytic bone lesions (Fig. 21.9)
d. Suppression of normal immunoglobulins (IgG < 6 g/l, IgA < 1 g/l or IgM < 0.5 g/l)

Diagnosis based on:
I or II plus one of b, c, or d
III plus a, c or d
a and b with either c or d

Features of disease remission
Serum paraprotein reduced by 75%
Bence Jones proteinuria reduced by 95%
Less than 5% plasma cells in bone marrow

Table 21.2 **Tests in the diagnosis and management of myeloma**

Test	Interpretation
Serum immunoglobulin levels	Evidence of immune paresis
Serum electrophoresis	Identify and quantify paraprotein; paresis of other Ig isotypes
Immunofixation	Paraprotein type
Urine electrophoresis	Bence Jones proteinuria
Bone marrow examination	Percentage plasma cells; plasma cell clonality
Skeletal radiology	Lytic bone lesions
Calcium, urea and electrolytes	Hypercalcaemia; renal function
Levels of β_2-microglobulin	Prognostic marker
Full blood count	Anaemia; leukopenia; thrombocytopenia; rouleaux; increased background staining

are diagnosed per year and multiple myeloma is twice as common in black Americans than in their white compatriots. Median age of onset is 60 years, men and women are equally affected, and the median survival from diagnosis is 3 years, with a range up to 10 years. Environmental factors are presumed to have an influence on the development of this, as of other neoplasms, and some have been identified (see box: 'Growth factors in multiple myeloma'). Agricultural workers and those exposed to benzene and radiation have a higher incidence, but the major factors have yet to be identified.

Patients typically present with symptoms arising from lytic bone disease (Fig. 21.9), anaemia, renal failure or secondary antibody deficiency. Approximately 20% of patients with multiple myeloma are diagnosed by chance, usually when liver function tests on a blood sample reveal an excessive concentration of total protein or gammaglobulins, caused by excessive immunoglobulin production. There are strict criteria for the diagnosis of multiple myeloma (Table 21.1). There are a number of tests that can be made to determine which criteria are present both for initial diagnosis and for subsequent management of the disease (Table 21.2).

Once the diagnosis is made, it is generally accepted that patients with symptoms should commence treat-

if the paraprotein has the physicochemical properties of a cryoglobulin (see p. 227) or cold agglutinin (see p. 289). The high levels of paraprotein can also interfere with the function of other plasma proteins, such as those of the clotting cascade, producing a coagulopathy, with nose bleeds and bruising being common signs at presentation. Anaemia is typically present and often more severe than in multiple myeloma. Bence Jones proteinuria is only found in 10% of patients, and bone lesions are rare.

Therapy for Waldenström's macroglobulinaemia involves the use of the alkylating agents chlorambucil and cyclophosphamide, administered with corticosteroids and accompanied by regular monitoring of paraprotein levels. Younger patients may be suitable for more aggressive therapy, with autologous or allogeneic bone marrow transplantation.

MONOCLONAL GAMMOPATHY OF UNKNOWN SIGNIFICANCE

Frequently, high levels of gammaglobulins or total protein detected in routine screening result in the identification of a paraprotein, but the diagnostic criteria for multiple myeloma are not met. In these cases, a diagnosis of monoclonal gammopathy of unknown significance (MGUS) may be made if the patient is asymptomatic; the paraprotein levels are below 35 g/l for IgG and 20 g/l for IgA; there are no Bence Jones proteins in the urine (<1 g/24 hours free light chains); there are <10% plasma cells in the bone marrow; and there are no bone lesions. Estimates of the frequency of MGUS go as high as 3% of the population over the age of 50 years. In some cases, the condition is pre-malignant and the conversion rate to frank myeloma is of the order of 1% of patients per year. A similar proportion of MGUS patients will progress to Waldenström's macroglobulinaemia or amyloidosis (see below). For this reason, regular monitoring of these patients for evidence of marrow suppression, increasing level of paraprotein and depression of normal immunoglobulin production is advisable.

One interesting complication of MGUS is the presence of a monoclonal paraprotein with specificity for the peripheral nerve component **myelin-associated glycoprotein** (see p. 251), giving rise to peripheral neuropathy.

HEAVY CHAIN DISEASE

There are rare B lymphocyte lymphoproliferative disorders in which only heavy chains are produced by the malignant cells. Typically it is the Fc region alone that is produced, and in the majority of patients described to date, this has been the α heavy chain. There are approximately 100 reported patients with γ heavy chain disease and even fewer involving production of μ chains. In most patients, the level of paraprotein is very low and the diagnosis difficult to make. The α heavy chain disease is the best characterised and appears to

be a pre-malignant syndrome in which young patients of Mediterranean origin present with upper gastrointestinal symptoms (pain, diarrhoea, fever and weight loss). The condition may respond to antibiotics or may progress to a lymphomatous condition. A high degree of intestinal infestation with microorganisms has been suggested as the aetiological factor in this condition, but no single organism has been identified to date.

AMYLOIDOSIS

Amyloidosis is a descriptive pathological term, reserved for conditions in which there is a tissue accumulation of insoluble fibrillar proteins, arranging themselves as non-branching β-pleated sheets that are resistant to proteolysis and phagocytosis. Deposition in the kidneys, heart, adrenal glands, spleen, liver, peripheral nerves and joints give rise to the multiorgan failure seen in the disease, most frequently typified by renal failure and cardiomyopathy.

There are several different forms of amyloidosis, two of which are pertinent to a discussion of immune-mediated disease. **Primary amyloidosis** is the most common form of amyloidosis. Light chains of immunoglobulin molecules are excessively produced by a neoplastic clone of plasma cells, either as an idiopathic disease or as part of frank multiple myeloma. The particular nature of these light chains is presumed to favour the production of the insoluble fibrillar proteins characteristic of the disease. Of relevance here may be the fact that the κ:λ ratio is reversed in primary amyloidosis in favour of λ chains.

In the other immunological form of the condition, termed **secondary amyloidosis**, there is deposition of a serum protein (serum amyloid A). Serum amyloid A is an acute-phase reactant, and this condition is usually seen in chronic infectious (e.g. tuberculosis) or inflammatory (e.g. rheumatoid arthritis) diseases characterised by prolonged acute-phase responses.

Patients with amyloidosis usually present with multisystem symptoms and signs and the diagnosis is easily made from tissue (e.g. rectal) biopsies: the abnormal proteins stain distinctively with Congo red. Up to 80% of patients with primary amyloidosis may have a low-level paraprotein in the serum or urine. Reversal of the tissue deposition is difficult to achieve, and management may rest upon cessation of further light chain production using melphalan and corticosteroids or, in the case of secondary amyloidosis, abrogation of the acute-phase response by treatment of the underlying condition.

CHRONIC LYMPHOCYTIC LEUKAEMIA AND NON-HODGKIN'S LYMPHOMA

Although these tumours are not discussed in detail here, it is important to note that such malignancies of mature circulating or lymph node B lymphocytes may manifest immune complications. Autoimmune phenomena are more commonly seen than paraproteinaemias, which accompany less than 5% of cases. In both disorders, paraproteins with the properties of cryoglobulins or cold agglutinins are occasionally found, giving rise to vasculitic lesions and cold autoimmune haemolysis, respectively.

Neoplastic disease of B cells

- Autoimmune disease and immunodeficiency states are the major complications of malignancies of cells of the B cell lineage. By far the most common malignancy is multiple myeloma.
- A distinctive feature of myeloma is the production of a monoclonal antibody by the malignant clone.
- A greater understanding of the cell biology of mature B cell malignancies may lead to harnessing immune-based therapies in haematological malignancies, such as myeloma and non-Hodgkin's lymphoma.

IMMUNE-BASED TREATMENT OF HAEMATOLOGICAL CANCERS

Two recent advances in the approach to treating haematological cancers are the use of monoclonal antibodies directed against malignant cells and insertion of genes into cancer cells to enhance antitumour immune responses (so-called 'immune gene therapy'). The treatment of haematological malignancies with these approaches is particularly attractive. Most haematological cancer cells (malignant plasma cells being a notable exception) bear surface markers typical of their lineage. For example, B cell tumours express CD19 and CD20; some T cell leukaemias express CD25 at high levels. These surface molecules are well characterised, and different monoclonal antibodies with varying characteristics are in plentiful supply. This is important, since the effectiveness of the therapy may depend upon the ability of an antibody to recruit complement or Fc receptor-bearing effector cells. Conjugation of antibodies to toxins (e.g. ricin; see p. 306) has also been used to enhance cytotoxicity.

When discussing the insertion of genes to enhance antitumour immune responses, an obvious question is whether there is any evidence that the immune system recognises and eradicates tumour cells. For haematological malignancies, there are two pieces of evidence that support the existence of such responses. First, there is the graft-versus-leukaemia effect in allogeneic bone marrow transplantation (see p. 151), indicating the capacity of an intact immune system to identify and kill tumour cells. Second, there is the evidence from studies looking at the effect of long-term immunosuppressive treatment (e.g. following transplantation) on the incidence of tumours. One might expect that, if the immune system has an important role in 'immune surveillance' against tumours, immunosuppression would lead to an increased incidence of malignancy. Indeed, immunosuppression is associated with increased susceptibility to tumours, *especially* those of haematological origin (e.g. lymphomas, leukaemias), suggesting that there are protective immune responses to these cancers.

MONOCLONAL ANTIBODIES IN TREATMENT OF B CELL LYMPHOMA

Several recent clinical trials have evaluated the use of monoclonal antibodies to treat B cell lymphomas with poor cure rates, namely intermediate and high-grade non-Hodgkin's lymphoma. In two studies, murine anti-CD20 antibodies were conjugated to radiolabelled iodine (^{131}I), to deliver high doses of radioactivity directly to the site of the tumour. There are several advantages to this approach. First, gamma camera imaging can be used to establish that the therapy has targeted the lymph nodes involved. Second, suppression of normal bone marrow function appears to be minimal. Despite the fact that the studies were actually phase I trials (i.e. evaluating the dose and delivery of the treatment) four out of ten patients in one and 16 out of 19 in the other underwent complete remission of their tumours. The future of 'radioimmunotherapy' appears promising, and as more monoclonal antibodies become available in 'humanised' forms (see p. 304), the treatments will become more refined.

IMMUNE GENE THERAPY

The evidence presented above that an immune response to haematological cancers can be generated brings two questions to mind. First, what is the nature of the antitumour response and, second, why do these malignancies still arise? The two questions can be answered in concert. It seems probable that there is an immune response made to some cancer cells that involves the recognition of tumour-specific antigens presented by HLA molecules on the tumour surface (Fig. 21.12). The immune response is presumably initiated by an interaction between APCs and T_H cells, with cytotoxic T cells the major effectors. Macroscopic tumours probably develop when malignant cells are allowed to escape from this immune surveillance. This may be the result of a failure to express tumour-specific antigens, loss of surface HLA molecules, or the development of anergy (i.e. a failure to respond) amongst the reactive T cells. Anergy, for example, could develop if a tumour cell presents antigen to a T_H cell without the obligatory co-signals (Fig. 21.13).

Immune gene therapy aims to overcome these escape mechanisms (Fig. 21.14). Briefly, the tumour is removed and cultured, and appropriate genes inserted into the progeny cells. One approach might be to insert HLA molecules to enhance immune recognition. Along similar lines, genes for known tumour antigens could

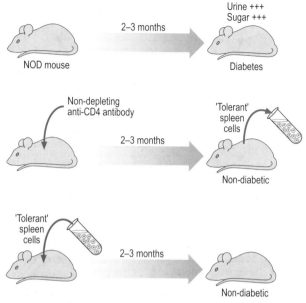

Fig. 22.6 Use of non-depleting antibodies to modulate damaging autoantigen-specific immune responses in an animal model of insulin-dependent diabetes.

When antibodies are being used therapeutically to remove cell populations (e.g. tumour cells, autoreactive lymphocytes), reliance on complement or ADCC mechanisms may be insufficient. The therapeutic antibody can be conjugated to a more harmful reagent: either a radioactive substance such as ^{131}iodine (**radio-immunotherapy**) or a toxin such as ricin, *Pseudomonas* exotoxin, or diphtheria toxin (**immunotoxins**). Ricin A chains kill cells they have entered by interfering with the function of the 60S ribosomal subunits in protein synthesis. (Incidentally, it was ricin contained in the tip of an umbrella that was used to stab and poison the Bulgarian broadcaster Giorgi Markov in London in the 1980s.) Diphtheria toxin and *Pseudomonas* exotoxin both interfere with protein synthesis by irreversibly modifying elongation factor 2.

At present, the problem of unwanted, systemic toxicity with therapeutic immunotoxins is considerable. Xenogeneic antibodies are likely to be concentrated at high levels in the liver and spleen as they are removed from the circulation by the mononuclear phagocyte system. In addition, glycosylated proteins such as ricin are absorbed selectively in the liver, though severe hepato-toxicity may be avoided by using non-glycosylated

forms of the toxin. Vascular leakage, with severe peripheral and lung oedema, is also a problem to be addressed before these approaches are adopted widely, though the mechanism of this complication is unknown. Several clinical trials of immunotoxin therapy are currently under way, in the treatment of melanoma, ovarian cancer, non-Hodgkin's lymphoma and severe graft-versus-host disease. Phase I trials of radioimmuno-therapy have also been completed recently in the treatment of high-grade non-Hodgkin's lymphoma (see p. 299).

Monoclonal antibody therapy

- Monoclonal antibodies allow immune responses to be directed against a specific target.
- Accessories, such as toxins, drugs or radioisotopes, can be linked to monoclonal antibodies.
- Monoclonal antibody therapy is still at a developmental stage, although in certain life-threatening conditions, such as organ graft rejection, it is indispensible.
- Advances in technology indicate that 'humanised' monoclonal antibodies will become viable therapeutic options.

IMMUNOSUPPRESSIVE DRUGS

CORTICOSTEROIDS

Glucocorticosteroids (cortisone, hydrocortisone, prednisone and prednisolone) are the most commonly used steroids. They have been used extensively to control damaging inflammatory immune responses in clinical practice for many years and appear to have a variety of effects on immune function (Table 22.1). Hydrocortisone succinate is water soluble and may be given intravenously; prednisone is given orally and is metabolised to prednisolone by liver enzymes. Endogenous glucocorticoid concentrations in plasma vary five-fold diurnally and may rise by up to 20 times in stressful situations, such as surgery (in the patient, not the surgeon). Therapeutic doses of steroids may increase plasma concentrations by up to 100 times.

Table 22.1 **Major mechanisms of steroid anti-inflammatory actions**

Target cell	Effect	Consequences
Monocyte	Block IL-1 production	Inhibition of T cell activation
	Block TNF-α production	Inhibition of activation and recruitment of monocytes, endothelial cells, neutrophils
	Reduced chemotaxis	Inhibition of migration to inflammation
T lymphocyte	Block IL-2 production	Inhibit T cell activation
	Block IFN-γ production	Inhibit monocyte activation, reduce antiviral effect
	Redistribution out of circulation	Reduced migration of lymphocytes (especially CD4⁺) to inflammation

Steroid effects are mediated through cytoplasmic receptors that translocate to the nucleus and modify gene expression. The recorded effects of steroids on immune function are legion. Difficulties in interpreting many of these data centre around the relevance of in vitro studies, while species differences in steroid physiology call into question data from many animal studies. What is clear is that steroid-mediated immune effects do not relate to a single mechanism. The major effects of steroids on immune function can be divided into effects on cytokine networks, direct effects on cells and effects on compartmentalisation within the immune system.

At pharmacological doses, glucocorticoids inhibit release of TNF-α and IL-1 from monocytes and reduce production of IFN-γ and IL-2 by T lymphocytes. These effects are apparent when monocytes or T cells are maximally stimulated, for example by incubation with bacterial lipopolysaccharide or with allogeneic lymphocytes in a mixed lymphocyte reaction. Overall, the summated effect of such reductions in cytokine secretion would be to inhibit monocyte and T cell activation. This is likely to have a profound effect on antigen-specific T cell responses, particularly those mediated by T_H1 cells.

Direct effects of steroids on lymphocytes and monocytes are more difficult to assess. In general, suprapharmacological doses will inhibit T cell proliferation in vitro. B cell activity appears to be enhanced, in that immunoglobulin secretion rises in the presence of steroids. This is probably the result of an inhibitory effect on the T cells controlling B cell function. Direct effects on monocyte function are difficult to assess. In vitro, pharmacological doses of steroids inhibit monocyte chemotaxis, but monocytes from patients on long-term high-dose therapy have normal chemotactic responses. Suprapharmacological doses are required to demonstrate inhibitory effects on monocyte phagocytosis and bacterial killing in vitro. Equally, most neutrophil functions appear steroid resistant.

An observation made in the 1970s regards the effects of steroids on circulating immune cell populations. Quite small doses of glucocorticoids reduce the circulating white blood cell count within 6 hours: CD4$^+$ T lymphocytes are particularly affected. Similar effects in animals are accompanied by redistribution of cells to the bone marrow and spleen. In contrast, circulating monocyte and neutrophil numbers appear to increase.

The side effects of steroid therapy should not be forgotten. Some of these are predictable from the mode of action (e.g. increased susceptibility to infection) but equally important are impaired wound healing, growth suppression in children, depression, hyperglycaemia and hypertension.

CYCLOSPORIN AND TACROLIMUS (FK506)

Cyclosporin is the product of the fungus *Tolypocladeium inflatium* and was first identified in 1976 during screening for novel antibiotic agents. It was adopted widely in clinical practice in the mid-1980s and has revolutionised many areas of medical and surgical practice. Much is now known about its mode of action, and within the last few years a drug of completely different structure, but similar *modus operandi*, has also entered clinical practice. This is tacrolimus, (previously called FK506), which is derived from the fungus *Streptomyces tsukubaensis*.

Cyclosporin is an undecapeptide containing one unique amino acid, whilst tacrolimus is a macrolide lactone antibiotic. Therefore, they have quite different structures, but both act as pro-drugs, only becoming active when complexed to intracellular binding proteins termed **immunophilins**. In early in vitro studies, cyclosporin was noted to have a profound effect on T cell activation, inhibiting it with a high degree of specificity and potency. Initially its use was restricted to prophylaxis against graft rejection, but in recent years it has undergone trials in autoimmune diseases, asthma and psoriasis. It is indicated as a potential therapy in any disease in which activation of T cells has a pathogenic role, though toxicity is a major drawback. Cyclosporin therapy not only results in a propensity to opportunistic infections but also has major toxic effects on the liver (fatty change and necrosis) and kidney (reduced glomerular filtration and tubular interstitial fibrosis).

Initial studies on the mode of action of cyclosporin revealed that it enters T cells and binds to an intracellular protein. The cytosolic binding protein for cyclosporin was originally called **cyclophilin** and has now been identified as the enzyme **peptidyl prolyl cis–trans isomerase** or **rotamase**. First discovered in 1984, rotamase accelerates the interconversion of *cis* and *trans* rotamers of proline-containing peptides or proteins, which is believed to be the rate-limiting step during protein folding. The binding protein for tacrolimus is termed just that (TBP) and collectively this and cyclophilin go under the term immunophilins. Intriguingly, the drug-binding protein complex in both cases (tacrolimus–TBP and cyclosporin–cyclophilin) has affinity for the same target, a Ca^{2+}-dependent protein phosphatase called **calcineurin**. Calcineurin receives the second messenger signal generated by the rise in intracellular Ca^{2+} concentration after TCR-mediated activation. Calcineurin then dephosphorylates a nuclear transcription factor present in the cytoplasm NF-AT$_c$ (for nuclear factor of activated T cells$_{cytoplasm}$, see p. 97), which is thus enabled to translocate from the cytoplasm to the nucleus and there initiate transcription of the IL-2 gene in concert with a similar nuclear transcription factor (NF-AT$_n$) (Fig. 22.7). Blocking of calcineurin function within the T cell by the complex of drug and binding protein has obvious consequences for TCR-mediated T cell activation.

A drug with a similar structure to tacrolimus is **rapamycin** (also known as sirolimus). Although rapamycin binds TBP, it appears to mediate its anti-IL-2/IL-2 receptor effect by inhibiting phosphorylation of a

Promoting IL-2-mediated activation of immune effector cells has been most widely applied in cancer immunotherapy. An approach pioneered by Steven Rosenberg, in the USA was to take peripheral blood lymphocytes from patients with tumours and activate and expand these in vitro with IL-2 over several days. Under these conditions, there is a preferential expansion of non-T lymphocytes with a large granular lymphocyte (LGL) morphology. In animal experiments, these cells have greatly enhanced cytotoxic potential against experimental tumours, and are termed lymphokine-activated killer (LAK) cells. LAK cell therapy has been shown to induce partial and complete remissions in up to 20% of patients with certain tumours, notably malignant melanoma and renal cell carcinoma. The effectiveness of the IL-2 activation in vitro is presumed to result from the high doses achievable, and the preferential expansion of cells with LGL morphology is put down to their constitutive low-level expression of IL-2 receptor β and γ chains. In contrast with LAK cell therapy, direct administration of IL-2 is unable to achieve such high cytokine levels, because of toxicity. However, intravenous IL-2 does induce a lymphocytosis and enhances natural killer and 'LAK-cell'-type activity. In subsequent trials of IL-2 therapy with and without generation of LAK cells ex vivo, there was only a marginal improvement with the addition of LAK cells and hence IL-2 is generally now used alone. Partial and complete remission rates of 10–20% are found in malignant melanoma and renal cell carcinoma, which remain the most responsive tumours, and for which IL-2 is now licenced both in the UK and USA. Side effects of IL-2 are considerable, with a death rate of 4% during the above studies. The side effects are similar to IL-1, with a capillary leak syndrome and cardiac failure being the major clinical problems. Therefore, therapy is advised for fit patients and must take place in adequate facilities.

INTERFERON-α

IFN-α has been one of the most successful therapeutic cytokines in clinical practice. It has activity against chronic viral infections and certain haematological malignancies. Whilst natural leukocyte-derived IFN-α is actually a cocktail of interferon proteins (there are multiple genes for this cytokine), human recombinant proteins from the IFN-α2 gene are available commercially (IFN-α-2a and IFN-α-2b, which differ at amino acid position 23). In addition, a leukocyte-derived interferon-α is produced by exposure of white blood cells to chronic viral infection in vitro.

There are several possible mechanisms for antiviral activity of IFN-α. It can directly inhibit synthesis of viral proteins, increase the possibility of immune recognition of virally infected cells by enhancing or inducing MHC class I and II protein expression and it also has some stimulatory effect (although less than IFN-γ) on monocytes, natural killer cells, and T lymphocytes.

The most notable haematological malignancy for which IFN-α is a recognised therapy is **hairy cell leukaemia**, an uncommon B lymphocyte tumour. The characteristic 'hairy cells' of the tumour express four to eight times more IFN-α receptors on their surface than normal B cells. The beneficial effect of IFN-α in this tumour appears to be in reducing DNA and protein synthesis in the tumour cells. The therapy induces clinical improvement and haematological remission in the majority of patients, and the effect is usually maintained for 1–2 years. After relapse, IFN-α is unlikely to be of further use, but its overall effect is to enhance survival (97% at 1 year compared with 70% in conventionally treated patients). Adverse effects are not as severe as for IL-1 and IL-2, centring on the induction of a 'flu-like' illness.

Other tumours in which early clinical trials suggest a beneficial response to IFN-α include Kaposi's sarcoma, renal cell carcinoma and malignant melanoma, although its use in these disorders remains controversial.

Approximately half of the patients acquiring acute hepatitis C virus infection will develop a chronic illness, of whom 20% will become cirrhotic. Trials with IFN-α in chronic hepatitis C infection have demonstrated an objective remission (e.g. biochemical evidence of improved liver function) in 40–50% of patients, although relapse is common upon cessation of therapy, indicating that the infection is not cleared. In a similar vein, IFN-α treatment in chronic hepatitis B virus infection induces remission in 40–50% of patients.

MANIPULATING THE T$_H$1/T$_H$2 BALANCE

Considerable advances in understanding the physiological role of the T helper cell subsets, which have distinctive cytokine secretion profiles, has enabled the identification of several diseases in which the balance of T$_H$1/T$_H$2 cells is disturbed. These include infectious diseases (e.g. lepromatous leprosy), autoimmune diseases (e.g. type 1 diabetes; see p. 185) and allergy (see p. 134) (Table 22.3). In leprosy, there is widespread invasion of skin and nerves by *Mycobacterium leprae* in the lepromatous form of the disease. Activation of macrophages is required to kill the intracellular

Table 22.3 **Diseases with putative T$_H$1/T$_H$2 imbalance, and possible corrective therapy**

Disease	T helper imbalance	Proposed therapy
Infectious diseases		
Lepromatous leprosy	T$_H$2 > T$_H$1	IFN-γ
Leishmaniasis	T$_H$2 > T$_H$1	IFN-γ
Autoimmune disease		
Animal models of insulin-dependent diabetes	T$_H$1 > T$_H$2	IL-4
		Anti-IFN-γ antibody
		Adoptive transfer of T$_H$2 cells
Allergy		
Severe pollen or bee sting allergy	T$_H$2 > T$_H$1	IFN-γ
		Anti-IL-4 antibodies

organisms and there is evidence that in patients with lepromatous leprosy, an ineffective T_H2 response is dominant, when a T_H1 response is required.

Evidence that the T_H1 and T_H2 subsets are mutually exclusive and mutually inhibitory has also been obtained (i.e. T_H1 cytokines block T_H2 responses and vice versa). This offers the potential therapeutic strategy, currently being evaluated, that restoration of the optimal T_H1/T_H2 balance may be achievable, and therapeutically desirable.

Cytokines and anticytokines

- Cytokines can have both beneficial effects and pathogenic effects: anticytokines can reduce the latter.
- Reducing levels of IL-1 can reduce its inflammatory action, e.g. in rheumatoid arthritis and toxic shock.
- IL-2 is involved in T cell activation and antibodies blocking IL-2 action (anti-Tac) are effective (in severe GVHD and renal transplant rejection) but are too immunogenic in themselves for general use.
- IL-2 is also used to enhance immune responses against malignant melanoma and renal cell carcinoma.
- IFN-α is used in therapy against viral infections and haematological malignancies.

OTHER THERAPEUTIC APPROACHES

INTERFERENCE IN T CELL–APC INTERACTIONS

The elements required in establishing a T cell response to antigen processed and presented by a professional APC are: T cell receptor, peptide antigen, class II MHC molecule, accessory molecules (e.g. CD4) co-stimulatory molecules (e.g. B7) and adhesion molecules (e.g. ICAMs). All of these essential components are open to manipulation, and interference in these processes is actively being attempted in order to devise new therapeutic immune suppressive strategies. These could then be applied in autoimmune disease and transplant rejection. Some of the approaches are likely to be antigen specific (e.g. interference in TCR–peptide–MHC interactions) whilst others will be more broadly immunosuppressive (e.g. interference in accessory or adhesion molecule function). The different approaches are shown in Figure 22.9. The majority of these have shown efficacy in animal models, and therapeutic trials are likely before the end of the 1990s.

LYMPHOCYTE VACCINATION

The concept of lymphocyte vaccination is particularly appealing, since it employs immunological principles that have been applied in the past to develop some of the most effective vaccines in use. The principle is illustrated using animal models, such as the non-obese diabetic (NOD) mouse (model of type 1 diabetes) or adjuvant arthritis in rats (model of rheumatoid arthritis). In these diseases, T lymphocytes obtained from affected animals are capable of adoptively transferring the disease to unaffected animals (Fig. 22.10). It has been suggested that such pathogenic T lymphocytes might be exploited to cure autoimmune disease using the principle of vaccination, in which an attenuated form of the damaging agent is presented to the immune system: during this 'safe' encounter, protection is acquired against subsequent infections. In the mouse model of diabetes or the rat model of arthritis, the T cells that could transfer the disease were treated to attenuate them and then the same cells were used as a

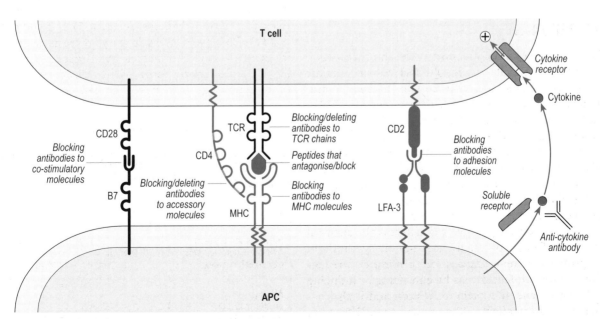

Fig. 22.9 **Potential sites and strategies for immune intervention in T cell–APC interactions.**

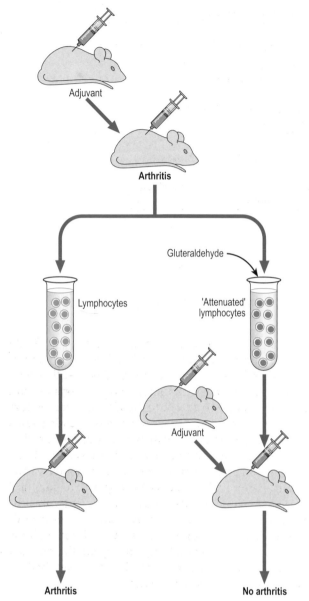

Fig. 22.10 **Principle of lymphocyte vaccination.**
A rat model of human rheumatoid arthritis is generated by injection of adjuvant. Lymphocytes from rats with 'adjuvant arthritis' can adoptively transfer the disease, making them a 'pathogenic agent'. Gluteraldehyde-attenuated lymphocytes do not transfer the disease but act like a vaccine, protecting the rat from disease induction.

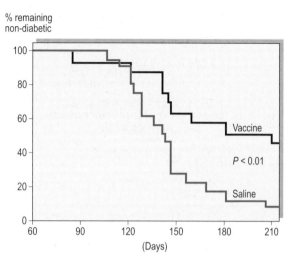

% remaining
non-diabetic

Fig. 22.11 **Survival of lymphocyte-vaccinated non-obese diabetic mice.**
Mice vaccinated with gluteraldehyde-treated lymphocytes derived from a diabetic mouse are protected from developing diabetes and have a 50% lower incidence of the disease than the sham-vaccinated group.

vaccine. In the NOD mice model, the animals receiving the lymphocyte vaccine did not become diabetic — quite the opposite, they were protected from the disease (Fig. 22.11). Clinical trials of lymphocyte vaccination are currently in progress in patients with multiple sclerosis and rheumatoid arthritis.

INTRAVENOUS IMMUNOGLOBULIN

IVIG is a therapeutic preparation of poly-specific IgG chemically purified from plasma pools of large numbers (approximately 20 000) of healthy donors. With such a large donor number, IVIG represents a wide spectrum of the expressed normal human IgG repertoire, includ-

ing antibodies to external agents, as well as autoantibodies (see p. 229). IgG subclasses are present in physiological proportions, and the IgG has an approximate half-life of 3 weeks (compared with 4 weeks for physiological IgG). IgA and IgM are present only in trace amounts.

IVIG therapy can be viewed as a replacement strategy, for primary and secondary antibody deficiencies; as a blocking agent, to prevent Fc-mediated effector mechanisms, such as destruction of IgG-coated erythrocytes; or as a therapy that has subtle effects on the balance of an immune response: so called **immunomodulation**. In replacement IVIG, the rationale and the indications for use are straightforward and have been dealt with elsewhere (see Ch. 19). Similarly, the use of IVIG in preventing splenic and hepatic destruction of antibody-coated blood cells in the circulation has been discussed (see Ch. 21). In contrast, use of IVIG as an immunomodulator is controversial. Many therapeutic benefits are claimed: few are backed up with randomised double-blind controlled clinical trials. To examine and pronounce on this area of controversy, the US National Institutes of Health have attempted to produce some guidelines for therapeutic use of IVIG (Table 22.4).

Proposed mechanisms of action of IVIG include:

- blockade of Fc receptors on mononuclear or polymorphonuclear phagocytes
- feedback inhibition of autoantibody synthesis by autoreactive B cells
- anti-idiotypic neutralisation of pathogenic autoantibodies
- inhibition of complement consumption by pathogenic autoantibodies
- interference with T cell regulation and cytokine release.

Table 22.4 **Guidelines on the use of IVIG replacement therapy in immunodeficiency.**

Indication	Comments
Primary immunodeficiency	
X-linked hypogammaglobulinaemia	Maintain IgG levels at 5 g/l or above
Common variable immunodeficiency	Maintain IgG levels at 5 g/l or above
Secondary immunodeficiency	
Chronic lymphocytic leukaemia	When hypogammaglobulinaemia present
Bone marrow transplantation	Benefits proven in adults
Paediatric AIDS	Proven benefit
Low-birthweight babies	Controversial
Myeloma	Reduces infections; long-term benefits unknown
Inflammatory conditions	
Kawasaki's disease	Proven benefit (Kawasaki's disease is probably caused by bacterial superantigens, which are neutralised by IVIG)
Idiopathic thrombocytopenic purpura	Use in children when disease self-limiting; in adults to cover splenectomy
Controversial uses as an immunomodulator	
Guillain–Barré syndrome and other inflammatory demyelinating polyneuropathies	
Vasculitic disease	
Myasthenia gravis	

Adoptive cellular therapy

Adoptive immunotherapy implies the passive transfer of immunity from one individual to another. This is typified by the prophylactic use of immune globulin containing antibodies against an infective agent or toxin, in, for example, infection with hepatitis A virus, rabies virus or *Clostridium tetani*. In these cases, the adopted immunity has been acquired by another individual, through natural exposure or vaccination. New technology enables this approach to be applied to immune responses that require T cells, such as the killing of intracellular viruses. Patients undergoing allogeneic bone marrow transplantation are particularly prone to infection with agents such as cytomegalovirus during the lymphopenic period that follows reinfusion of marrow cells. In a recent study, peripheral blood T cells were harvested from the marrow donor before the transplant and cultured in vitro with a source of viral antigen and IL-2. Responding cytotoxic cells were expanded and introduced into the lympho-penic marrow recipient. Antiviral T cell responses in the peripheral blood during the period after this autologous T cell adoptive therapy were very high, and none of the treated patients became infected with cytomegalovirus. Although laborious, the therapy was clearly safe and may become one of the future approaches to protecting lymphopenic bone marrow transplant patients.

However, the actual mechanism by which IVIG works in most autoimmune and inflammatory conditions, apart from the immune cytopenias, is still unclear and its benefit in inflammatory polyneuropathy and vasculitis remains to be established. One theory is that large doses of extrinsic antibody block endogenous autoantibody production, which would be beneficial in inflammatory polyneuropathy and vasculitis. IVIG could also interfere with complement-mediated tissue damage, by providing excess Fc regions to 'soak up' complement components. Effects on T cell suppressor and cytokine-releasing mechanisms have been proposed, but with little corroborative data. A final possibility is that IVIG contains neutralising IgG antibodies directed against the autoantigen-binding site of autoantibodies: so called anti-idiotypic antibodies.

Other immunotherapies

- Trials of lymphocyte vaccination are currently in progress in patients with rheumatoid arthritis and multiple sclerosis.
- IVIG therapy can be used in primary and secondary immunodeficiencies and in inflammatory conditions.

Immunisation

The term 'immunisation' can be used to denote an artifical process whereby an individual is rendered immune. There are two broad categories of immunisation: active and passive (or adoptive). **Active immunisation** implies that a non-immune individual acquires long-lasting ability to respond to an organism or its toxic products by generating his or her own protective mechanisms. Active immunisation is largely synonymous with 'vaccination'. **Vaccination** (from the Latin *vacca*, meaning a cow) was the term originally used to describe the process of generating immunity to the lethal smallpox virus by injecting, under the skin, extracts from lesions of the cowpox virus, cause of a relatively harmless infection in humans. **Passive immunisation** denotes the process of conferring protective immunity without the need for an immune response on the part of the recipient, for example by giving injections of antibodies.

Active immunisation, or vaccination, is based upon exploitation of the characteristics of primary (slow, low-affinity, low-capacity IgM produced in antibody responses) and secondary (fast, high-affinity, high-capacity IgG and IgA) immune responses (see p. 41). The vaccine itself is an attenuated or inactivated infective agent, disabled toxin, or an inert subunit of an infective agent. It is introduced, usually by intradermal or intramuscular injection, or sometimes orally, to a non-immune individual. The characteristic of this process is that it is a *safe* encounter with an agent that mimics the natural primary infection. Immunity is acquired, and when the 'wild-type' agent is confronted, either protective immunity is in place (e.g. circulating neutralising antibody) or a rapid, high-affinity secondary response can be mobilised.

The history of immunisation begins in the 18th century. The observation had been made that individuals who recovered from certain diseases were protected from recurrences. This led to the introduction of a process known as variolation (*Variola major* is the smallpox virus), in which fluid extracts from the pustules caused by the smallpox virus were obtained from individuals who appeared to have recovered from the infection and injected under the skin of uninfected individuals. The procedure was hazardous but occasionally successful. There is a famous letter from Lady Mary Wortley Montagu, wife of the British Ambassador in Turkey in 1717, who is largely credited with introducing variolation to England, in which she wrote that 'The smallpox so fatal and so general among us, is here entirely harmless by the invention of ingrafting, which is the term they give it'. On her return, Lady Montagu had her daughters 'ingrafted', but only after it had been tried first on six condemned criminals in the local prison!

In a distinct approach, Edward Jenner, a country doctor with a practice in the West country in England, made the observation that milkmaids, who frequently suffered with disfiguring cowpox lesions, rarely contracted smallpox. He used extracts from the cowpox lesions to protect successfully against smallpox, and the science of immunisation was born. Many spectacular successes were witnessed in the 20th century. The introduction of modified toxins (toxoids) from *Corynebacterium diphtheriae* and *Clostridium tetani* had a dramatic effect on the incidence of these infections. Polio vaccine, produced as a killed virus by Salk in 1954 or as a live but attenuated virus by Sabin in 1956, rapidly eradicated the scourge that was poliomyelitis in many countries (Fig. 23.1). Hepatitis B vaccine, introduced in 1975 as a viral surface antigen (HBsAg) purified from the plasma of patients with chronic infection, was the first subunit vaccine and, subsequently, the first recombinant vaccine in 1986. It is chastening for modern immunologists to remember that the vast majority of the highly successful vaccines in current use were all developed before 1970.

VACCINES

GENERAL PRINCIPLES

Vaccines in current use are either whole or subunit. Whole vaccines may have been inactivated (attenuated) or killed, and each of these has relative advantages and disadvantages (Table 23.1).

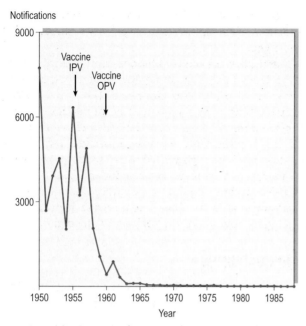

Notifications

Fig. 23.1 Annual notifications of polio infection in the UK between 1950 and 1987, demonstrating the powerful effect of the introduction of the injected (IPV) and oral (OPV) polio vaccines.

Not surprisingly, the choice of vaccine type involves trading off the advantages against the disadvantages. Administration of live, attenuated vaccines by their natural route is perhaps the optimal approach for the induction of immunity, but the least safe since there is a possibility of reversion of the organism to its pathogenic wild type. Choice of route is important: an agent typically encountered at a mucosal site (e.g. the enterovirus polio) requires good levels of specific secretory IgA for protection. This may not be generated as effectively when the killed vaccine is given by injection as when the attentuated virus is given by the natural, oral route.

Reversion to virulence is an important consideration. In the UK, almost all cases of polio infection acquired within this country are the result of reversion to virulence of an attenuated virus. One of the most recent cases, which illustrates this point, was in a father acquiring the virus from the nappy of his recently immunised daughter: the father was an immigrant to this country who had no immunity. However, this risk is balanced by the increase in so-called **herd immunity** obtained with a live attenuated virus. For example, with the Sabin live attenuated poliovaccine, the virus is still able to replicate, and some person–person passage takes place, increasing immunity even amongst non-immunised individuals. Therefore to achieve protection of the whole population, immunisation rates need not be 100%. This is in contrast with killed vaccines, which can only protect the recipient and for which immunisation rates must be nearer 100% to achieve population immunity. Legislative measures are usually required for such a high level of uptake, and in the USA, for example, school entry is often conditional upon production of the appropriate documentation to prove that immunisations have been carried out.

ADJUVANTS

The response to immunisation can be enhanced by a number of agents, and collectively these are termed adjuvants. These are a heterogeneous group of compounds, with several different mechanisms of action. In the history of immunisation, many compounds have been used empirically, with little knowledge about how they may work.

Several vaccines are composed of proteins that have been precipitated with **alum**, and others are **emulsified** in oil-based compounds. One of the best known emulsifying agents in vaccine studies is **Freund's complete adjuvant** (FCA), which contains mycobacterial derivatives. Amongst these, bacterial cell wall components such as lipopolysaccharide (LPS) are powerful immune stimulants, having a mitogenic and activating effect on macrophages and T cells (FCA produces such a vigorous local inflammatory reponse, however, that it cannot be used clinically). Manoeuvres such as the use of alum and oils are thought to retain antigen at the site of injection, prolonging the immune response, as well as providing relatively 'indigestible' antigenic compounds. This leads to chronic stimulation of APCs, which is likely in turn to enhance co-stimulation of T cells.

Knowledge about the nature of immune responses can now be put to use to design specific new adjuvants for particular types of immunopotentiation. An im-

Table 23.1 **Advantages and disadvantages of live and killed vaccines**

Vaccine type	Advantages	Disadvantages
Live attenuated vaccine	Reproduces natural infection	Possible reversion to virulent wild type
	Provides good level of protection, especially if administered by natural route (e.g. orally for Sabin poliovaccine)	Limited shelf-life and requires refrigeration for storage in tropics
	Usually only one dose required	Presence of viral growth media or culture cells produces adverse effects
	Person–person passage of attenuated virus enhances herd immunity: uptake levels need not be 100%	Contraindicated in T cell immunodeficiency states, pregnancy
Killed vaccine	Safe from reversion to virulence	Less effective than live vaccines
	More stable for transport and storage	More than one dose required
	Acceptable for immunocompromised recipients	No herd immunity induced: uptake levels must approximate 100%

portant goal is to identify adjuvants that specifically enhance cytotoxic T cell generation, or those that alter the T_H1/T_H2 balance in favour of the subset known to confer protection in a particular disease. For example, mice immunised with the same vaccine precipitated in alum, or emulsified in an oil-based adjuvant produce differing responses: alum mainly induces an antibody response (T_H2), whilst emulsification induces a cell-mediated response (T_H1). In addition, many of the potential vaccines produced during the current molecular biology revolution are protein subunits or even short peptides, which, on their own, are not inherently immunogenic. A new generation of adjuvants is being sought to complement the activity of the new vaccines.

Currently, there are three major approaches to the production of new adjuvants. The first is to place the immunogen inside a micelle-like structure, formed from a mixture of lipids (mainly cholesterol) and plant-derived detergents (saponin). This cage-like structure (actually a pentagonal dodecahedron!) is termed an **immunostimulating complex** or **ISCOM** and is 30–40 nm in size (Fig. 23.2). ISCOMs increase antibody and cell-mediated immune responses to a variety of antigens. In addition, there is some evidence that they can mimic viruses, entering cells directly. This leads to presentation of antigens through the endogenous pathway (see p. 89), with immunogenic peptides appearing in the class I MHC groove and activating CD8$^+$ cytotoxic T cells.

A second approach to the generation of adjuvants is to identify the smallest subunit of bacterial cell wall derivatives (e.g. those found in FCA) that retain immune stimulatory effects. Two of these are **monophosphoryl lipid A** (MLA) and **muramyl dipeptide** (MDP). These stimulate macrophages, as evidenced

by secretion of TNF-α, and also induce IFN-γ production, biasing immune responses towards a T_H1 phenotype.

The third approach is to harness the powerful effects of cytokines in up-regulating and influencing immune responses directly. Recombinant IL-1 and IFN-γ injected into animals simultaneously with an immunogen enhance immune responses. Clinical trials with IFN-α and IFN-γ given with hepatitis B vaccine have shown that they are both highly effective adjuvants, converting previous non-responders into responders. IL-2 may also be effective but requires continuous administration: a current goal is to obtain slow-release preparations, possibly by encasing the cytokine in a liposome.

VIRUS VACCINES

Virus vaccines have been produced that are live attenuated, killed or represent subunits:

- Live-attenuated vaccines: measles, mumps, polio (Sabin), rubella, varicella zoster.
- Inactivated (killed) vaccines: polio (Salk), influenza, rabies.
- Subunit vaccines: hepatitis B, influenza.

Attenuation is applicable only to viruses that are easily and reliably inactivated. In general, RNA viruses are easier to attenuate than DNA viruses, since RNA is more susceptible to inactivation. Countries differ in their choice of killed or attenuated vaccine for polio.

For the generation of subunit vaccines, some knowledge about the part of the virus that induces T cell responses and the targets of the most effective neutralising antibodies is required. As a generalisation, neutralising antibodies tend to target surface proteins, whilst T cell responses are directed against internal components. The other major consideration in the construction of viral subunit vaccines is to ensure that the subunit is represented in all strains of the virus (i.e. using group-specific rather than strain-specific subunits). T cell epitopes are likely to differ between different individuals in an HLA-dependent fashion, and the size of subunit should also take this constraint into consideration.

Influenza outbreaks occur as pandemics, with an unpredictable, periodic frequency. Four such pandemics have occurred this century, and during the 1918–19 outbreak, more people died within a few months than in the whole of the First World War. The pandemics result from antigenic shift in the influenza A strain, giving rise to virus with a previously unseen or resurgent haemagglutinin or neuraminidase subtype. Children and the elderly are at risk, along with those with known chronic respiratory or cardiac disease, diabetes, and immune suppression caused by disease or therapy. Each year, the Department of Health in the UK issues guidelines as to the use of the vaccines. Long-stay facilities, particularly nursing homes for the elderly, should also be targeted. Although annual vaccination is

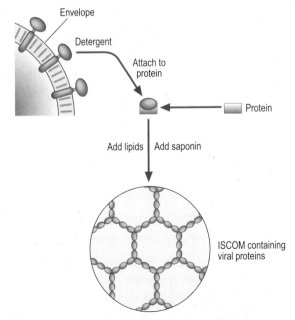

Fig. 23.2 **Construction of immunostimulating complexes.**

Envelope

Detergent

Attach to protein

Protein

Add lipids | Add saponin

ISCOM containing viral proteins

recommended for those at risk, there is some controversy as to whether this offers optimal protection. Keen public health surveillance is constantly in place to recognise outbreaks early. The antigenic composition of the vaccines available is also under constant review, and typically these contain haemagglutinin and neuraminidase from at least two influenza A subtypes and influenza B.

BACTERIAL VACCINES

As for viral vaccines, bacteria may be rendered as useful immunogens by killing or inactivation. Both of these approaches require the bacteria to be cultured in vitro, which is not possible with some organisms (e.g. *Treponema pallidum*, the cause of syphilis). Bacterial vaccines in common use include:

- Live-attenuated vaccine:
  — bacille Calmette–Guérin for tuberculosis.
- Inactivated (killed) vaccine:
  — *Bordetella pertussis* for whooping cough
  — *Salmonella typhi* and *S. paratyphi* for typhoid.
- Subunit/toxin vaccine:
  — chemically inactivated *Clostridium tetani* neurotoxin
  — Chemically inactivated *Corynebacterium diphtheriae* toxin
  — Cell wall polysaccharide from *Haemophilus influenzae* type b
  — Cell wall polysaccharides from *Neisseria meningitidis* A and C.

In general, bacterial vaccines are killed using heat treatment or agents such as formaldehyde and phenol. One of the best examples of an attenuated vaccine is that for tuberculosis, the bacille Calmette–Guérin. This was originally *Mycobacterium bovis* isolated from a cow, which through repeated culture passages (231 times in 3 years) lost its virulence and has now been administered to over 10^9 people worldwide.

Whole cell bacterial vaccines can be associated with problems related to production in cell culture, as well as with side effects that have made their use controversial. This has led to a shift towards the development of subunit vaccines, often termed **acellular vaccines**. For example, *Bordetella pertussis*, the aetiological agent in whooping cough, has a toxin and a surface fimbrial haemagglutinin that is thought to be important in attachment to host epithelial cells. A combined vaccine, based on purified, inactivated forms of these proteins has been developed recently and represents a novel step forward in bacterial vaccine design. Similarly, the traditional killed whole-cell typhoid vaccine is associated with unpleasant side effects, and an acellular vaccine based on the Vi capsular polysaccharide appears to confer adequate protection without this drawback.

A success in the new generation of acellular vaccines includes the **Hib vaccine** for *Haemophilus influenzae* type b. This is composed of capsular polysaccharide coupled to tetanus protein and has dramatically reduced the incidence of *Haemophilus* meningitis (which carried a mortality of almost 8%) since its introduction.

PARASITE VACCINES

Parasites pose some difficult problems for vaccine development. They are multicellular, frequently have more than one host organism and also colonise more than one organ during their life cycle. In addition, many of them have evolved some sophisticated mechanisms for evading host immune responses. Despite these problems, there is no doubting the need for parasite vaccines. Malaria (caused by *Plasmodium* spp.) kills 1.2 million people per year and annually infects an estimated 800 million worldwide. Other infections that cause considerable morbidity and for which vaccines are urgently sought are schistosomiasis (*Schistosoma* spp.; 200 million infected), Chagas' disease (*Trypanosoma cruzi*; 12 million), leishmaniasis (*Leishmania* spp.; 12 million) and sleeping sickness (*Trypanosoma gambiense/rhodesiense*; 1 million).

There are several well-documented immune evasion mechanisms exploited by the organisms causing these infections. Organisms may vary the antigens they present (e.g. *Plasmodium* spp., trypanosomes). The mastigote stage of trypanosomes can escape from macrophage lysosomes, negating attempts to kill them or establish an immune response. Schistosomes are able to camouflage their surface using host-derived antigens. An additional problem for the vaccinologist is the difficulty in culturing the organisms, which reduces the opportunity to study the life cycle and purify relevant antigens.

Nonetheless, certain facts indicate that immunisation against parasites is an achievable goal. First, for some of the infections (e.g. malaria) it is clear that individuals in endemic areas have some resistance to the parasite, indicating a state of protection. Second, passive immunisation of experimental animals with antibodies against the circumsporozoite antigens of malaria offers protection from challenge with the whole organism.

Important advances in malarial vaccines have been made in recent years. There is now evidence that cytotoxic T cells are capable of killing the liver stage of the organism. In this case, peptides derived from malaria that bind to class I MHC molecules offer some hope of protection if incorporated into a vaccine (see box: 'Prediction of peptides for malaria vaccine').

IMMUNISATION PROTOCOLS: PROTECTION FOR LIFE

The current UK immunisation programme is shown in Table 23.2. Diphtheria, tetanus and pertussis immunisation within the first 6 months of life is an important public health priority. Whooping cough is most dangerous when acquired at this age and early immunisation

Prediction of peptides for malaria vaccine

In 1991, evidence that protection from severe malaria in the Gambia was associated with possession of the HLA-B53 class I MHC molecule generated considerable interest. Following on from this work, Hill and colleagues in Oxford eluted antigenic peptides from the groove of B53 molecules and sequenced these to identify the characteristics of peptides that bind to this molecule. Having done so, they searched the peptide sequence of *Plasmodium falciparum* for candidate stretches that they predicted would bind to B53. The peptides obtained were then tested to see whether B53$^+$ individuals from malaria endemic areas had cytotoxic T cells that specifically recognised the B53–peptide complex. The results demonstrated the existence amongst Gambians in an endemic area of a B53-restricted cytotoxic T cell response to a nonameric peptide from the liver-stage-specific antigen-1 (LSA-1). This suggests that the basis for the protective effect of B53 in this population is the ability to generate a cytotoxic response to the malarial parasite when it is at the early, liver stage, thus avoiding extension of the infection. This also suggests that vaccines modelled on the production of peptides from the LSA-1 that bind MHC molecules could be successful. However, the key will be in identifying numerous peptides to cover the polymorphic nature of class I molecules.

for *Haemophilus influenzae* type b is an important recent addition to the protocol. The MMR triple vaccine was phased in during the late 1980s, and once uptake is complete, immunisation of schoolgirls with rubella will no longer be required as a routine practice.

Despite the existence of such a rigid programme, there is considerable flexibility within the public health systems of developed countries for rapid responses to real or potential risks. For example, the upsurge in reported diphtheria cases outside Western Europe and America has seen the adoption of a diphtheria booster

at school-leaving age in these countries. In addition, in the UK, an increase in measles notifications in early 1994 followed a reduction in uptake of the triple vaccine. Measles is a potentially fatal disease, and the prediction of an epidemic in early 1995 provoked the response of a massive public health campaign to encourage uptake of the measles vaccine.

FUTURE APPROACHES

The use of recombinant DNA technology to generate vaccines has several obvious advantages. First it is safe

Immunisation with genes

Some of the major problems with generating vaccines are in the identification and purification in sufficient quantities for widespread use of the appropriate immunogenic proteins from the organisms. A new approach, 'genetic immunisation' has recently been described, which may potentially side-step these obstacles. In genetic immunisation, the gene for the immunogenic protein is coated onto gold microspheres and injected directly into living cells within the host animal. In studies designed to assess the feasibility of this approach, mice were injected beneath the skin, but directly into skin cells, with a genomic copy of the DNA encoding human growth hormone (hGH), under the control of a promoter. An antibody response to hGH was seen, commencing some 3 weeks after the injection. It is presumed that the injected DNA is translated and transcribed in the injected cells and that the immunising protein is then produced and either exported or expressed on the cell surface. There are at least two major caveats: the procedure will require enhancement for clinical use since antibody levels were generally low; and we can only speculate on the public acceptability of injecting 'bug genes into babies'!

Table 23.2 **UK immunisation programme in 1994**

Age	Vaccine	Comments
2 months 3 months 4 months	1st dose DPT, polio and Hib 2nd dose DPT, polio and Hib 3rd dose DPT, polio and Hib	DPT is a triple vaccine containing diphtheria and tetanus toxoids, plus pertussis vaccine. Hib has recently been introduced for *Haemophilus influenzae* b protection
12–18 months	MMR	MMR is a triple vaccine for mumps, measles and rubella
4–5 years	Booster DT and polio	DT, diphtheria and tetanus
10–14 years	Rubella	Girls only[a]
10–14 years	BCG	Bacille Calmette–Guérin for tuberculosis[b]
15–18 years	Booster for DT and polio	Booster for diphtheria at this age only recently introduced because of increases in disease abroad
Adulthood	Rubella vaccine Polio and tetanus Hepatitis B, influenza	Women seronegative for rubella Non-immunised individuals (e.g. immigrants) High-risk groups

[a]Rubella vaccination of girls approaching menarche will continue until MMR (introduced 1988) has comprehensive uptake.
[b]BCG may be given to infants in high-risk groups.

Index